The KEY TOPICS Series

Advisors:

T.M. Craft *Department of Anaesthesia and Intensive Care, Royal United Hospital, Bath, UK*
C.S. Garrard *Intensive Therapy Unit, John Radcliffe Hospital, Oxford, UK*
P.M. Upton *Department of Anaesthetics, Royal Cornwall Hospital, Treliske, Truro, UK*

Anaesthesia, Second Edition
Obstetrics and Gynaecology, Second Edition
Accident and Emergency Medicine
Paediatrics, Second Edition
Orthopaedic Surgery
Otolaryngology
Ophthalmology
Psychiatry
General Surgery
Renal Medicine
Trauma
Chronic Pain
Oral and Maxillofacial Surgery
Oncology
Cardiovascular Medicine
Neurology
Neonatology
Gastroenterology
Thoracic Surgery
Respiratory Medicine
Orthopaedic Trauma Surgery
Critical Care

Forthcoming titles include:

Accident and Emergency Medicine, Second Edition

KEY TOPICS IN
CRITICAL CARE

TIM CRAFT
MB BS, FRCA

Consultant in Anaesthesia and Intensive Care Medicine,
Royal United Hospital, Bath, UK

JERRY NOLAN
MB BS, FRCA

Consultant in Anaesthesia and Intensive Care Medicine
Royal United Hospital, Bath, UK

MIKE PARR
MB BS, MRCP, FRCA, FANZCA

Consultant in Intensive Care Medicine, Liverpool Hospital
and Lecturer in Intensive Care, Anaesthesia and Emergency Medicine,
University of New South Wales, Sydney, NSW, Australia

βIOS
SCIENTIFIC
PUBLISHERS

BIOS Scientific Publishers Ltd
9 Newtec Place, Magdalen Road, Oxford OX4 1RE, UK
Tel. +44 (0)1865 726286. Fax +44 (0)1865 246823
World Wide Web home page: http://www.bios.co.uk/

Important Note from the Publisher
The information contained within this book was obtained by BIOS Scientific Publishers Ltd from sources believed by us to be reliable. However, while every effort has been made to ensure its accuracy, no responsibility for loss or injury whatsoever occasioned to any person acting or refraining from action as a result of information contained herein can be accepted by the authors or publishers.

The reader should remember that medicine is a constantly evolving science and while the authors and publishers have ensured that all dosages, applications and practices are based on current indications, there may be specific practices which differ between communities. You should always follow the guidelines laid down by the manufacturers of specific products and the relevant authorities in the country in which you are practising.

Production Editor: Andrea Bosher.
Typeset by Footnote Graphics, Warminster, UK.
Printed by TJ International Ltd, Padstow, UK.

Cover photograph kindly supplied by Mike Scott Photography

CONTENTS

CONTRIBUTORS

Tim Cook MB BS BA FRCA
Consultant in Anaesthesia, Royal United Hospital, Bath, UK

Bronwen Evans MB BS FANZCA
Visiting Fellow, Department of Anaesthesia, Royal United Hospital, Bath, UK

Stephen Fletcher MB BS MRCP FRCA FFICANZCA
Senior Registrar, Intensive Care Unit, Liverpool Hospital, Sydney, NSW, Australia

Claire Fouque MB BS FRCA
Resuscitation Registrar, Intensive Care Unit, Liverpool Hospital, Sydney, NSW, Australia

Alex Goodwin MB BS FRCA
Consultant in Anaesthesia and Intensive Care, Royal United Hospital, Bath, UK

Manivannan Gopalkrishnan MB BS FFICANZCA
Senior Registrar, Intensive Care Unit, Royal Prince Alfred Hospital, Darlington, NSW, Australia

Kim Gupta MB ChB FRCA
Senior Registrar in Intensive Care Medicine, Royal North Shore Hospital, Sydney, NSW, Australia

Jonathon Hadfield MB BS FRCA
Senior Registrar, Intensive Care Unit, Liverpool Hospital, Sydney, NSW, Australia

Jeff Handel MB BS MRCP FRCA
Consultant in Anaesthesia and Intensive Care, Royal United Hospital, Bath, UK

S. Kim Jacobsen MB ChB MSc MRCP MRCPath
Consultant Medical Microbiologist, Royal United Hospital, Bath, UK and UBHT, Bristol, UK

Myrene Kilminster MB BS FANZCA FFICANZCA
Director, Intensive Care Unit, Lismore Base Hospital, NSW, Australia

David Lockey MB BS Dip IMC RCS (Ed) FRCA
Senior Registrar in Intensive Care, Royal Perth Hospital, Perth, WA, Australia

James Low MB BCh DCH
Specialist Registrar in Anaesthesia, John Radcliffe Hospital, Oxford, UK

Susan Murray PhD FRCPath
Clinical Microbiologist, Royal United Hospital, Bath, UK

Cathal Nolan MB BCh BAO FFARCSI
Senior Registrar, Intensive Care Unit, Liverpool Hospital, Sydney, NSW, Australia

Andrew Padkin MB ChB BSc MRCP FRCA
Specialist Registrar in Anaesthesia, Royal United Hospital, Bath, UK

Richard Protheroe MB BS MRCS MRCP FRCA
Specialist Registrar in Anaesthesia, Royal United Hospital, Bath, UK

Martin Schuster-Bruce MB BS BSc MRCP FRCA
Specialist Registrar in Anaesthesia, Royal United Hospital, Bath, UK

Tom Simpson MB BS BSc FRCA
Specialist Registrar in Anaesthesia, Royal United Hospital, Bath, UK

Jas Soar BA MB BCh MA FRCA
Specialist Registrar in Anaesthesia, Frenchay Hospital, Bristol, UK

Antony Stewart MB BS FANZCA
Senior Registrar, Intensive Care Unit, Liverpool Hospital, Sydney, NSW, Australia

Minh Tran MB BS BSc
Registrar in Anaesthesia, Liverpool Hospital, Sydney, NSW, Australia

Jenny Tuckey MB ChB DCH FRCA
Consultant in Obstetric Anaesthesia, Royal United Hospital, Bath, UK

Cynthia Uy MB BS
Senior Registrar in Oncology, Royal North Shore Hospital, NSW, Australia

Angela White MB ChB
Senior House Officer in Surgery, Royal United Hospital, Bath, UK

ABBREVIATIONS

ACE	angiotensin converting enzyme
ACT	activated clotting time
ACTH	adrenocorticotrophic hormone
ADH	anti-diuretic hormone
AF	atrial fibrillation
ALI	acute lung injury
ALS	advanced life support
APACHE	acute physiology and chronic health evaluation
APPT	activated partial thromboplastin time
ARDS	acute respiratory distress syndrome
ATN	acute tubular necrosis
BiPAP	bilevel positive airway pressure
BLS	basic life support
CABG	coronary artery bypass grafting
CBF	cerebral blood flow
CHF	congestive heart failure
$CMRO_2$	cerebral metabolic rate of oxygen
CNS	central nervous system
COPD	chronic obstructive pulmonary disease
CPAP	continuous positive airway pressure
CPP	cerebral perfusion pressure
CPR	cardiopulmonary resuscitation
CSF	cerebrospinal fluid
CT	computerized tomography
CVP	central venous pressure
CVS	cardiovascular system
CXR	chest X-ray
DDAVP	d'-8-amino arginine vasopressin or desmopressin
DIC	disseminated intravascular coagulation
DPL	diagnostic peritoneal lavage
DVT	deep venous thrombosis
$ECCO_2R$	extracorporeal CO_2 removal
ECF	extracellular fluid
ESBL	extended spectrum beta-lactamase
FBC	full blood count
FDPs	fibrin degradation products
FFP	fresh frozen plasma
FOB	fibreoptic bronchoscopy
FRC	functional residual capacity
GALT	gut associated lymphoid tissue
GBS	Guillain–Barré syndrome
GCS	Glasgow coma scale
GFR	glomerular filtration rate
GI	gastrointestinal

GTN	glyceryl trinitrate
GvHD	graft versus host disease
HDU	high dependency unit
ICF	intracellular fluid
ICP	intracranial pressure
ICU	intensive care unit
IDDM	insulin dependent diabetes mellitus
IHD	intermittent haemodialysis
IMV	intermittent mandatory ventilation
ISS	injury severity score
IVC	inferior vena cava
LMA	laryngeal mask airway
LMWH	low molecular weight heparin
LRTI	lower respiratory tract infections
LV	left ventricular
LVEDP	left ventricular end diastolic pressure
MAP	mean arterial pressure
MH	malignant hyperthermia
MI	myocardial infarction
MILS	manual in-line cervical stabilization
MODS	multiple organ dysfunction syndrome
MOF	multiple organ failure
MRSA	methicillin resistant *Staphylococcus aureus*
MRTB	multi-resistant *Mycobacterium tuberculosis*
NGT	nasogastric tube
NIDDM	non-insulin dependent diabetes mellitus
NIPPV	non-invasive positive pressure ventilation
NSAID	non-steroidal anti-inflammatory drugs
PAOP	pulmonary artery occlusion pressure
PCA	patient controlled analgesia
PCP	*Pneumocystis carinii* pneumonia
PE	pulmonary embolism
PEEP	positive end expiratory pressure
PEEPi	intrinsic positive end expiratory pressure
PEF	peak expiratory flow
pHi	intramucosal pH
PND	paroxysmal nocturnal dyspnoea
PSV	pressure support ventilation
PT	prothrombin time
ROSC	return of spontaneous circulation
RTAs	road traffic accidents
RVEDV	right ventricular end diastolic volume
SAGM	saline, adenine, glucose and mannitol
SAH	subarachnoid haemorrhage
SDD	selective decontamination of the digestive tract
SIMV	synchronized intermittent mandatory ventilation
SLE	systemic lupus erythematosus

SIRS	systemic inflammatory response syndrome
SVC	superior vena cava
SVR	systemic vascular resistance
TBW	total body water
TIA	transient ischaemic attack
TISS	therapeutic intervention scoring system
TNF	tumour necrosis factor
TOE	transoesophageal echocardiography
t-PA	tissue plasminogen activator
UTI	urinary tract infections
V/Q	ventilation perfusion scan
VAS	visual analogue scale
VF	ventricular fibrillation
VRE	vancomycin resistant enterococcus

PREFACE

Critical care in acute hospitals is developing perhaps faster than any other clinical specialty. The pace of change is driven both by an ever increasing ability of medicine to offer the chance of survival from critical illness and the expectations of our patients. At the same time we have a responsibilty to ensure that our critical care resources are directed only at those patients who will benefit from them. The importance of critical care medicine is recognized, too, by many of the Royal Colleges in their exam structure. Critical care now forms a part of the examinations for Fellowship of the Royal College of Anaesthetists, Membership of the Royal College of Physicians, and Fellowship of the Royal Colleges of Surgeons, amongst others.

Key Topics in Critical Care provides a framework for candidates of postgraduate medical examinations as well as a footing for all those expected to care for critically ill patients. Care of the critically ill involves clinicians working together as teams across some of the more traditional professional boundaries. *Key Topics in Critical Care* has been written by clinicians from a variety of different backgrounds working in two different continents. As usual with the Key Topics format, each topic presents a succinct overview of its subject and is referenced with current publications for further reading. Wherever possible, these references are to major review articles in widely available journals.

T. Craft, J. Nolan, M. Parr,
(Bath and Sydney, 1999)

FOREWORD

Intensive care has travelled a long way in the last 20 years or so. From being a sub speciality where it was practised in corners of the hospital, mainly by anaesthetists whose main task was seen to be adjusting knobs on ventilators, it has expanded enormously to now become the focal point of most hospitals. In so doing it has lead to a growing body of research which has focused on the problems of acutely sick patients, usually with multi-organ failure. It is now on the verge, at least in the United Kingdom, of becoming a speciality in its own right, with a training programme now in place leading to a Diploma of Intensive Care Medicine. It has become apparent that there are many young doctors from both anaesthesia and internal medicine wanting training in intensive care, some of whom will become either part-time or even full-time intensive care specialists. Those practising this discipline require a wide knowledge of a variety of subjects and the humility to ask when they need further advice.

This book will be very useful for those young trainees who are now embarking upon an intensive care career and who will need to take a diploma of one sort or another in the next 2 or 3 years. It is presented as immediately accessible, with clear statements of fact and a logical flow that makes it easy to read and to absorb. It is wide ranging, covering most aspects of intensive care, with a useful guide to further reading and related topics of interest. It will also be useful as a reference book to be looked at quickly on the 'shop floor', giving clear didactic information which is so essential in an emergency situation. It is also accessible for senior nursing staff, physiotherapists and technicians and is, I believe, a very interesting addition to the literature of intensive care medicine.

Professor E. D. Bennett

ADMISSION AND DISCHARGE CRITERIA

One of the most difficult aspects of critical care medicine is the identification of the patients who are most likely to benefit from intensive and high dependency care. These resources are scarce and expensive. Patients who are not ill enough to require critical care and those unlikely to benefit because they are too ill must be excluded. The Department of Health's publication 'Guidelines on admission to and discharge from Intensive Care and High Dependency Units' provides useful advice for doctors in the United Kingdom.

Definitions

Intensive care may be defined as 'a service for patients with potentially recoverable conditions who can benefit from more detailed observation and invasive treatment than can safely be provided in general wards or high dependency areas'. Intensive care is typically provided for patients with threatened or established organ failure. This may have arisen from an acute illness, trauma, or during planned treatment. High dependency care provides a level of care immediate between that on a general ward and intensive care. Patients with, or at risk of developing, single organ failure are candidates for high dependency care. Patients requiring mechanical ventilation will need admission to an intensive care unit (ICU).

1. Characteristics of intensive care
The characteristics of intensive care are:
(a) A designated area where there is a minimum nurse:patient ratio of 1:1, together with a nurse-in-charge, throughout 24 hours;
(b) Twenty-four hour cover by resident medical staff;
(c) The ability to support organ system failures; ventilator haemofilter
(d) Intensive care is appropriate for:
- Patients requiring, or likely to require, advanced respiratory support alone;
- Patients requiring support of two or more organ systems;
- Patients with co-morbidity (see below) who require support for an acute reversible failure of another organ system.

2. Characteristics of high dependency care
The characteristics of high dependency care are:
- A designated area where there is a minimum nurse:patient ratio of 1:2, together with a nurse-in-charge, throughout 24 hours;
- Continuous availability of medical staff from either the admitting specialty or from intensive care;
- Appropriate monitoring and other equipment.

3. Categories of organ system monitoring and support
The Department of Health has defined categories of organ system monitoring and support:
1. Advanced Respiratory Support:
    1.1. Mechanical ventilatory support [excluding mask continuous positive airways pressure (CPAP) or non-invasive ventilation].

1.2. The possibility of a sudden deterioration in respiratory function requiring immediate tracheal intubation and mechanical ventilation.
2. Basic Respiratory Monitoring and Support:
    2.1. The need for more than 40% oxygen.
    2.2. The possibility of progressive deterioration to the point of needing advanced respiratory support.
    2.3. The need for physiotherapy to clear secretions at least 2-hourly.
    2.4. Patients recently extubated after a prolonged period of intubation and mechanical ventilation.
    2.5. The need for mask CPAP or non-invasive ventilation.
    2.6. Patients who are intubated to protect the airway, but not needing ventilatory support.
3. Circulatory Support:
    3.1. The need for vasoactive drugs.
    3.2. Support for circulatory instability due to hypovolaemia from any cause and which is unresponsive to modest volume replacement.
    3.3. Patients resuscitated following cardiac arrest where intensive or high dependency care is considered clinically appropriate.
4. Neurological Monitoring and Support:
    4.1. Central nervous system depression sufficient to prejudice the airway and protective reflexes.
    4.2. Invasive neurological monitoring.
5. Renal support:
    5.1. The need for acute renal replacement therapy.

Admission to intensive care

1. Referral. When considering referral for intensive care, when possible, it is essential to consult with the patient and the patient's family and to determine their wishes. The referral must be on a consultant to consultant basis. The Department of Health has published a flow chart for admission to intensive care and high dependency units (HDUs) (*Fig. 1*).

2. Reversibility of illness. The potential benefits of intensive care will, to a large extent, depend on whether or not the patient has a reversible condition. This is not always easy to determine and in some cases it is necessary to admit the patient and assess the response to a trial of appropriate treatment. The potential benefit of intensive care, in terms of quality and length of life, must be discussed at length with the patient (where possible) and with the patient's family. Subjecting a patient who is near to death to mechanical ventilation solely for the purposes of organ donation is considered unlawful in the UK.

3. Co-morbidity. Co-morbidity is a chronic impairment of one or more organs sufficient to restrict daily activities. Intensive care cannot reverse chronic ill health and significant co-morbidity will weigh against a patient's admission to an ICU. However, patients often adapt to their co-morbidity and happily accept a quality of life which others would find unacceptable. Thus, denying ICU admission to a patient with significant co-morbidity may not be in their best interests. This represents the great weakness of the flow chart in *Fig. 1*.

2 ADMISSION AND DISCHARGE CRITERIA

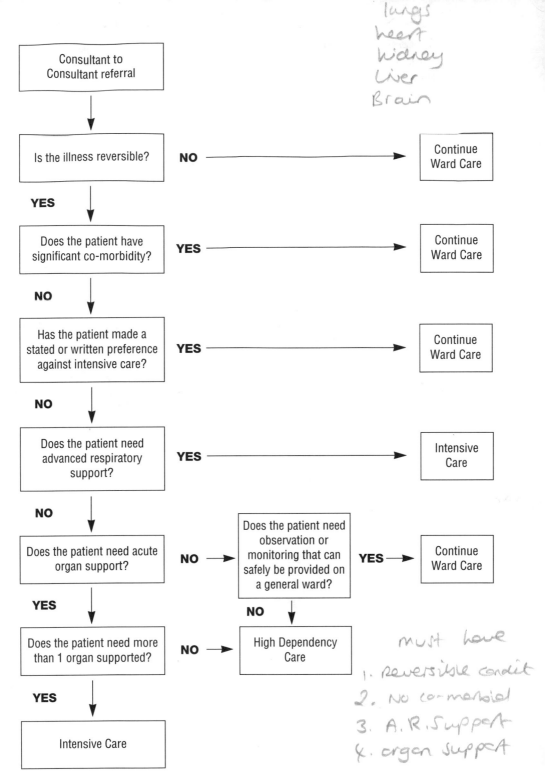

Fig. 1. Flow chart for admission to intensive care and high dependency care.

4. Admission to high dependency care. High dependency care is appropriate for patients requiring support of one organ system (excluding advanced respiratory support) or who need close monitoring. ICUs in hospitals without HDUs may have to admit patients who need only high dependency care. Most hospitals with HDUs will have local guidelines on indications for admission. The criteria may depend on the number of HDU beds available. In the UK, many patients fulfilling standard criteria for high dependency care are nursed on general wards.

5. Discharge from intensive care and high dependency care. A patient should be discharged from the ICU when the condition that led to the admission has been adequately reversed or when the patient is no longer benefiting from the treatment available. If it is clear that there is no chance of survival with a quality of life that would be acceptable to the patient, it may be appropriate to limit or withdraw aggressive therapy. Unless a patient's death is imminent, it is appropriate to transfer the patient to another area of the hospital and allow death with dignity. Bed management policies should prevent patients being inappropriately detained in intensive care or high dependency care. This ideal is becoming increasingly difficult to achieve as acute general hospitals run on the absolute minimum number of ward beds. Intensive care patients may be discharged to high dependency care or to the general ward, as appropriate.

Further reading

Department of Health NHS Executive. Guidelines on admission to and discharge from Intensive Care and High Dependency Units, Department of Health 1996

ACUTE RESPIRATORY DISTRESS SYNDROME

Tim Cook

Acute respiratory distress syndrome (ARDS) is a syndrome of respiratory failure associated with severe hypoxia and low respiratory compliance. The characteristic radiological changes are of widespread pulmonary infiltrates. Pulmonary artery occlusion pressure (PAOP) measurements may be low or normal. The plasma oncotic pressure is usually normal. The reported annual incidence of ARDS is variable, 5:100 000 being quoted in the UK, but 75:100 000 in the USA. This reflects differing thresholds for diagnosis.

ARDS is usually the pulmonary manifestation of the systemic inflammatory response syndrome (SIRS). Sepsis and trauma are the commonest causes. Other causes include haemorrhage with hypotension, transfusion, obstetric emergencies, cardiopulmonary bypass, pancreatitis, disseminated intravascular coagulation (DIC), fat embolus and following cardiac arrest or head injury. Local insults such as aspiration or smoke inhalation may also result in ARDS. Onset of the disease is rapid; most cases develop within 24 hours of the initial insult. The clinical presentation is one of tachypnoea, laboured breathing, and cyanosis.

The pathophysiological features of ARDS are due initially to epithelial injury and include a severe protein-rich alveolar oedema with inflammatory infiltrates (principally neutrophils), although ARDS may occur in the neutropenic patient. Surfactant denaturation by protein leaking into the alveolus leads to atelectasis, a reduced functional residual capacity (FRC) and hypoxia. Type I alveolar cells are damaged and type II cells proliferate. Later, fibroblast infiltration and collagen proliferation lead, in some cases, to an accelerated fibrosing alveolitis, and microvascular obliteration. This disease process does not affect the lung in a uniform fashion; there may be considerable functional variation between different lung regions.

Diagnosis

There are strict definitions for the diagnosis of acute lung injury (ALI) and ARDS. The triad of hypoxia, low lung compliance and widespread infiltrates on chest X-ray (CXR) should be accompanied by a known precipitant of the syndrome and a normal left atrial pressure (measured indirectly by the PAOP). A PaO_2/FIO_2 40 kPa defines ALI and a PaO_2/FIO_2 27 kPa defines ARDS.

Prognosis

The reported mortality for ARDS is variable. This is, in part, related to a lack of consistency in diagnosis. Sepsis is associated with the greatest mortality at any stage of the disease whilst fat embolism alone is associated with a low mortality (90% survival). ARDS associated with bone marrow transplant or liver failure has negligible survival. Over 80% of deaths in ARDS are not as a result of respiratory failure. The presence of other organ failure thus has great bearing on the prognosis. Recent studies suggest that the mortality rate has fallen in the past decade from ~60% to 40%.

Management

Inspired O_2 concentrations greater than 0.5, high tidal volumes (> 10 ml kg^{-1}) and high plateau airway pressures (> 35 cm H_2O), may cause lung damage. Avoiding these risk factors may improve outcome.

Treatment is supportive, but control of infection is vital. Bacteriological specimens should be cultured and every effort made to prevent nosocomial infection. Prevention of gastric colonization by avoiding the use of H_2 receptor antagonists may reduce the incidence of nosocomial pneumonia. Nursing and medical hygiene must be scrupulous. Positive blood cultures should be followed by an extensive search for the site of infection.

Ventilation

The principles of mechanical ventilation are to provide adequate oxygenation and CO_2 removal while minimizing the risk of barotrauma and volutrauma. Dependent, collapsed alveoli should be recruited using positive end expiratory pressure (PEEP) of 5–18 cm H_2O. The use of prolonged inspiratory times (i.e. inverse ratio ventilation) will increase intrinsic PEEP (PEEPi) and may be beneficial. Relatively small tidal volumes (< 7 ml kg^{-1}) will minimize peak inspiratory pressures and reduce the potentially damaging shear forces in the alveoli. Inspired O_2 concentrations should be reduced to 0.5 as soon as possible by setting targets for acceptable hypoxaemia (e.g., $SaO_2 > 88\%$). Arterial pCO_2 may therefore be allowed to rise to 10 kPa or higher, providing renal compensation minimizes the accompanying acidosis (permissive hypercarbia). Prospective controlled studies of protective ventilation strategies and permissive hypercarbia have produced conflicting results. Refractory hypoxia is often improved by the use of reversed I:E ratios and/or nursing the patient prone. Although extracorporeal membrane oxygenation (ECMO) with CO_2 removal is of benefit in infantile ARDS, its use in adults remains controversial.

Pulmonary artery catheterization may be valuable initially to exclude cardiogenic pulmonary oedema, in assessing optimum preload, and to guide inotrope, vasodilator and vasopressor therapy. Measurement of cardiac output, mixed venous saturation, and lactate or base deficit help to assess oxygen consumption. Extravascular lung water may be controlled by judicious administration of fluids to prevent high left atrial pressures. Controversy still surrounds the choice between colloid and crystalloid.

Specific treatment

The exact role of prostaglandin inhibitors, anti-tumour necrosis factor antibodies, surfactant therapy, and oxypentifylline is uncertain in this condition. Steroid therapy may be beneficial during the fibrosing stage of ARDS (late steroid rescue). This benefit appears to be limited to a narrow therapeutic window of between 7 and 15 days after the onset of ARDS.

Nitric oxide

Nitric oxide is a potent vasodilator. When it is inhaled it enters only ventilated areas of the lung and causes appropriate vasodilation so improving ventilation:perfusion matching and oxygenation. This is in contrast to intravenous vasodilators that tend to do the converse and so increase shunt. It has a great affinity for haemoglobin (15000 times that of carbon monoxide) and combines rapidly with it on entering the blood stream. As a result it does not cause systemic vasodilation. It is given directly into the ventilated gas mixture at a concentration of 5–20 ppm. The use of nitric oxide has not been shown to improve outcome from ARDS.

Survivors

The outlook for survivors is good. At 1 year 50% of survivors have abnormal lung function but few have functional respiratory disability. Late deaths in ARDS are secondary to pulmonary fibrosis (55%) and sepsis/multiple organ failure (69%).

Further reading

Bernard GR, Artigas A, Brigham KL, *et al*. Report of the American-European Consensus Conference on ARDS: definitions, mechanisms, relevant outcomes and clinical trial corordination. *Intensive Care Medicine*, 1994; **20**: 225–232.

Kollef MK, Shuster DP. The acute respiratory distress syndrome. *New England Journal of Medicine*, 1995; **332**: 27–37.

Related topics of interest

Pneumonia – hospital acquired, p. 177; Respiratory support – invasive, p. 205; Respiratory support – weaning from ventilation, p. 210; SIRS, sepsis and multiple organ failure, p. 228

1. Give H₂ antag
2. No Acid

___

1. Acid H₂ antag
2. Acid there + so kills bacteria so if aspirate no bacteria inhaled
3. Less chance of 'nosocomial' HAP

Peep ↑
Insp time (↑ Peep)
Small TV
Low O₂ (>88%) – allow met acid to compensate "permissive hypercarbia"

ADRENAL DISEASE

The adrenal cortex produces glucocorticoid, mineralocorticoid and sex hormones (mainly testosterone). Cortisol, the principal glucocorticoid, modulates stress and inflammatory responses. It is a potent stimulator of gluconeogenesis and antagonizes insulin.

Aldosterone is the principal mineralocorticoid. It causes increased sodium reabsorption, and potassium and hydrogen ion loss at the distal renal tubule. Adrenal androgen production increases markedly at puberty, declining with age thereafter. Androstenedione is converted by the liver to testosterone in the male and oestrogen in the female. Cortisol and androgen production are under diurnal pituitary control (adrenocorticotrophic hormone – ACTH). Aldosterone is released in response to increased circulating angiotensin II, itself produced following renal renin release and subsequent pulmonary conversion of angiotensin I to angiotensin II.

Clinical diseases result from relative excess or lack of hormones. The conditions below are relevant to critical care.

Adrenocortical excess

Cushing's syndrome
May result from steroid therapy, adrenal hyperplasia, adrenal carcinoma or ectopic ACTH.

Cushing's disease
Is due to an ACTH secreting pituitary tumour.

Clinical features of adrenocortical excess include moon face, thin skin, easy bruising, hypertension (60%), hirsutism, obesity with a centripetal distribution, buffalo hump, muscle weakness, diabetes (10%), osteoporosis (50%), aseptic necrosis of the hip and pancreatitis (especially with iatrogenic Cushing's syndrome).

Problems
- Control of blood sugar (insulin may be required).
- Hypokalaemia resulting in arrhythmias, muscle weakness and postoperative respiratory impairment.
- Hypertension, polycythaemia, CHF. The patient may require central venous and/or PAOP monitoring.

Adrenocortical insufficiency

Primary adrenocortical insufficiency
Is commonly due to an autoimmune adrenalitis (Addison's disease) and may be associated with other autoimmune disorders. Females are affected more often than males. Other causes include adrenal infiltration with tumour, leukaemia, infection (TB, histoplasmosis) and amyloidosis.

Secondary adrenocortical insufficiency

Results from a deficiency of ACTH. It may occur as a result of administration of corticosteroid in sufficient dose to suppress ACTH release, or as a consequence of hypothalamic or pituitary dysfunction.

Adrenocortical insufficiency may present as either an acute disease or slowly progressive chronic condition.

1. *Acute (Addisonian crisis).* This may follow sepsis, pharmacological adrenal suppression or adrenal haemorrhage associated with anti-coagulant therapy, especially in the sick patient. Post-partum pituitary infarction (Sheehan's syndrome) may also present as acute adrenocortical insufficiency.

Clinical features include apathy, hypotension, coma, and hypoglycaemia. Circulatory failure and shock may be present as may a history of recent infection. The diagnosis should be considered in all shocked patients in whom the cause is not immediately apparent. Adrenocortical insufficiency may be more common in the critically ill than previously suspected.

2. *Chronic* deficiency may follow surgical adrenalectomy, autoimmune adrenalitis, or be secondary to pituitary dysfunction.

Clinical features include, fatigue, weakness, weight loss, nausea and hyperpigmentation. Hypotension, hyponatraemia, hyperkalaemia, eosinophilia and occasionally hypoglycaemia may also occur.

Investigations

- Biochemistry to exclude hyponatraemia, hypochloraemia, hyperkalaemia, hypercalcaemia, hypoglycaemia, and a raised blood urea.
- Haematology may reveal an elevated haematocrit (dehydration) and possible eosinophilia.
- Endocrine investigations. A low cortisol level supports the diagnosis. An ACTH assay will differentiate between primary and secondary disease, being high in the former and low or normal in the latter.
- Arterial blood gas analysis may show a metabolic acidosis with additional respiratory contribution in the presence of severe muscle weakness.
- Immunology may reveal autoantibodies.

Management

Patients presenting with an acute crisis should be admitted to an appropriate critical care unit to permit invasive monitoring of circulatory pressures and arterial blood gases.

Circulatory shock is managed in the usual way with initial attention to the critical elements covered by the ABC scheme of assessment/treatment. Large volumes (6–8 l in 24 hours) of isotonic saline and inotropic support may be required in the first few hours of treatment.

Corticosteroids are given without waiting for confirmatory laboratory results.

Hydrocortisone is administered as a slow intravenous bolus (100–200 mg) before commencing an infusion every 6 hours.

Infection is treated with appropriate antibiotics.

Investigation and determination of the precipitating cause will guide further management.

Steroid withdrawal

Withdrawal of corticosteroid therapy may cause an acute Addisonian-type crisis. Patients who have been taking steroids (more than 10 mg daily) for periods in excess of 1 year are at particular risk, though the critically ill may show similar signs after much shorter treatment periods. Withdrawal of steroids should thus be gradual. If there is doubt about a patient's ability to restore normal adrenocortical function an ACTH stimulation test (Synacthen test) should be performed.

- Administer tetracosactrin [synthetic 1-24-ACTH (Synacthen)] 250 μg i.m.
- Measure blood cortisol levels at 30 and 60 min following injection.

Diminished or absent cortisol response indicates insufficient endogenous adrenocortical activity.

Hyperaldosteronism

Primary (Conn's syndrome)

This is caused by an adenoma in the zona glomerulosa secreting aldosterone. Clinical features include, hypokalaemia, muscle weakness and hypertension.

Problems

- Hypokalaemia may result in cardiac arrhythmias, post-operative muscle weakness and ventilatory impairment.
- Hypertension.
- Hormone replacement required following adrenalectomy.

Further reading

Breslow MJ, Ligier B. Hyperadrenergic states. *Critical Care Medicine* 1991; **19**: 1566–1578.
Nicholson G, Burrin JM, Hall GM. Peri-operative steroid supplementation. *Anaesthesia* 1998; **53**: 1091–1104.

Related topics of interest

Calcium, magnesium and phosphate, p. 56; Fluid therapy, p. 122; Potassium, p. 180; Sodium, p. 231

AIDS

Cynthia Uy

The Acquired Immunodeficiency Syndrome (AIDS) is caused by the Human Immuno-deficiency Virus (HIV). It causes a range of illnesses some of which are reversible with aggressive management. HIV is a retrovirus. It infects the CD4 T-lymphocyte by attaching to the CD4 receptor and introducing its RNA into the cell. The enzyme reverse transcriptase, which is contained in the virus, uses this RNA to generate DNA which is then incorporated in the host's DNA. This 'provirus' may remain inactive (latent) or manifest high levels of gene expression with production of virus and infection of other cells, resulting in impairment and eventually destruction and depletion of the patient's CD4 cells.

The 1993 Centers for Disease Control surveillance case definition for AIDS includes all HIV-infected persons who have CD4 T-lymphocyte count < 200 ml^{-1} of blood or a CD4 T-lymphocyte percentage of total lymphocytes < 14. Indicator diseases of AIDS include: *Pneumocystis carinii* pneumonia (PCP); pulmonary tuberculosis; Kaposi sarcoma; extra-pulmonary cryptococcosis; HIV encephalopathy; non-Hodgkin's lymphoma; infection with cytomegalo or herpes simplex virus, coccidioidomycosis, toxoplasmosis, candidiasis and salmonella; (non-typhoid) septicaemia.

HIV can be transmitted by sexual contact (homosexual or heterosexual), blood or blood products (e.g., haemophiliacs and intravenous drug users) and by mother to child intra-partum, perinatally or through breast milk. It has been established that there is a small but definite risk of HIV transmission among health care workers who work with HIV infected specimens. At present, the risk of transmission from an infected health care worker to a patient is too low to be measured.

Since AIDS was first reported in 1981 there has been an exponential rise in the number of seropositive people infected with HIV worldwide. The World Health Organization estimate that by the year 2000, there will be approximately 40 million people infected with the virus. With the rise in the number of cases of AIDS, there has been increasing use of critical care resources by HIV infected patients. There is concern, however, that HIV patients receiving treatment in a critical care setting do not have an altered outcome, have prolonged suffering and the treatment is not cost-effective.

The commonest reason for HIV infected patients to be admitted to a critical care unit is for ventilatory support for respiratory failure secondary to PCP. Other causes for admission are: respiratory failure secondary to non-specific interstitial pneumonitis; cardiac arrhythmia; CHF; hypotension due to sepsis or adrenal insufficiency; seizures; gastrointestinal bleeding; upper airway obstruction, syncopal episodes; drug toxicity and suicide attempts.

Pneumocystis carinii pneumonia

1. Presentation. This usually includes fever, dry cough and a characteristic pleuritic retrosternal pain. Shortness of breath on exertion, lethargy and weight loss are seen in more advanced cases. Findings on examination are minimal. The CXR is either normal or, as severe PCP resembles ARDS, can show a faint bilateral interstitial infiltrate.

2. Laboratory evaluation is usually unhelpful. Studies of oxygen saturation and diffusing capacity for carbon monoxide are sensitive but not specific for PCP. A definitive diagnosis is made when the organism is identified in samples obtained from induced sputum, bronchoalveolar lavage (BAL), transbronchial or open lung biopsy.

3. **Complications.** Pneumothorax occurs in approximately 2% of cases, more so in patients who have had previous episodes of PCP or in patients who have received prophylactic nebulized pentamidine. The mortality of PCP associated with pneumothorax is 10%. Sclerotherapy or surgical intervention may be indicated.

4. **Treatment** is chiefly with intravenous co-trimoxazole or pentamidine isethionate. The main problem with therapy is the high incidence of side effects, exceeding 50% in most series. Adverse reactions to co-trimoxazole include: nausea, vomiting, diarrhoea, rashes, glossitis, erythema multiforme, epidermal necrolysis, pancreatitis, blood dyscrasias, pseudomembranous colitis, jaundice and hepatic necrosis. Adverse reactions to pentamidine isethionate include: hypoglycaemia, pancreatitis, cardiac arrhythmias, renal dysfunction, hypocalcaemia, blood dyscrasias, hyperglycaemia, rashes, bronchoconstriction and orthostatic hypotension.

Patients on treatment do not begin to improve until the end of the first week. Some patients clinically deteriorate during the first few days of treatment, presumably due to the deaths of large numbers of organisms in the lung resulting in increased capillary permeability and oedema formation.

Glucocorticoids used as adjuvant therapy with standard anti-pneumocystis treatment have been shown to reduce the risk of respiratory failure and death in patients with AIDS. The National Institute of Health/University of California Expert Panel recommend that 40 mg of oral prednisone twice a day be given to patients with a $PaO_2 < 9.3$ kPa or an arterial/alveolar gradient > 4.66 kPa. After 5 days, the dose should be tapered gradually over 3 weeks. It has not been established whether adjuvant steroids alter mortality in patients already in respiratory failure.

5. **Prognosis.** Seventy-five per cent of patients with HIV experience at least one episode of PCP and 20% die as a consequence despite treatment. Recent reports suggest an improvement in survival following admission to critical care units in AIDS patients with PCP despite initial concerns over the validity of such measures.

Prevention

1. **Universal precautions,** which assume that all patients may be infected are recommended to minimize the chances of transmission of HIV. Guidelines include:

- The use of gloves when there is any risk of contact with infective body fluids.
- The wearing of masks and protective eyewear when infective fluids may become airborne and gowns made of impervious material if there is any chance of being splashed.
- Open or exudative wounds should be covered and contact with potentially infective fluids avoided. If any contact with body fluids occurs, the affected part should be washed immediately.
- Needles must not be resheathed or passed from one person to another.
- Contaminated waste must be segregated, placed in a suitable leak proof container and contained at the place it is generated before being disposed of in an appropriate manner.

- It is advisable, given the high prevalence of hepatitis B and pulmonary tuberculosis in HIV patients, for staff to be immunized/vaccinated.

2. *In addition, to protect other patients:*

- All blood and blood products should be screened for antibodies to HIV. Transmission can occur in the 3 month 'window period' between infection and seroconversion, or due to clerical errors in reporting results or labelling blood. This risk is less than one in a million per transfused unit of blood.
- Disposable equipment should be used for infected patients. Reusable devices employed in invasive procedures must be disinfected and sterilized.
- In HIV infected patients with undiagnosed respiratory illness, tuberculosis must be considered and patients nursed in a single room. Mechanical ventilators should be fitted with exhaled gas scavenging systems.
- The isolation of seropositive patients is not appropriate unless the patient is bleeding or requires isolation due to immunosuppression or a contagious secondary infection.

Needlestick and surgical knife accidents are the likeliest causes of seroconversion. The data from several studies suggest that the risk of HIV infection following a percutaneous injury with an HIV contaminated needle is approximately 0.3%. The wound should be washed and zidovudine prophylaxis commenced. An individual who thinks they may be infected should seek confidential expert advice. HIV infected individuals should not carry out procedures where their hands are not completely visible.

Further reading

Notterman DA. Acquired immunodeficiency syndrome, *Pneumocystis carinii* pneumonia and futility. *Critical Care Medicine* 1996; **24:** 907–909.
Rosen MJ, De Palo VA. Outcome of intensive care for patients with AIDS. *Critical Care Clinics* 1993; **9:** 107–114.

Related topics of interest

Infection control, p. 140; Infection in critical care, p. 143

ANALGESIA – BASIC

Bronwen Evans

The International Society for the Study of Pain defines pain as 'an unpleasant sensory and emotional experience associated with actual or potential tissue damage or described in terms of such damage'.

Problems

- Assessment of pain is difficult in critical care patients. Injury, intoxication or sedation may impair their conscious state. Intubated and paralysed patients cannot respond verbally. There may be multiple foci for pain from injury, surgery, invasive monitors and indwelling catheters. It may be difficult to distinguish pain from anxiety; the two will often coexist.
- Haemodynamic instability, renal and hepatic failure will influence the pharmacodynamics and pharmacokinetics of analgesic strategies. Coagulopathy will preclude the use of regional catheter techniques.
- The need for sedation (and sometimes paralysis) coexists with the need for analgesics.
- Prolonged infusions of opioids lead to tolerance, and accumulation of the drug and its metabolites especially in renal or hepatic failure.
- Misunderstanding of the importance of analgesia may lead to under prescribing and underdosing of drugs. A majority of patients discharged from critical care units (60–70%) recall being in pain. Coronary patients may minimize and under-report their pain. The early administration of effective analgesia to patients with abdominal pain does not interfere with diagnosis.

Pain assessment

It is difficult to make an objective measure of a subjective experience. Tools of assessment include adjective, numeric or behaviour and physiological parameters.

1. Adjective scale. None, mild, moderate, severe, intolerable.

2. Visual Analogue Scale (VAS). Pain is indicated on a 10 cm scale continuum or expressed as a numeric value from 0 to 10.

3. Happy and sad faces. A qualitative scale for paediatric patients.

4. Poker chips. A quantitative measure in paediatric patients.

5. Observer scale. For non-communicative or intubated patients. This scores a series of behavioural and physiological parameters including vital signs, non-vocal communication, facial expression, posture and agitation.

Pain assessment must be continuous and should include the response to an intervention and subsequent adjustments in therapy.

Non-pharmacological pain management

- Attention to aspects of nursing with repositioning and pressure area care. Positioning of catheters and invasive monitors so that they do not drag.

Elevation of limbs assists venous drainage and prevents stasis oedema. Circulatory assessment of covered limbs. Relief of urinary retention. Correct posture for optimal ventilation.

- Physiotherapy, both passive and active.
- Relaxation techniques have been shown to reduce distress and use of analgesic medication and to increase comfort. Cognitive-behavioural interventions are time consuming but may have a positive effect on pain management and, despite pragmatic considerations, should not be considered invalid.
- Psychological support is important so that talking to and explaining procedures even to sedated or unconscious patients may reduce overall stress. Appropriate involvement of relatives and friends is helpful.
- TENS: *see* Analgesia – advanced (p. 19)

Pharmacological pain management

1. Non-steroidal anti-inflammatories

(a) Paracetamol. Paracetamol is an analgesic and anti-pyretic. It inhibits central and peripheral prostaglandin synthesis. It is a poor anti-inflammatory. It has few irritant side effects and is renally excreted following hepatic conjugation. Paracetamol has a ceiling effect and is used for mild pain. It is administered orally (or NGT) or rectally. A parenteral form is available in some countries. It should be given regularly if it is to have an opioid sparing effect.

(b) Other NSAIDs. These non-opioids are reversible inhibitors of cyclo-oxygenase, reducing levels of prostaglandin, prostacyclin and thromboxane A_2 pain mediators. They have both a central and peripheral role in blocking the prostaglandin mediated lowering of pain receptor thresholds. Salicylates are non-reversible inhibitors of prostaglandins. They are useful for the management of mild to moderate pain. They can be used in combination with opioids and regional analgesic techniques.

(c) Side effects of NSAIDs.

- Gastrointestinal erosions are due to local irritation, reduced gastric blood flow, and increased acid secretion mediated by prostaglandin inhibition. Rectal and parenteral routes may lessen the risk. H_2 antagonists and proton pump inhibitors may reduce the risks also.
- Platelet aggregation homeostasis is mediated by a balance between the platelet derived thromboxane A_2 (promotes aggregation) and endothelial derived prostacyclin (a vasodilator which inhibits aggregation). Aspirin induced inhibition of platelet function is irreversible, prolonging bleeding time for the life of the platelet (8–11) days. Other NSAIDs will affect bleeding time for five times the half-life of the drug.
- Aspirin-induced asthma may occur in some adult asthmatics. Cross sensitivity with other NSAIDs does exist.
- Renal failure may be precipitated when prostaglandin dependent intrarenal blood flow is reduced in patients with reduced intravascular volume. In volume depleted states, compensatory humoral and sympathetic homeostatic responses will reduce renal blood flow in an effort to conserve water and sodium. The only remaining vasodilatory mechanism which maintains renal blood flow is prostaglandin dependent. Prostaglandin inhibition by NSAIDs,

alone, or in combination with the administration of other renal toxins (aminoglycoside antibiotics, contrast media) or pre-existing renal impairment may precipitate ATN. NSAIDs may promote sodium, potassium and water retention, causing oedema.

2. *Opioid analgesics.* Opioids are those analgesics with morphine-like actions. They may be opiates; derivatives of the opium poppy *Papaver somniferum* (morphine and codeine) or synthetic analogues (pethidine, fentanyl, methadone). They are agonists at opioid receptors in the central and peripheral nervous systems.

Opioid receptors are subclassed as mu, kappa and delta. Opioid analgesics are primarily mu receptor agonists. They produce both excitatory and inhibitory phenomena including: analgesia, respiratory depression, euphoria, bradycardia, pruritis, meiosis, nausea and vomiting (via the chemoreceptor trigger zone) and inhibition of gut motility.

In equianalgesic doses and in most patients, the incidence of side effects is similar regardless of the opioid used.

(a) Side effects of opioids

- Respiratory depression, with direct depression of the respiratory centre in the medulla results in reduced respiratory rate and tidal volume and reduced sensitivity to hypercapnoea. Suppression of cough reflex reduces sputum clearance and may risk airway soiling. The best early sign of opioid induced respiratory depression is sedation. Decreased respiratory rate is a late and unreliable sign. Sedation may be due to the combined effect of opioid and elevated $PaCO_2$. Thus, respiratory depression can coexist with a normal respiratory rate and if the patient is receiving supplemental oxygen, then a normal PaO_2 does not preclude hypoventilation.
- Cardiovascular side effects due to direct arterial and venous smooth muscle relaxation and histamine release (morphine, diamorphine, pethidine and codeine) result in vasodilatation. Postural hypotension may occur. Significant supine hypotension suggests hypovolaemia that is unmasked by opioids. Vagally mediated bradycardia can occur. Pethidine however has atropine-like effects and mediates a tachycardia.
- Pruritis may be histamine or non-histamine mediated. Mast cell histamine release localized to the site of injection or along the vein of injection may cause localized or generalized pruritis and is not indicative of opioid allergy. Centrally mediated pruritis is possibly mu receptor mediated and is more commonly associated with epidural or intrathecal opioid, especially morphine. Pruritis may be treated with antihistamines or naloxone.
- Bowel motility is reduced by local and central mechanisms and causes constipation and aggravates ileus. Sphincter of Oddi spasm and urinary retention can be reversed by naloxone.

True opioid allergy is not common. It is mediated by the immune system resulting in rash, urticaria, bronchoconstriction, CVS collapse and angioedema.

In general, dosage varies inversely with age (not size). There is still a ten-fold variation in dose requirements between individuals of the same age. The initial dose should be based on patient age and subsequent doses titrated to suit the individual with respect to renal and hepatic function and cardiorespiratory function.

(b) Equianalgesic doses

Opioid	i.m./i.v. (mg)	oral (mg)	$t_{1/2}\beta$ (elimination half life; h)
Morphine	10	30–60	2–3
Pethidine	100	400	3–4
Fentanyl	0.1	N/A	3–4
Codeine[a]	130	200	3–4
Oxycodone	15	10–20	2–3
Diamorphine	5	60	0.5 (rapidly hydrolyzed to morphine)
Methadone	10	20	15–40

[a]The metabolic conversion of codeine to morphine is subject to wide pharmacogenetic variation. It is a poor choice of analgesic in critical care.

(c) Adjuvant therapy
- *Anxiolysis.* Hypnotic medication providing sedation will reduce distress and form adjuvant therapy to analgesics.
- *Antidepressants.* Useful during long-term critical care admissions for mood elevation. They can be weaned following recovery. Tricyclic antidepressants are commonly used.

(d) Drug tolerance and withdrawal. Tolerance results when, over time, more drug is needed to produce the same effect. It occurs with long-term administration of opioids. It may be due to altered drug receptor affinity and may be minimized by using the lowest dose possible to achieve analgesia.

Withdrawal phenomena will be experienced when drugs to which the patient is tolerant are ceased abruptly. Such drugs should be withdrawn slowly. Substitution with drugs with a long half-life may be of benefit.

Addiction is a behavioural phenomenon and occurs rarely in a clinical setting. Addicts demonstrate tolerance and suffer withdrawal.

Further reading

McQuay H, Moore A, Justins D. Treating acute pain in hospital. *BMJ* 1997; **314**: 1531–1535.

Related topic of interest

Analgesia – advanced, p. 18

ANALGESIA – ADVANCED

Bronwen Evans

Epidural analgesia

Infusion of a combination of local anaesthetics and/or an opioid into the epidural space will block and modify the conduction of pain impulses.

1. Benefits

- Selective sensory nerve blockade.
- High quality analgesia.
- The reduced or absent systemic plasma concentration of opioid reduces or avoids opioid-related side effects.
- The quality of comfort is beneficial for physiotherapy, positioning and nursing.
- Weaning from ventilation is assisted by the absence of opioid-related sedation and respiratory depression.

2. Disadvantages and complications

- Expertise required to site the epidural catheter.
- Hypotension due to sympathetic nerve blockade.
- Risk of infection in the epidural space increases with the duration of catheter placement.
- Small risk of nerve root or cord damage, epidural haematoma, infection with neurological sequelae (transient: ~ 1:4000; permanent: ~ 1:35 000).
- Catheter misplacement into subarachnoid space causing massive subarachnoid block with bradycardia, hypotension and loss of consciousness.
- Catheter misplacement into a vessel causing systemic local anaesthetic toxicity with CNS and then CVS collapse.
- Dural puncture headache which may be confused with meningism.

3. Drug actions

(a) **Local anaesthetics** block sodium channels, preventing neural transmission. Higher concentrations are required to block motor nerves which have the thickest myelin sheath. Unmyelinated and lightly myelinated C and A delta pain and temperature fibres are blocked at low concentrations. Autonomic nerves are also blocked thus, vasodilatation and hypotension are side effects. Intravenous fluid loading and vasopressors are used to combat hypotension. Blockade at the level of cardioaccelerator fibres T_1–T_4 will cause bradycardia and hypotension.

(b) **Opioids** act at opioid receptors in the dorsal horn to provide analgesia. Highly lipid-soluble fentanyl will act near the site of absorption across the dura. Less lipid-soluble morphine has a longer half-life in the CSF, and may circulate up to the medulla, causing respiratory depression. This risk persists for 18–24 hours. Morphine and fentanyl do not block sensory autonomic or motor nerves.

Extensive cover is provided by larger volumes or by simultaneous epidurals at two levels (lumbar and thoracic).

4. Contraindications to epidural analgesia

- Patient refusal.
- Infection at the site of insertion.
- Coagulopathy (risk of epidural haematoma).
- Septicaemia (theoretical risk of epidural abscess).

Patient controlled analgesia (PCA)

Some patients receiving critical care may be orientated and motivated enough to utilize PCA. A drug delivery system (syringe driver) delivers a bolus dose of opioid analgesic upon demand by the patient. The patient should be reassured about addiction and overdosage. They should be instructed to anticipate pain (e.g., prior to physiotherapy) and advised to use regular dosing rather than allow severe pain to develop.

TENS

Low-frequency pulses of electricity from electrodes placed over the dermatome of pain, stimulate large nerve fibres which in turn transmit to the dorsal horn substantia gelatinosa cells. Input from large fibres produces negative feedback in the substantia gelatinosa, preventing onward transmission of nociceptive signals.

Ketamine

This phencyclidine derivative may be used in conjunction with benzodiazepines for short painful procedures. It provides good analgesia without respiratory depression at subanaesthetic concentrations. Its unpleasant psychological sequelae are minimized by concomitant benzodiazepines.

Further reading

Kroll W, List WF. Pain treatment in the ICU: intravenous, regional or both? *European Journal of Anaesthesiology* Suppl. 1997; **15**: 49–52.

Related topics of interest

Analgesia – basic, p. 14; Sedation, p. 223

ANAPHYLAXIS

Adverse immunological responses may be anaphylactic (IgE mediated) or anaphylactoid (non-IgE mediated and often following first exposure to the trigger agent). Anaphylactic reactions occur following 'classical' pathway complement activation. Previous exposure to the antigen with antibody formation is required. 'Alternative' pathway activation occurs when the trigger activates the cascade directly; previous exposure to the antigen is not necessary (e.g., reactions to drugs, dextrans or contrast media). Reactions to drugs may also occur as a consequence of direct activation of mast cells by the drug (pharmacological histamine release) and do not involve complement activation (e.g., after administration of certain muscle relaxants).

The manifestations and management of severe anaphylactic and anaphylactoid reactions are similar. The distinction is thus less important in the acute phase, though it may aid follow-up management.

Clinical signs and symptoms

Typically, patients present with angioedema, urticaria, dyspnoea, and hypotension. Features include:

- Cardiovascular collapse due to vasodilatation and loss of plasma from the circulating compartment. It is present in 90% of patients and is the only feature in 10%.
- Bronchospasm, present in 50% and the only feature in 3%.
- Acute upper airway obstruction due to laryngeal oedema.
- Skin erythema (urticaria), conjunctivitis, rhinitis.
- Gastrointestinal symptoms including nausea, vomiting, abdominal pain, and diarrhoea.

Anaphylactic reactions vary in severity and progression. The onset may be rapid, slow, or (unusually) biphasic.

Treatment considerations

- Adrenaline is the most important drug for the treatment of severe reactions. Its alpha-adrenoceptor agonism reverses peripheral vasodilatation and reduces oedema. Its beta-adrenoceptor activity dilates the airways, increases the force of myocardial contractility, and suppresses the release of mediators such as histamine and leukotrienes. Adrenaline works best when given shortly after the onset of a reaction. Its use is not without risk, however, especially when given intravenously. Rarely, adrenaline may fail to reverse the signs of a severe reaction, especially if given late or to a patient already being treated with beta-blockers. Under such circumstances aggressive volume replacement may be life saving.
- Anti-H_1 antihistamines should be given to all patients suffering an anaphylactic reaction. They help combat histamine mediated vasodilatation and control symptoms such as urticaria.
- Corticosteroids are slow onset drugs whose action may take 4–6 hours to develop even after intravenous administration. They are not life saving drugs in

anaphylaxis. They may be useful, however, in preventing recurrent or short-ening protracted reactions and should thus be given to all victims of a severe reaction.

Management

A. **Airway.** 100% oxygen by face mask.

B. **Breathing.** Bag and mask ventilation if assistance needed. Intubate if there is serious airway obstruction or in cardiac arrest.

C. **Circulation.** Intramuscular adrenaline requires an effective circulation. Administer intravenous fluids.

(a) Adrenaline should be administered intramuscularly to all patients with signs of shock, airway swelling, or breathing difficulty.

- Adults: Give 0.5 ml of a 1:1000 solution adrenaline i.m. (i.e., 500 µg).

In the critical care unit it is more appropriate to titrate 0.5–1 ml of a 1:10 000 solution of adrenaline intravenously i.e., 50–100 µg. Intravenous adrenaline should not be given without continuous ECG monitoring.

It should be repeated after 5 min if there are no signs of improvement or the patient deteriorates.

Caution: Patients receiving monoamine oxidase inhibitors should be given only 25% of the dose of adrenaline at a time due to a potentially dangerous interaction.

- **Children**

> 11 years	up to 500 µg i.m. (0.5 ml 1:1000 solution)
6–11 years	250 µg i.m. (0.25 ml 1:1000 solution)
2–5 years	125 µg i.m. (0.125 ml 1:1000 solution)
< 2 years	62.5 µg i.m. (by additional dilution of 1:100 solution)

If anaphylaxis is thought to have been precipitated by a drug or infusion, its administration should be discontinued immediately.

(b) An antihistamine (e.g. chlorpheniramine 10–20 mg) should be given.

(c) Hydrocortisone (100–500 mg i.m or by slow i.v. injection) should be administered for severe attacks especially in asthmatics.

(d) Inhaled or intravenous β_2 agonists may be helpful in patients with persisting bronchospasm.

Investigation

Once the patient has recovered from the immediate life threatening reaction, they should be investigated for the cause.

1. Non-specific tests. Take blood samples for measurement of complement and tryptase. An elevated blood C3 and C4 complement level indicates an immune mediated response. Elevation of C3 alone suggests alternative pathway activation. Total IgE antibody levels may also be measured. Blood histamine levels may be elevated for a short time only, but its metabolite methylhistamine has a longer half-life and is measurable in urine up to 2–3 hours following a reaction. Tryptase, a mast cell specific protease released during degranulation, may also remain in the blood for about 3 hours.

2. *Specific tests.* Drug specific antibodies may be quantified using labelled anti-human IgE antibody by radioallergosorbant tests (RAST).

3. *Skin testing.* These tests should be performed only where full resuscitation facilities are immediately available. The optimum time for testing is 6 weeks following a reaction. The patient should not be taking drugs which may interfere with the response (e.g. corticosteroids, antihistamines).

Intradermal testing utilizes dilute solutions of potential antigens. Solutions of the test agents are diluted to 1:1000 and 1:100 and a control solution (e.g. saline) prepared. A 1 mm weal of each solution is then raised on the forearm of the patient. A positive result occurs when a weal > 10 mm persists for more than 30 min.

Skin prick testing is safer, quicker and easier to perform (the test agent does not require dilution). A drop of solution is placed on the skin and a puncture made through it (< 1 mm). A wheal > 3 mm after 15 minutes is considered a positive result.

Further reading

Brown AFT. Anaphylactic shock: mechanisms and treatment. *Journal of Accident and Emergency Medicine* 1995; **12**: 89–100.

Chamberlain D, *et al.* The emergency medical treatment of anaphylactic reactions. *Project Team of The Resuscitation Council (UK)*, 1999.

Whittington T, Fisher MM. Anaphylactic and anaphylactial reactions. *Ballière's Clinical Anaesthesiology* 1998; **12**: 301–323.

Related topics of interest

Asthma, p. 31; Resuscitation–cardiopulmonary, p. 213

ARTERIAL BLOOD GASES – ACID–BASE PHYSIOLOGY

Alex Goodwin

A biochemical milieu maintained within a narrow range is required for the normal function of enzymes within the cells of the body. The concentration of hydrogen ions (H^+) is low but crucial for normal enzyme function.

The following definitions are essential to the understanding of acid–base physiology:

Acid	Proton donor
Base	Proton acceptor
Strong acid	Fully dissociates in solution
Weak acid	Partially dissociates in solution
Buffer	A chemical substance that prevents large changes in hydrogen ion concentration when an acid or base is added to a solution
Acidaemia	Decrease in pH
Acidosis	Increase in hydrogen ion concentration

The normal plasma concentration of sodium is 140 mmol l^{-1} whilst that of H^+ is 0.00004 mmol l^{-1}. Thus, hydrogen ion concentration is represented as pH, which is the negative Log_{10} of the hydrogen ion concentration. The normal extracellular pH is 7.4, venous blood 7.35, red blood cells 7.2, muscle cells 6.8 – 7.0 (in anaerobic metabolism 6.40) and that of CSF 7.32

Aerobic metabolism produces 1400 mmols of carbon dioxide per day. This is termed volatile acid because it is excreted via the lungs. Amino acid metabolism results in the production of approximately 80 mmols day^{-1} of non-volatile acid.

Anaerobic metabolism results in the production of lactic acid. The abnormal metabolism of fats results in the production of keto-acids (e.g., diabetic ketoacidosis).

The body's defence against a hydrogen ion load involves the following compensatory mechanisms:

Dilution

Acid produced in cells is diluted in total body water because it diffuses into the extracellular fluid and into other cells. Each ten-fold dilution increases the pH by 1 unit.

Buffers

An acid–base buffer is a solution of two or more chemical compounds that prevents marked changes in hydrogen ion concentration when an acid or a base is added. The pK of a buffer system defines the pH at which the ionized and unionized forms are in equilibrium. It is also the pH at which the buffer system is most efficient.

Important buffer systems are found in:

Plasma
Bicarbonate: $CO_2 + H_2O \rightleftharpoons H_2CO_3 \rightleftharpoons H^+ + HCO_3^-$ ($pK = 6.1$)
Phosphate: $H_2PO_4^- \rightleftharpoons H^+ + HPO_4^{2-}$ ($pK = 6.8$)

Blood and intracellular

Protein: Hprotein $\rightleftharpoons$ H$^+$ + Protein$^-$ (*pK* = 7.3)

Haemoglobin: HHb $\rightleftharpoons$ H$^+$ + Hb$^-$ (*pK* = 7.3)

The Henderson Hasselbalch equation considers the relationship of a buffer system to pH.

pH = pKa + Log$_{10}$ Base/Acid

For the bicarbonate system: pH = 6.1 + Log$_{10}$ HCO$_3^-$/PaCO$_2$

Hence at plasma bicarbonate of 24 mmol l^{-1} and a PaCO$_2$ of 40 mmHg the equation becomes: pH = 6.1 + Log$_{10}$ 24/0.03 × 40

(0.03 = solubility coefficient of carbon dioxide, mmol mmHg^{-1})

pH = 7.4

Respiratory compensation

The respiratory system is able to regulate pH. An increase in CO_2 concentration leads to a decrease in pH and a decrease in CO_2 leads to a rise in pH. If the metabolic production of CO_2 remains constant the only factor that affects CO_2 concentration is alveolar ventilation. The respiratory centre in the medulla oblongata is sensitive to hydrogen ion concentration and changes alveolar ventilation accordingly. This affects hydrogen ion concentration within minutes. Thus, the respiratory system is a 'physiological buffer'.

Renal control

The kidneys control acid–base balance by controlling the secretion of hydrogen ions relative to the amount of filtered bicarbonate.

1. ***Tubular secretion of hydrogen ions.*** Hydrogen ions are secreted throughout most of the tubular system. There are two quite distinct methods of secretion:

- Secondary active transport of hydrogen ions occurs in the proximal tubule, thick segment of the ascending loop of Henle, and the distal tubule. Within the epithelial cell carbon dioxide combines with water under the influence of carbonic anhydrase to form carbonic acid. This then dissociates into a hydrogen ion and bicarbonate. The hydrogen ion is secreted into the tubular lumen by a mechanism of sodium/hydrogen counter-transport.
- Primary active transport occurs in the latter part of the distal tubules all the way to the renal pelvis. This transport system accounts for less than 5% of the total hydrogen ions secreted. However, it can concentrate hydrogen ions 900-fold compared to four-fold for secondary active transport. The rate of hydrogen ion secretion changes in response to changes in extracellular hydrogen ion concentration.

2. ***Interaction of bicarbonate and hydrogen ions in the tubules.*** The bicarbonate ion does not diffuse into the epithelial cells of the renal tubules readily because it is a large molecule and is electrically charged. However, it combines with a secreted hydrogen ion to form carbon dioxide and water and is, effectively, 'reabsorbed'. The CO_2 diffuses into the epithelial cell and combines with water to form carbonic acid, which immediately dissociates to bicarbonate and hydrogen ion. The bicarbonate ion then diffuses into the extracellular fluid.

The rate of hydrogen ion secretion is about 3.5 mmol min^{-1} and the rate of filtration of bicarbonate is 3.46 mmol min^{-1}. Normally, the hydrogen ions and bicarbonate titrate themselves. The mechanism by which the kidney corrects either acidosis or alkalosis is by incomplete titration. An excess of hydrogen ions in the urine can be buffered by phosphate and ammonia.

The liver

The liver assists in acid–base balance by regulating ureagenesis. Amino acid metabolism leads to the generation of bicarbonate and ammonia. These combine to form urea, CO_2 and water:

$$2NH_4^+ + 2HCO_3^- \rightleftharpoons NH_2\text{-}CO\text{-}NH_2 + CO_2 + 3H_2O$$

The lungs remove the CO_2 and there is no net acid or base production. The liver is able to regulate the metabolism of ammonia and bicarbonate to urea. In alkalosis ureagenesis increases, consuming bicarbonate. In acidosis ureagenesis decreases, increasing available bicarbonate

Bone

Extracellular hydrogen ions can exchange with cations from bone and cells (e.g., sodium, potassium, magnesium and calcium). This is a slow process and may take hours or days.

Further reading

Gluck SL. Acid-base. *Lancet* 1998; 352: 474–479.

Related topic of interest

Arterial blood gases – analysis, p. 26

ARTERIAL BLOOD GASES – ANALYSIS

Alex Goodwin

An understanding of arterial blood gases (ABGs) is fundamental to the management of critically ill patients. Having processed an arterial blood sample, the blood gas analyser will typically display the following information.

PaO_2 – partial pressure of oxygen in arterial blood

This is measured directly. Its relationship with the fractional inspired oxygen concentration (FIO_2), is described by the alveolar gas equation:

$$PaO_2 = FIO_2 (P_b - P_{H_2O}) - PaCO_2/RQ$$

PaO_2 = Alveolar oxygen pressure	FIO_2 = Inspired oxygen fraction
P_b = Atmospheric pressure	Pa_{H_2O} = Water vapour pressure
$PaCO_2$ = Alveolar CO_2 pressure	RQ = Respiratory quotient

When breathing air at an atmospheric pressure of 100 kPa, the partial pressure of inspired oxygen is 20.9 kPa. Having become fully saturated with water in the upper respiratory tract the partial pressure of oxygen falls to 19.5 kPa. At the alveolus, oxygen is taken up and replaced by CO_2, which reduces the PaO_2 to 14 kPa. Because of shunt, the arterial oxygen pressure is always slightly lower than that in the alveolus. When breathing air, the normal PaO_2 is 12.5 kPa at the age of 20 years and 10.8 kPa at 65 years.

$PaCO_2$ – partial pressure of carbon dioxide in arterial blood

This is measured directly and is normally 5.3 kPa.

pH

This is the negative Log_{10} of the hydrogen ion concentration and is measured directly. The normal pH is 7.35–7.45.

Standard bicarbonate

This is calculated from the CO_2 and pH using the Henderson Hasselbach equation. It is the concentration of bicarbonate in a sample equilibrated to 37°C and $PaCO_2$ 40 mmHg. Thus, the metabolic component of acid–base balance can be assessed. The normal value is 21–27 mmol l^{-1}.

Actual bicarbonate

This reflects the contribution of both the respiratory and metabolic components. The normal value in venous blood is 21–28 mmol l^{-1}.

Base excess and base deficit

This is a measure of the amount of acid or base that needs to be added to a sample, under standard conditions (37°C and $PaCO_2$ 40 mmHg), to return the pH to 7.4. It is traditionally reported as 'base excess'. The normal range is +2 mmol l^{-1} to −2 mmol l^{-1}.

Interpretation of blood gas data

When evaluating respiratory and acid–base disorders arterial blood gas data must be considered within the context of the wider clinical picture. Having noted the FIO_2 and PaO_2, the ABG results should be assessed as follows:

1. Assess the hydrogen ion concentration.
   - pH > 7.45 – alkalaemia
   - pH < 7.35 – acidaemia
   - 7.35–7.45 no disturbance or mixed disturbance
2. Assess the metabolic component
   - HCO_3 > 33 mmol l^{-1} – metabolic alkalosis
   - HCO_3 < 23 mmol l^{-1} – metabolic acidosis
3. Assess the respiratory component
   - $PaCO_2$ > 45 mmHg – respiratory acidosis
   - $PaCO_2$ < 35 mmHg – respiratory alkalosis
4. Combine the information from 1,2 and 3 and determine if there is any metabolic or respiratory compensation.
5. Consider the anion gap. This indicates the presence of non-volatile acids (lactic acid, keto-acids and exogenous acids). The normal anion gap is 10–18 mmol l^{-1} and can be estimated using the following equation:

$$[(Na^+) + (K^+)] - [(Cl^-) + (HCO3^-)]$$

Disorders of acid–base balance are divided into acidosis and alkalosis and into those of metabolic and respiratory origin. They can be subdivided by the presence or absence of an abnormal anion gap.

Disorders of acid–base balance

1. *Metabolic acidosis (with a normal anion gap)*
- Increased gastrointestinal bicarbonate loss (e.g., diarrhoea, ileostomy, ureterosigmoidostomy).
- Increased renal bicarbonate loss (e.g., acetazolamide, proximal renal tubular acidosis (type 2), hyperparathyroidism, tubular damage e.g., drugs, heavy metals, paraproteins).
- Decreased renal hydrogen secretion [e.g., distal renal tubular acidosis (type 1), type 4 renal tubular acidosis (aldosterone deficiency)].
- Increased HCl production (e.g., ammonium chloride ingestion, increased catabolism of lysine, arginine).

2. *Metabolic acidosis with abnormal anion gap.* Accumulation of organic acids
- Lactic acidosis. L-lactic acid – Type A (anaerobic metabolism, hypotension/cardiac arrest, sepsis, poisoning – ethylene glycol, methanol). Type B (decreased hepatic lactate metabolism, insulin deficiency, metformin accumulation, haematological malignancies, rare inherited enzyme defects). D-lactic acid (fermentation of glucose in the bowel e.g., in blind loops).
- Ketoacidosis (e.g., insulin deficiency, alcohol excess, starvation).
- Exogenous acids (e.g., salicylates).

3. Metabolic alkalosis

- Loss of acid (e.g., hydrogen on loss from GI tract – vomiting, nasogastric suction, hydrogen loss from kidney – diuretics, hypokalaemia, excess mineralocorticoid, low chloride states – diuretic therapy).
- Addition of alkali (e.g., sodium bicarbonate (paradoxical intracellular acidosis), addition of substance converted to bicarbonate – citrate, lactate, acetate).

4. Respiratory acidosis

- Respiratory depression (e.g., drugs, cerebral injury).
- Muscle weakness (e.g., Guillain-Barre, myasthenia, polio, muscle relaxants).
- Trauma (e.g., flail chest, lung contusion).
- Pulmonary insufficiency (e.g., pulmonary oedema, pneumonia, ARDS).
- Airway obstruction.
- Artificial ventilation (e.g., inadequate minute volume, excessive PEEP).

5. Respiratory alkalosis

- Excessively high minute volume.
- Hypoxaemia.
- Pulmonary embolism.
- Asthma.
- Impairment of cerebral function (e.g., meningo-encephalitis).
- Respiratory stimulants (e.g., salycilate overdose).
- Sepsis.
- Parenchymal pulmonary disorder (e.g., oedema).

6. Mixed disorders

- Metabolic acidosis and respiratory acidosis (e.g., cardiac arrest, respiratory failure with anoxia).
- Metabolic alkalosis and respiratory alkalosis (e.g., CCF and vomiting, diuretics and hepatic failure, diuretic therapy and pneumonia).
- Metabolic alkalosis and respiratory acidosis (e.g., COPD and diuretics, COPD and vomiting).
- Metabolic acidosis and respiratory alkalosis (e.g., salycilate overdose, septic shock, sepsis and renal failure, CCF and renal failure).
- Metabolic alkalosis and metabolic acidosis (e.g., diuretics and ketoacidosis, vomiting and renal failure, vomiting and lactic acidosis).

Further reading

Armstrong RF. The interpretation of arterial blood gases. *Current Anaesthesia and Intensive Care* 1994; 5: 74–80.

Related topic of interest

Arterial blood gases – acid–base physiology, p. 23

ARTERIAL CANNULATION

Peripheral arterial cannulation is a common procedure performed in critical care units. The radial artery at the wrist is the most popular site but there are a number of other suitable arteries: the ulnar, dorsalis pedis, and posterior tibial arteries are, like the radial artery, relatively small distal vessels, but each has a collateral vessel. The brachial, femoral, and axillary arteries do not have collaterals but are much larger and less likely to thrombose.

Indications

1. Continuous monitoring of arterial blood pressure:
(a) Where haemodynamic instability is anticipated:
- Major surgical procedures e.g., cardiac, vascular.
- Large fluid shifts e.g., major trauma.
- Medical problems e.g., heart valve disease.
- Drug therapy e.g., inotropes.

(b) For neurosurgical procedures.
(c) Where non-invasive blood pressure monitoring is not possible e.g., burns.
2. Sampling:
- Blood gases.
- Repeated blood sampling (to prevent the need for multiple punctures).

Contraindications

- Local infection.
- Coagulopathy is a relative contraindication.

Technique

A modified Allen's test may be performed to assess the adequacy of collateral blood flow to the hand before cannulating the radial artery. However, ischaemia may occur despite a normal result and an abnormal result does not reliably predict this complication. Consequently, most clinicians have discarded the Allen's test; if there is any doubt about the perfusion of the hand after radial cannulation, remove the cannula immediately. A 20 gauge arterial cannula may be inserted under local anaesthesia in the same way as a venous cannula, although on occasions it can be easier to transfix the vessel first.

Alternatives to radial artery cannulation

1. Ulnar artery. The ulnar artery can be cannulated using the position and technique described above. If multiple attempts at cannulation of the radial artery have been unsuccessful, do not attempt to cannulate the ipsilateral ulnar artery.

2. Brachial artery. The brachial artery may be cannulated just proximal to the skin crease of the antecubital fossa, medial to the biceps tendon and lateral to pronator teres.

3. Dorsalis pedis. If perfusion to the foot is satisfactory, the dorsalis pedis or posterior tibial arteries may be cannulated safely with a 20 gauge catheter.

4. ***Femoral artery.*** The femoral artery may be cannulated 1–2 cm distal to the inguinal ligament at the midpoint of a line drawn between the superior iliac spine and the symphysis pubis. Insert an 18 gauge central venous cannula into the artery using a Seldinger technique. A standard 20 gauge arterial cannula is too short for reliable femoral access.

Sources of error

An over-damped trace will under read the systolic pressure and over read the diastolic pressure. Causes of over-damping include a kinked cannula, partial obstruction of the cannula by blood clot or by the vessel wall, and air bubbles in the manometer line or transducer. An under-damped trace will over read the systolic and under read the diastolic pressure. The usual cause of this is resonance in long manometer lines. The mean arterial pressure should remain accurate even in the presence of damping or resonance.

Complications

The most significant complications are ischaemia and infection but overall, the incidence of serious complications is low. Thrombosis is more likely to occur when the cannula is large relative to the artery, particularly if it is left in place for longer than 72 hours. In some series, 50% of radial artery cannulations have resulted in thrombosis but few of these cause ischaemia. Thrombi at the catheter tip can embolize peripherally. Flushing the arterial catheter can cause retrograde emboli of thrombus or clot.

Disconnection can cause extensive haemorrhage, and bleeding around the catheter site can cause haematomas, particularly in patients with a coagulopathy. Infection is extremely rare in patients who have arterial catheters solely for intra-operative monitoring, but it is a significant risk in the critical care unit, particularly after about 4 days. An arterial catheter should be removed immediately there is any local inflammation. Accidental injection of drugs may cause distal gangrene. Aneurysm and pseudoaneurysm formations are rare, late complications.

Further reading

Cohen NH, Brett CM. Arterial catheterization. In: Benumof JL (ed.), *Clinical Procedures in Anesthesia and Intensive Care*. Philadelphia; J.B. Lippincott Company, 1992, pp. 375–390.

Related topics of interest

Arterial blood gases – analysis, p. 26; Cardiac output – measurement of, p. 77; Central venous pressure monitoring, p. 87

ASTHMA

Asthma is a chronic disease characterized by increased responsiveness of the tracheobronchial tree to various stimuli (e.g., inhaled allergens, infection, exercise, anxiety, cold or drugs). It manifests as widespread airway narrowing with mucosal oedema and a cellular infiltrate. Reversibility of airway obstruction is characteristic and distinguishes asthma from the fixed obstruction of chronic bronchitis and emphysema. The severity of airflow obstruction varies widely over short periods but airway resistance may be normal for long periods. Acute severe asthma may be a life threatening condition.

Features of acute severe asthma
- Peak expiratory flow (PEF) < 50% of predicted.
- Unable to complete sentences in one breath.
- Respiratory rate > 25 breaths min^{-1}.
- Pulse rate > 110 beats min^{-1}.

and in children
- Too breathless to talk or too breathless to feed.

Features of life threatening asthma
- PEF < 33% of predicted.
- Silent chest, cyanosis, or feeble respiratory effort.
- Bradycardia or hypotension.
- Exhaustion, confusion, or coma.

If the oxygen saturation according to a pulse oximeter (SpO_2) is less than 92% or there are any life threatening features an arterial blood gas analysis should be undertaken urgently. (Blood gas measurements are rarely helpful in deciding initial management in children.)

Arterial blood gas markers of life threatening asthma
- Severe hypoxia (PaO_2 < 8 kPa) irrespective of FiO_2.
- Low pH (or high H^+).
- Normal or high $PaCO_2$.

No other investigation is required for the immediate management of acute severe asthma.

Treatment – immediate
- Oxygen. High concentration.
- β-agonist via oxygen driven nebulizer (salbutamol 5 mg or terbutaline 10 mg – halve doses in very young children).
- Steroids. Prednisolone 30–60 mg orally or hydrocortisone 200 mg i.v. or both. (Prednisolone 1–2 mg kg^{-1} to a maximum of 40 mg in children.)
- NO SEDATION.
- CXR to exclude a pneumothorax.

If life threatening

- Add ipratropium 0.5 mg to nebulized β-agonist (0.25 mg in children or 0.125 mg in the very young).
- Aminophylline. Load with 250 mg over 20 min (5 mg kg^{-1} in children) Do not give bolus aminophylline to patients already taking oral theophyllines. Continue with aminophylline infusion (1 mg kg^{-1} h^{-1}). Measure blood concentrations if continued for over 24 hours.
- Intravenous infusion of salbutamol or terbutaline is an alternative to aminophylline. Give 250 μg salbutamol or terbutaline over 10 min then continue with an infusion.

Monitoring treatment

- Repeat measurement of PEF 15–30 min after starting treatment.
- Maintain SpO$_2$ > 92%.
- Repeat blood gas measurement if initial PaO_2 < 8 kPa, $PaCO_2$ normal or raised, or there is any possibility that the patient may have deteriorated.

Transfer the patient to a critical care unit accompanied at all times by a doctor prepared to intubate if there is:

- Exhaustion, feeble respirations, confusion, or drowsiness.
- Deteriorating PEF, worsening or persisting hypoxia, or hypercapnoea.
- Coma or respiratory arrest.

Mechanical ventilation of a patient with acute severe asthma

This is a procedure of last resort. It should only be considered when maximal medical therapy has failed to improve the patient. Serious life threatening complications of ventilation are not uncommon under such circumstances. The decision to ventilate should be based on the patient's degree of exhaustion.

Dehydration is common in the asthmatic *in extremis*. Oral fluid intake will have been low, the patient may have been sweating, and tachypnoea will have increased fluid loss. High positive intrathoracic pressures during mechanical ventilation will reduce venous return to the right heart. Before induction of anaesthesia and intubation 500 ml of i.v. fluid should be infused rapidly.

Ventilator settings must be optimized for individual patients. The appropriate settings will vary considerably over time. It is important not to over ventilate or aim for normocarbia. Permissive hypercarbia should be tolerated providing the pH > 7.2. This will help limit inspiratory pressures and thus barotrauma and cardiovascular depression. A slow inspiratory flow rate may be optimal for low intrathoracic pressures but may not deliver an adequate tidal volume or allow sufficient time for expiration. As much time as possible should be allowed for expiration. Dynamic hyperinflation is common. Peak inspiratory pressures should be kept below 50 cm H$_2$O and muscle relaxation in addition to sedation may be required to prevent the patient from coughing.

The patient and a current CXR should be examined regularly for evidence of extensive alveolar rupture (mediastinal emphysema, subcutaneous emphysema, or pneumothorax). Maximal medical therapy should be continued throughout the period of ventilation.

Further reading

Corbridge TC, Hell JB. The assessment and management of adults with status asthmaticus. *American Journal of Respiratory Critical Care Medicine* 1995; **151**: 1296–1316.

The British Guidelines on Asthma Management. *Thorax* 1997; **52(suppl 1)**: 12–13.

Related topics of interest

Anaphylaxis, p. 20; Chronic obstructive pulmonary disease, p. 91; Respiratory support – weaning from ventilation, p. 210

BLOOD COAGULATION

Coagulation failure is common in critically ill patients. Normal haemostasis requires an equilibrium between the fibrinolytic system and the clotting cascade, the vascular endothelium and platelets. The reasons for coagulation failure in critical care are often multifactorial and include:

- Surgical and non-surgical vessel trauma.
- Acquired deficiencies of clotting factors (e.g., major trauma, massive transfusion, DIC, extracorporeal circuits, liver disease).
- Thrombocytopenia: [e.g., drug induced (heparin), anti-platelet antibodies, idiopathic thrombocytopaenic purpura (ITP), heparin induced thrombotic thrombocytopaenic syndrome (HITTS), sepsis].
- Hypothermia which impairs clotting factor activity.
- Anticoagulants: (e.g., heparin, warfarin, aspirin, thrombolytics).
- Congenital coagulation factor deficiency.

Coagulation tests

Prothrombin time (PT) tests the extrinsic pathway, with vitamin K-dependent factors (II, VII and X). Factor VII is the first to decrease with warfarin therapy. A normal result is 12–14 s for clot formation, the test sample should clot within < 3 s of control. Prolonged PT is found in factor VII deficiency, liver disease, vitamin K deficiency or oral anticoagulant therapy.

Activated partial thromboplastin time (APTT) tests the intrinsic pathway (XII, XI, IX, VIII and X) activated by kaolin or cephaloplastin. The normal is 39–42 s and test samples which clot > 6 s longer than control are abnormal. APPT is prolonged in the presence of heparin, the haemophilias, von Willebrand's disease, severe fibrinolysis and DIC.

Activated clotting time (ACT) is performed when whole blood is activated with diatomaceous earth. Clot formation normally occurs 90–130 s later. It predominantly tests the intrinsic pathway and is used as a bedside test for the action of heparin but is also prolonged by thrombocytopaenia, hypothermia, fibrinolysis and high dose aprotinin.

Thrombin time. Both the PT and APPT include the final common pathway in their tests. This is specifically tested by the addition of thrombin to plasma (thrombin time). A normal result is 9–15 s. Unlike a reptilase test it is affected by heparin and fibrin degradation products (FDPs).

Bleeding time (normal range: 3–9 min) tests primary haemostasis of platelets and vessels. A blood pressure cuff is inflated to 40 mmHg and a standardized skin incision is made distal to it. If bleeding stops within 9 min then this is considered normal.

Platelet count (normal range: 150–400 $\times$ 10^9 l^{-1}), specific platelet function tests are rarely used in practice but thromboelastography allows some functional assessment.

All factors can be assayed, but factor VII components and fibrinogen are the ones most commonly performed.

Normal fibrinogen level is 2–4.5 g l⁻¹. Factor Xa assays are used to monitor the anticoagulant effect of low molecular weight heparins (LMWH) that do not affect APTT.

D-dimers and fibrinogen degradation products (FDPS). FDPS released by plasminolysis can be assayed and are often measured to confirm disseminated intravascular coagulation. Levels of 20–40 μg ml⁻¹ are seen following surgery and trauma and may also accompany sepsis, thromboembolism and renal failure. Assay of the D-dimer fragments is more specific but less sensitive for fibrinolysis. Minor elevations of D-dimer may also be seen post-surgery, trauma, sepsis, venous thrombosis and renal impairment. High D-dimer levels suggest excessive fibrinolysis (e.g. DIC).

Euglobulin lysis time (ELT). ELT reflects the presence of plasminogen activators. With fibrinolytic activation the ELT time is shortened (normal range > 90 min).

Specific problems

1. Haemophilias. Haemophilia A (classical haemophilia) is a sex-linked disorder due to a deficiency of factor VIII. Haemophilia B or Christmas disease is due to factor IX deficiency, and is less common than haemophilia A. Treatment is with factor VIII and IX.

2. von Willebrand's disease. Autosomal dominant and the commonest hereditary coagulation disorder. Prophylactic infusion of DDAVP 0.3 μg kg⁻¹ augments factor VIII, increases release of von Willebrand's factor and reduces the risk of haemorrhage. Crypoprecipitate and FFP will also correct the defects

3. Haemostatic failure associated with liver disease. Cholestatic liver disease is associated with deficiencies of the vitamin K-dependent coagulation factors (II, VII, IX and X). This is reversed rapidly with vitamin K therapy. In the presence of extensive hepatocellular damage vitamin K may be ineffective. Liver disease is also associated with thrombocytopenia secondary to splenomegaly.

4. Oral anticoagulant agents. Oral anticoagulants result in deficiencies of vitamin K-dependent clotting factors (II, VII, IX, X). FFP will provide short term reversal of anticoagulation (factor VII has a half life of around 7 hours) while vitamin K provides long term antagonism of warfarin.

5. Heparin. Heparin potentiates the action of anti-thrombin III which inhibits coagulation and can be measured by APTT prolongation. Protamine sulphate is a direct antagonist of heparin and is effective in a dose of 1 mg protamine to neutralize 100 units of heparin. Protamine in overdose is anti-coagulant and administration needs to be slow because of hypotension due to pulmonary vasoconstriction. The LMWH do not affect APPT but anti-Xa levels can be used for monitoring. Their effect may not be fully reversed by protamine.

6. Antiplatelet agents. Aspirin and other NSAIDs have platelet-inhibitory effects. Platelet function effects are largely irreversible lasting up to 10 days after administration. Platelet transfusion may be required despite a normal platelet count.

Disseminated intravascular coagulation (DIC)

DIC occurs when a powerful or persistent trigger activates haemostasis. The release of free thrombin leads to widespread deposition of fibrin and a secondary fibrinolytic response.

The major problem and presenting feature of DIC is bleeding. Thrombotic, haemorrhagic or mixed manifestations in various organ systems may coexist. DIC is associated with numerous underlying problems:

- Sepsis (bacterial, especially Gram-negative organisms, viral, protozoal especially malaria).
- Shock, burns and trauma. Snake bite, heat stroke.
- Eclampsia, placental abruption, amniotic fluid embolism, retained products of conception, purperal sepsis.
- Hepatic failure and autoimmune diseases.
- Malignancy (promyelocytic leukaemia and mucin secreting adenocarcinomas).
- Surgery (cardiac, vascular neurosurgery, prostatic).
- Incompatible blood transfusion.
- Extensive intravascular haemolysis.
- Extracorporeal circuits.

1. Diagnosis. The diagnosis is usually based on the clinical picture with a supportive pattern of laboratory tests. A PT > 15 s, a prolonged APPT, fibrinogen level 1.6 g l^{-1} and platelet count < 150 $\times 10^9 l^{-1}$ with high levels of FDPs (D-dimers) are confirmatory although they may not be present in all cases. The blood film may show fragmentation of the red cells (microangiopathic haemolytic anaemia), which is more commonly seen in chronic DIC associated with malignancy.

2. Management
- Treatment of the precipitating cause.
- Replacement of deficient clotting factors and platelets.
- Heparin may be useful in theory but is rarely used in practice.

Thrombocytopaenia

Thrombocytopaenia results from decreased production, increased consumption or extracorporeal loss of platelets. Sepsis is probably the most common association in critical care where a combination of these factors result in thrombocytopaenia.

1. Decreased production. Leukaemias, drug-induced thrombocytopaenia (thiazides, quinine, anti-tuberculous drugs, carbamazepine, chloroquine, chlorpropamide, gold salts, methyldopa, chloramphenicol, high dose penicillin, chemotherapy agents), marrow depression or infiltration by malignancy.

2. Increased consumption. Sepsis. ITP due to anti-platelet IgG autoantibodies, thrombotic thrombocytopaenic purpura (TTP), haemolytic uraemic syndrome (HUS), shock, DIC, hypersplenism due to splenomegaly, HITTS.

3. *Extracorporeal loss.* Due to haemorrhage and haemodilution, extracorporeal circuits (cardiopulmonary bypass, renal replacement therapy, plasmaphoresis). Treatment is directed at the underlying cause. Platelet transfusion if count $< 10–20 \times 10^9 \, l^{-1}$. Prophylactic platelets are given prior to surgery or an invasive procedure.

Aprotinin

Aprotinin is a naturally occurring serine protease inhibitor with a half-life of around 2 hours. Aprotinin given during cardiopulmonary bypass preserves platelet function and reduces peri-operative blood loss. It may have a role in other situations such as repeat neurosurgery and multitrauma. The loading dose is 2 million units followed by $500\,000 \, U \, h^{-1}$.

Bleeding related to thrombolysis

With increasing use of thrombolytic agents there are increasing numbers of haemorrhagic complications. The majority of haemorrhages occur from cannula sites, the urinary or gastrointestinal tract. Less than 1% of bleeding complications are intracranial but the mortality rate is high. The risk of bleeding increases with dose and is increased if heparin is also administered. In the presence of serious bleeding the infusion of thrombolytic agents should be stopped and clotting normalized by giving FFP and platelets.

Management of abnormal bleeding

- Prevent hypovolaemia and hypoxia.
- Exclude surgical bleeding: large vessel bleeding, external haemorrhage may be controlled initially by pressure but usually requires surgical haemostasis. Non-surgical haemostasis should be used where appropriate (e.g., fracture immobilization, vessel embolization under X-ray control).
- Take blood samples for coagulation studies and platelet count.
- Give blood to maintain an adequate circulating haemoglobin.
- Give fresh frozen plasma to replace lost coagulation factors.
- Give platelets to maintain a platelet count of $> 50–100 \times 10^9 \, l^{-1}$ in the presence of active bleeding.
- In the absence of active bleeding a platelet count of $> 20 \times 10^9 \, l^{-1}$ is tolerated in most patients.
- Give platelets to those patients who are bleeding with known recent aspirin or non-steroidal anti-inflammatory drug (NSAI) use.
- Give cryoprecipitate to replace fibrinogen.
- Give other specific clotting factors as indicated (e.g., VIII, IX for the haemophilias).
- Give vitamin K in liver failure and to reverse the effects of warfarin. One milligramme of vitamin K will reverse warfarin effects within 12 hours while 10 mg will saturate liver stores and prevent warfarin anticoagulation for weeks.
- Give protamine to reverse the effects of heparin.
- Consider the use of aprotinin, or alternative agents such as epsilon-aminocaproic acid.

Further reading

Parker RI. Etiology and treatment of acquired coagulopathies in the critically ill adult and child. *Critical Care Clinics* 1997; **13**: 591–609.

Mannucci PM. Hemostatic drugs. *New England Journal of Medicine* 1998; **339**: 245–253.

Related topics of interest

Blood and blood products, p. 39; Blood transfusion, p. 43

BLOOD AND BLOOD PRODUCTS

Myrene Kilminster

Improvements in the safety of the blood supply have been achieved but cost has increased substantially.

Screening

All donors are screened carefully. Those considered to be a risk are excluded from donating and all blood is screened for the following:

- HIV 1 and 2 antibodies.
- Hepatitis B surface antigen.
- Hepatitis C antibody.
- CMV.
- HTLV1.
- Syphilis serology.

Collection and storage

Approximately 430 ml of whole blood is collected into a closed triple pack containing CPD-A (citrate, phosphate, dextrose-adenine) anticoagulant. Platelets and plasma are separated off and the remaining red cells are resuspended in optimal additive [e.g., SAGM (saline, adenine, glucose and mannitol)]. The shelf life of SAGM blood is up to 42 days.

Continuing metabolic activity causes the following biochemical and cellular changes (referred to as storage lesion):

- Depletion of 2,3 DPG, ATP, PO_4^{2-}, platelets and factors V and VIII.
- Accumulation of CO_2, H^+, activated clotting factors, denatured and activated proteins, microaggregates of platelets, white cells and fibrin.
- The Hb–O_2 dissociation curve is shifted to the right by acidosis which is offset by the left shift due to reduced 2,3 DPG and hypothermia.
- The P_{50} is less than 18 mmHg after 1 week.
- A reduction in red cell membrane integrity causes an increase in extracellular K^+, increased osmotic fragility, and an increase in free haemoglobin.

Blood components

1. Blood. Fresh blood is less than 5 days old. It is rich in clotting factors and platelets. It is inefficient to store blood as whole blood. Most patients will require red cells only and the separation off of platelets and plasma allows these products to be targeted at the needs of individual patients. The shelf life of whole blood is shorter than packed cells. There is more microaggregate formation and a higher risk of haemolysis and GvHD because of larger amounts of plasma and white cells. Packed cells have a haematocrit of 0.5–0.6.

Leukocyte depleted red cells are indicated in patients with a history of non-haemolytic febrile transfusion reactions (NHFTR) which are due usually to recipient antibody to donor white cells. Following theoretical concerns about the transmission of prions in white cells, all donated blood in the UK is now leukocyte depleted.

Frozen red cells are used for rare blood groups or autologous storage in large amounts.

2. Platelets. One unit of platelet concentrate will increase the platelet count by approximately $7 \times 10^9 \, l^{-1}$. The shelf life is up to 7 days, but they need to be stored on a horizontal shaker. The presence of some red cells can result in sensitization if ABO-Rh incompatible platelets are transfused. This can cause Rhesus sensitization in Rhesus negative females, low grade haemolysis and a positive Coombs test.

3. Fresh frozen plasma. The fractionated volume of fresh frozen plasma (FFP) is approximately 200 ml. It can be spun further into cryoprecipitate and supernatant. FFP contains all the clotting factors, and components of the fibrinolytic and complement systems.

Large volumes (4–8 units) are required to produce clinically important increases in serum levels of clotting factors. It carries infectious risks, and donor plasma antibodies can cause haemolysis. There are methods of reducing the infectious risk:

- Photochemical inactivation with methylene blue is effective against enveloped viruses (hepatitis B, hepatitis C and HIV) and partially effective against non-enveloped viruses (hepatitis A, parvoviruses). Approximately 70–80% of clotting factor activity is retained.
- Detergent methods require pooling of at least 2000 l and are not effective against non-enveloped viruses, the factor retention is 73–97%.
- Pasteurization also requires pooling but is more effective against non-enveloped viruses with 75–90% factor retention rate.

4. Cryoprecipitate. Cryoprecipitate is prepared from FFP. It contains factor VIII (FVIII:C), fibrinogen, factor XIII, von Willebrand's factor and fibronectin. It is indicated in fibrinogen deficiency/depletion, particularly in DIC and massive transfusion.

Pre-operative autologous donation

In an attempt to avoid the hazards of homologous transfusion, patients undergoing elective procedures that are likely to require transfusion can pre-donate their own blood. Collections can occur weekly for up to 4 weeks pre-surgery. This autologous blood is subject to the same screening tests as the homologous supply. The process is relatively expensive because unused autologous blood cannot be returned to the homologous blood bank. The risk of administrative errors is the same as for homologous blood.

Peri-operative red cell salvage

Salvage techniques are used widely in trauma, cardiothoracic, vascular and orthopaedic surgery. Post-operatively, cardiac surgical patients can receive both re-transfused pump blood and blood from thoracic drains. Intraoperative cell saver blood consists of washed red cells without platelets or clotting factors. Problems with these techniques include traumatic haemolysis, air emboli, microemboli, infusion of irrigants, and hyperkalaemia.

Other plasma products

Albumin, immunoglobulins, and factor VIII are all derived from large plasma pools. Recipients are thus exposed to multiple donors. The sterilization processes for albumin and immunoglobulin products may not be sufficient to inactivate non-enveloped viruses, but are thought to be safe for enveloped viruses. The theoretical risk of prion transmission has forced the UK to use albumin sourced only from outside the country

1. Albumin. Albumin is made by fractionation followed by heating to 60° for 10 hours to inactivate viruses. It is supplied as 4–5% or 20% albumin solution, each with varying constituents. Albumin infusion does not improve outcome in critically ill patients.

2. Factor VIII. The current sterilization processes for factor VIII are thought to inactivate viruses completely. However, human factor VIII exposes each recipient to 20 000 donors. In the UK, the theoretical risk of disease transmission has provoked legislation dictating the use of genetically engineered product only in new haemophilia patients and those under the age of 16. Recombinant factor VIII is derived from genetically engineered Chinese hamster ovary cells. It is structurally similar with the same biological activity to human AHF. It is indicated for bleeding in patients with haemophilia A, but is not useful in von Willebrand's disease.

Red cell substitutes

A number of red cell substitutes are at advanced stages of investigation but, as yet, none are licensed for this use clinically. They can be divided in to two groups: haemoglobin solutions and perfluorocarbons.

1. Haemoglobin solutions. Haemoglobin solutions are produced from three sources: out of date human blood, animal blood, or by recombinant techniques. These solutions have a high O_2-affinity due to lack of 2,3-DPG and a variable haemoglobin content (usually 60–80 g l^{-1}). The short intravascular half-life of free haemoglobin has been increased by polymerization or linkage to large molecules. Oxygen affinity has been reduced in some preparations by the addition of pyridoxal phosphate. A polymerized bovine haemoglobin is under investigation but concerns with prion transmission persist. A genetically engineered recombinant haemoglobin solution is likely to enter phase 3 trials in the near future.

2. Perflurocarbons. Perflurocarbons are hydrocarbons with F^- replacing H^+. This increases the solubility for oxygen. They are chemically inert and immiscible in water, but can be emulsified with surfactant. Fluosol-DA 20% can carry 1–2 ml O_2 per 100 mmHg ($3\times$ plasma). It requires a high FiO_2 for efficacy. Studies in Jehovah's Witnesses have failed to demonstrate an improvement in survival. Its low viscosity improves perfusion and oxygen delivery to ischaemic tissue. It has a half-life of 10 hours and side effects include anaphylaxis. Similar agents are being used for partial liquid ventilation in patients with severe hypoxia and ARDS.

Further reading

Goodenough LT, Brecher ME, Kanter MH, AuBuchon JP. Transfusion medicine. Blood transfusion. *New England Journal of Medicine* 1999; **340**: 438–447.

Related topics of interest

Blood coagulation, p. 34; Blood transfusion, p. 43

BLOOD TRANSFUSION

Myrene Kilminster

Guidelines on transfusion practices have been published in an attempt to minimize the incidence of adverse reactions and reduce costs. In the UK and Ireland, the Serious Hazards of Transfusion (SHOT) enquiry monitors the adverse effects of blood transfusion. Exposure to homologous blood and blood products should be minimized and autologous blood should be used where possible. The cause of anaemia must be sought aggressively and treated. Blood restoration (haematopoesis) should be optimized with the use of iron supplementation, folic acid, vitamin B_{12}, vitamin C, erythropoietin (EPO), and adequate nutrition.

Causes of anaemia in the critically ill

Critically ill patients become anaemic for many reasons:

(a) Overt or occult bleeding may occur from within the GI tract, intra-abdominal or intrathoracic cavities, or pelvis. Orthopaedic injuries may continue to bleed into tissues.

(b) Frequent blood sampling.

(c) Anaemia of critical illness:

- Bone marrow suppression.
- Reduced EPO production by impaired kidneys.
- Inhibition of marrow response to EPO.
- Altered iron metabolism.

Inflammatory mediators, many of which work via inducible nitric oxide synthetase (iNOS) pathways, probably induce these responses.

Compatibility testing

Clerical error remains the most common cause for an ABO incompatible transfusion reaction. The risks of immunological reaction are small if ABO-compatible blood is used. There are more than 30 common antigens and hundreds more rare antigens, but apart from ABO and Rhesus (Rh) D they rarely cause problems with matching.

Donor and recipient blood is grouped using direct antiglobulin testing with the addition of A, B, and RhD antisera to a suspension of donor red cells. This determines the ABO and RhD status and takes 5 min. There are two types of cross-match:

- An immediate spin cross-match involves the addition of recipient serum to donor cells and observing immediate agglutination. It confirms ABO compatibility and will take about 5 min to perform. It will not reliably detect unexpected antibodies.

- A full cross-match requires incubation of donor cells and recipient sera for at least 15 min and observing for agglutination. A Coombs' test is then performed to detect antibody on donor red cells. The full cross-match test takes about 45 min.

An antibody screen may be performed in conjunction with a cross-match or as part of a 'type and screen'. The recipient's serum is added to red cells from several normal group O blood samples expressing known antigens. Once a blood sample has been typed and screened if, later on, blood is required urgently, it can be released following a just spin cross-match to confirm ABO compatibility. Thus, fully compatible blood is available in just 15 min.

The risk of a major incompatible reaction varies with the extent of compatibility testing undertaken:

- Randomly selected (untyped donor and recipient)   35.6%
- Group   0.8%
- ABO - compatible   0.6%
- ABO and Rhesus compatible   0.2%
- ABO, Rhesus and negative antibody screen   0.06%
- Complete compatibility testing   0.05%

In an emergency, Group O positive (for males and post-menopausal females) and Group O negative for pre-menopausal females (to reduce the risk of sensitization to Rhesus D antigen) has been established to be safe. Patients who are Group O are most at risk for an incompatible transfusion reaction due to the presence of anti-A and anti-B in their plasma; they are implicated in 70% of incompatible reactions while representing only 45% of the population. Patients who receive large transfusions of Group O cells should undergo full cross-matching before receiving blood of their original group; they may have received a large amount of anti-A and anti-B in the sera of the previous transfusions.

Blood transfusion triggers

The safe lower limit of haemoglobin concentration in critically ill patients is controversial. There is no doubt that anaemia is tolerated considerably better than hypovolaemia. However, patients with fixed perfusion defects of vital organs and serious co-morbidity are far less likely to tolerate such a dramatic reduction in oxygen delivery without adverse consequences.

With restoration of an adequate circulating volume there are a variety of mechanisms to compensate for acute anaemia and maintain oxygen delivery. Cardiac output is increased as a result of lower viscosity, lower SVR, and auto-regulation in regional capillary beds. Most tissues (except the myocardium and renal medulla) can increase oxygen extraction substantially. Tolerance to reduced oxygen content will depend on the individual's ability to compensate, and maintain a favourable oxygen supply to oxygen demand. This will vary from patient to patient and organ to organ. Blood transfusion may not always improve oxygen delivery; increased viscosity may reduce cardiac output and, in combination with a reduced P_{50}, any increase in O_2 content may be negated.

Critically ill patients have increased O_2 demand due to a catabolic state, pain, fever, increased work of breathing, use of inotropes, and sepsis. Their ability to compensate may be impaired by myocardial dysfunction, respiratory failure, renal failure, coronary artery, cerebrovascular or renovascular disease, and co-morbidity.

There is no single criterion to trigger transfusion. The decision must be based on:

- Haemoglobin concentration.
- Likelihood of continuing blood loss.
- Chronicity of anaemia.
- Presence of fixed perfusion defects in vital organs.
- Cardiopulmonary reserve (which declines at extremes of age).
- Catabolic state.
- Evidence of impaired tissue oxygenation.

A haemoglobin of 7 g dl^{-1} may be tolerated in a fit young post-operative patient without anticipated further blood loss, whereas a haemoglobin > 10 g dl^{-1} may be required for a patient with severe coronary artery disease. A recent multicentre, randomized controlled trial supports a more restrictive practice for red cell transfusion in the critically ill. This demonstrated that maintaining a haemoglobin of 7–9 g dl^{-1} was as effective and possibly superior to a liberal transfusion strategy of maintaining a haemoglobin of 10–12 g dl^{-1}.

Control of haemorrhage

Control of haemorrhage may require surgical or radiological intervention, cessation or reversal of anticoagulation. Antifibrinolytics (e.g., tranexamic acid) may be indicated in patients who have received recent fibrinolytic therapy. Correction of clotting abnormalities and thrombocytopaenia may be enough to control the bleeding and reduce the need for ongoing transfusion.

Massive transfusion

Packed cells and resuspended cells are deficient in platelets and factors V and VIII. During massive transfusion, coagulation and platelet counts must be assessed. Indications for their replacement are described on p. 37.

Complications of blood transfusions

1. Immediate immune reactions

- Acute haemolytic transfusion reaction is usually due to an ABO, Lewis, Kell or Duffy incompatible transfusion. IgM complement mediated cytotoxicity or IgG mediated lysis of red cells results in liberation of anaphylotoxins, histamine, and coagulation activation. There may be fevers, rigors, chest pain, back pain, dyspnoea, headache, urticaria, cyanosis, bronchospasm, pulmonary oedema, and cardiovascular collapse. Acute renal failure (secondary to hypotension, microvascular thrombosis and haemoglobin plugging of tubules) is common. The transfusion must be ceased while appropriate organ support is started. Investigations include a Coombs' test, LDH and haptoglobin, LFTs, baseline coagulation studies, electrolytes, urea, creatinine, and FBC.
- NHFTR account for 75% of all reactions (1–5% of all transfusions) and are due to recipient antibody to donor white cell/platelet HLA antigens. Patients may require washed or leukocyte depleted red cells subsequently.
- Allergy is more common after whole blood or plasma transfusions. The reaction is usually mild but can be severe with hypotension, angioedema, bronchospasm, urticaria, and fever.

- Transfusion related acute lung injury (TRALI) is non-cardiogenic pulmonary oedema caused by recipient antibody to donor leucocyte HLA antigens. It occurs usually within 6 hours and can occur with minimal volumes.

2. Delayed immune reactions. Delayed haemolytic transfusion reactions (4–14 days after transfusion) are due to undetected antibody. They can be similar to acute reactions but are generally more benign. Alloimmunization to cellular or protein antigens is common, and rarely affects the patient until the next time they need a blood transfusion. GvHD is due to donor lymphocytes in blood products that react against host tissue. It is more likely in immunocompromised individuals, or those with some shared HLA antigens (family member donors).

3. Non-immune immediate reactions
- The risk of microbial contamination of blood is related directly to the length of storage. The most commonly implicated organism is *Yersinia enterocolitica* but a number of other organisms have been described.
- There is considerable evidence that homologous transfusion has an immuno-suppressive effect and increases the risk of infection that is independent of bacterial contamination. Whether blood transfusion increases the risk of recurrence of cancer is still controversial.
- Volume overload is more likely with a normovolaemic transfusion in the elderly and those with impaired cardiac function.
- Haemolysis due to red cell trauma, osmotic lysis and senescent red cells can occur but is rarely of great clinical significance.
- Microaggregates of white cells, platelets and fibrin are associated with lung sequestration and ALI and the potential for ARDS.
- Massive transfusion (> 10 units or > 1 blood volume) may cause coagulopathy, hypothermia, DIC, hyperkalaemia, hypoalbuminaemia, and acidosis. The coagulopathy of massive transfusion is multifactorial (deficiencies of factors V and VIII and platelets, DIC, hypothermia). FFP and platelets should be given empirically after 10 bags if non-surgical bleeding is a problem and hypothermia has been corrected.
- Metabolic abnormalities resulting from a storage lesion are rarely a clinical problem except during rapid administration or massive transfusion. It is more likely with older blood. Hyperkalaemia, metabolic acidosis, and metabolic alkalosis (citrate metabolism) may occur. Citrate toxicity, resulting in hypocalcaemia, is exceedingly rare.

4. Non-immune delayed reactions
- Viral infections. The current estimated infection risks (per unit transfused) associated with voluntary donor programmes are approximately: HIV 1:1 000 000, hepatitis B 1:100 000, hepatitis C 1:100 000, CMV 1:2. The risk of transmitting non-A, non-B, non-C hepatitis is unknown.
- Iron overload is a complication of multiple transfusions over a long period of time. It results in haemosiderin deposition with myocardial and hepatic damage.

Further reading

Goodenough LT, Brecher ME, Kanter MH, AuBuchon JP. Transfusion medicine. Blood transfusion. *New England Journal of Medicine* 1999; **340**: 438–447.

Hebert PC, Wells G, Blajchman MA, *et al.* A multicenter, randomised, controlled clinical trial of transfusion requirements in critical care. *New England Journal of Medicine* 1999; **340**: 409–417.

Related topics of interest

BRAIN STEM DEATH AND ORGAN DONATION

Brain stem death is defined as the irreversible cessation of brain stem function, but not necessarily the physical destruction of the brain. In the UK, it has been agreed that brain stem death = death (i.e. despite the presence of a beating heart). Prior to the diagnosis of brain stem death it is necessary to consider certain preconditions and exclusions. Head injury and intracranial haemorrhage account for approximately 80% of cases. Brain stem death has been the subject of two joint Royal College reports and a recent Department of Health publication.

Preconditions

- Apnoeic coma requiring ventilation.
- Irreversible brain damage of known cause.

Exclusions

- Hypothermia (temperature < 35°C).
- Drugs (no depressant or muscle relaxant drugs present).
- Acid/base abnormality.
- Metabolic/endocrine disease, e.g., uncontrolled diabetes mellitus, uraemia, hyponatraemia, Addison's disease, hepatic encephalopathy, thyrotoxicosis.
- Markedly elevated $PaCO_2$.
- Severe hypotension.

The brain stem death tests

These should be performed by two doctors but not necessarily at the same time. Neither should belong to the transplant team and both should have been registered for 5 years or more. One must be a consultant. More than 6 hours should have elapsed since the event that caused the suspected brain stem death. Two sets of tests must be performed. They may be carried out by the doctors separately or together. The tests are often repeated to eliminate observer error, although this is not required by law. Careful records should be kept.

1. Pupillary responses. There are no direct or consensual reactions to light. This tests the 2nd cranial nerve and the parasympathetic outflow.

2. Corneal reflex. No response to lightly touching the cornea. This tests the 5th and 7th cranial nerves.

3. Painful stimulus to the face. A motor response in the cranial nerve distribution of the stimulus is looked for. Tests the 5th and 7th cranial nerves.

4. Caloric tests. After visualizing both ear drums (wax may need to be removed first), 30 ml of ice cold water is injected into each external auditory canal. No response is seen if the 8th nerve and brain stem are dead. Nystagmus occurs if the vestibular reflexes are intact. (Tests 8th, 3rd, and 6th cranial nerves.)

5. Gag reflex. Tests the 9th and 10th cranial nerves.

6. *Apnoea test.* The patient is ventilated with 100% O_2 and then disconnected from the ventilator, while observing for respiratory effort. A tracheal catheter supplies $6\,l\,min^{-1}$ of O_2. The patient is left disconnected for 10 minutes or until the $PaCO_2$ is > 6.65 kPa. If marked bradycardia or haemodynamic instability occur the test is discontinued. The SpO_2 should not fall below 90%. It may help the patient's realtives come to terms with the concept of brain death if they witness the apnoea test.

Other tests

Doll's eyes movement. The head is moved rapidly from side to side. If the brain stem is dead the eyes remain in a fixed position within the orbit. This is the oculocephalic reflex and tests the 8th cranial nerve. If the cortex is dead but the brain stem is intact the eyes appear to move to the opposite side and then realign with the head. It does not form part of the legally required brain stem death tests.

Some countries require other tests for the diagnosis of brain death. These include EEG, 'four vessel' cerebral angiography, radioisotope scanning, and transcranial Doppler ultrasound. There is no evidence that these tests increase the accuracy of diagnosis. Their use may be limited but they may be helpful in situations where the clinical testing described above cannot be undertaken (e.g., local cranial nerve injuries, an inability to perform the apnoea test because of severe hypoxia).

Potential problems

- Spinal reflexes may be present. However, decerebrate posturing means some brain stem activity exists.
- The presence of drugs or other unresponsive states may lead to a false diagnosis of brain death.
- Communication with relatives. The discussion of a 'hopeless prognosis' being misinterpreted as brain stem death. A subsequent survival may then be ascribed to an incorrect diagnosis of brain stem death.
- Death of the cortex leading to a vegetative state is not brain death.
- Elective ventilation. A patient who is dying should not commence assisted ventilation simply to allow organ donation where this ventilation is of no therapeutic benefit to the dying patient. This practice is considered to be unlawful in the UK.

Organ donation

The question of organ donation is often raised with relatives after the first set of brain stem death tests. This process may be eased if the potential donor had already registered with the NHS Organ Donor Register as an individual willing to donate. If consent is given, blood should be sent for tissue typing, HIV, hepatitis B and CMV testing. In 1993 the United Kingdom Transplant Support Authority divided the UK into a number of zones for the retrieval and allocation of donor organs. The local transplant co-ordinator should thus be contacted. If the second set of brain stem death tests confirm death, then the patient is prepared for the operating theatre. The 5 year survival after first heart transplantation is currently 64% but approximately 10% of transplanted organs fail early after transplantation from causes not related to acute rejection or infection. It is thus essential to optimize the function of donor organs in order to make optimal use of this scarce resource.

Potential complications in brain stem dead organ donors
- Cardiovascular instability.
- Hypoxaemia.
- Diabetes insipidus.
- Endocrine abnormalities (e.g., thyroid, adrenal, or pancreatic function).
- Electrolyte imbalances.
- Acid-base disorders.
- Hypothermia.
- Hyperglycaemia.
- Coagulopathy.

Organ retrieval takes place in the operating theatre. Organ perfusion is maintained, with fluids and inotropes if necessary. High dose inotropes are, however, detrimental to subsequent organ function. During surgery the mean arterial pressure (MAP), SVR and pulmonary artery occlusion pressure (PAOP) increase initially and then fall below preoperative levels. A pulmonary artery catheter should be considered for multi-organ donors. Ventilation to keep the $PaO_2 > 10$ kPa is continued.

Suggested minimum criteria for organ donation
- MAP > 60 mmHg.
- Central venous pressure < 12 mmHg.
- PAOP < 12 mmHg.
- Cardiac index $> 2.1 \, \mathrm{l \, m^{-2}}$.

Spinal reflexes and autonomic haemodynamic responses require neuromuscular blockers and opioids for control. Once the organs have been harvested ventilation is stopped. The emotional needs of the relatives and staff must not be forgotten, particularly if a child is involved.

Further reading

Criteria for the diagnosis of brain stem death. *Journal of the Royal College of Physicians*, 1995; **29**: 381–382.
Milner QJW, Vuylsteke A, Ismail F, Ismail-Zade I, Latimer RD. ICU resuscitation of the multi-organ donor. *British Journal of Intensive Care*, 1997; **7**: 49–54.
Working Party for the Department of Health. A code of practice for the diagnosis of brain stem death. Department of Health, March 1998.

Related topics of interest

Death certification, p. 103; Head injury, p. 128; Subarachnoid haemorrhage, p. 245

BURNS

Tom Simpson

Temperatures greater than 40°C cause burns to the human skin. In England and Wales 10 000 burns patients are admitted to hospital each year, 500–600 of whom die. The mortality is falling with patients surviving burns greater than 90% body surface area (BSA).

Initial assessment and resuscitation

Burns are classified by BSA, depth, and presence of inhalational injury.

1. BSA. The affected area can be estimated in adults by the rule of nines. Lund and Browder charts are age specific, more accurate and they take into account the disproportionate distribution of BSA in children (larger heads and smaller arms, legs and torso).

2. Depth

- First degree (superficial) burns are confined to the epidermis and will heal spontaneously.
- Second degree (partial thickness) burns involve the epidermis and extend into the upper dermis, in which case they heal spontaneously, or the deep dermis where excision and grafting is required for return of function.
- Third degree (full thickness) burns involve both dermis and epidermis and even with wound excision and grafting there will be some limitation of function and scar formation.
- Fourth degree burns involve muscle, fascia and bone and will always result in disability.

First and second degree burns form watery blisters within hours of the injury. They are hypersensitive with moist, pink underlying tissue, which blanches when pressed. Third degree burns are firm, dry and leathery, and have decreased sensation. There may be coagulated vessels present.

All major burns (defined as full thickness > 10% BSA, partial thickness > 25% and burns involving the face, hands or perineum) should be referred to a specialist centre.

3. Fluid and electrolyte management. Intravenous fluid resuscitation is required in adults if the burn involves more than 20% BSA or 15% with smoke inhalation. The objectives are to avoid end organ ischaemia, preserve viable tissue by restoring tissue perfusion and minimize tissue oedema. The type of fluid used is unimportant as long as assessment of fluid status is ongoing. Crystalloid-only regimes are becoming increasingly popular as albumin and hypertonic saline solutions have not been shown to improve outcome.

Formulae have been devised to aid fluid administration. For example, the Parkland formula suggests giving Ringers lactate 4 ml kg^{-1} per %BSA burn in the first 24 hours, with 50% being given in the first 8 hours. Such formulae are only guides and fluid resuscitation should be titrated against clinical assessment, invasive haemodynamic monitoring and urine output, aiming for at least 0.5–1.0 ml $kg^{-1} h^{-1}$. Insensible losses should be replaced with low sodium containing solutions.

Hypokalaemia, hypophosphataemia, hypocalcaemia and hypomagnesaemia are common and should be treated appropriately.

Intensive care management

1. **Cardiovascular responses.** 'Burn shock' is due to loss of plasma from the circulation and decrease in cardiac output. Macrophages, neutrophils and endothelial cells release arachadonic metabolites that cause vasoconstriction and local damage (thromboxone A_2, thromboxone B_2). Failure of cell membrane Na^+/K^+ ATPase increases microvascular permeability and microvascular leak. Locally released inflammatory mediators produce widespread effects if they pass into the systemic circulation. Systemic vascular resistance (SVR) is increased, increasing myocardial work.

In the first 24–48 hours following resuscitation the hormonal response (increased cotisol, glucagon and catecholamine release) and inflammatory mediators (TNF, O_2 free radicals, endothelin and interleukins) cause hypermetabolism, immunosupression and SIRS with increased cardiac output and decreased SVR.

2. **Airway and breathing**

- **Inhalational injury.** The presence of a significant inhalational injury is associated with a 10% mortality, and is doubled in conjunction with a cutaneous burn. It should be suspected if there is a history of entrapment within a confined space, facial burns, carbonaceous sputum, respiratory distress or stridor. Arterial blood gases should be taken and carboxyhaemoglobin (HbCO) levels measured. Indirect laryngoscopy or fibreoptic assessment can confirm the diagnosis.

  Early intubation is advisable as it may be impossible later when tissue oedema occurs. Intubation should be undertaken by someone experienced in managing a difficult airway. A gaseous induction is often preferred. Suxamethonium can be used safely in the first 24 hours after injury.

  Airway injury from hot gases rarely extends distal to the trachea. Toxic compounds within smoke (NH_3, NO_2, SO_2, and Cl) dissolve in the upper airways to form highly toxic acids e.g., HCl. These can cause bronchospasm and epithelial ulceration. Deeper penetration into the bronchial tree will cause mucosal sloughing and alveolar damage leading to airway obstruction and pulmonary oedema.

  Supportive treatment is usually all that is required. Prophylactic antibiotics do not improve outcome. Nebulized N-acetyl cystine and heparin improves lung function by decreasing cast formation, small airway obstruction and barotrauma. High flow jet ventilation has been shown to decrease pneumonia and improve survival.

- **Carbon monoxide (CO) poisoning.** CO poisoning is responsible for 80% of deaths associated with smoke inhalation. CO has an affinity for haemoglobin that is 250 times that of O_2; it also shifts the oxyhaemaglobin (HbO_2) dissociation curve to the left. It therefore greatly reduces the amount of O_2 available for metabolism, causing tissue hypoxia and metabolic acidosis. Signs and symptoms depend on the amount present:

10–20%	tinnitus, headaches and nausea.
20–40%	weakness and drowsiness.
> 40%	coma, convulsions and cardiac arrest.

Direct co-oximeters using multiwavelength spectroscopy are required to differentiate Hb, HbO_2, and HbCO. Pulse oximeters and blood gas analysers will give an overestimation of HbO_2.

Treatment comprises high concentration O_2 therapy which decreases the half-life of CO from 2 hours to 30 min. The role of hyperbaric O_2 (HBO) in preventing long term neurological deficit is controversial. Patients should be considered for HBO treatment if there is CNS impairment and a HbCO level > 30%. There are great technical difficulties in the transfer and administration of HBO treatment to a severely burned patient.

- **Cyanide (CN) poisoning.** Hydrogen cyanide causes tissue asphyxia by inhibition of cytochrome oxidase activity and thus prevents mitochondrial O_2 consumption and arrests the tricarboxylic acid cycle. The only pathway left for ATP production is anaerobic metabolism of pyruvate to lactate and consequently metabolic acidosis. A raised lactate level in the presence of smoke inhalation correlates with CN levels and can be used as a diagnostic test. Signs and symptoms vary with concentration present:

  50 ppm; headache, dizziness, tachycardia and tachypnoea.
  100 ppm; lethargy, seizures and respiratory failure.

  Treatment is normally conservative but high CN levels and persisting metabolic acidosis should be treated with sodium thiosulphate (speeds hepatic metabolism to inactive metabolites), sodium nitrites (provides methaemaglobin which combines with CN to form inactive cyanomethaemaglobin) and dicobalt edetate (binds to CN to form inactive complex).

- **Indirect lung injury.** ARDS occurs secondary to the systemic inflammatory response triggered by the burn wound, infection and complications of burn therapy e.g., fluid overload. The combination of reduced plasma oncotic pressure, endothelial damage and pulmonary hypertension increase the risk of pulmonary oedema.

3. *Metabolism and nutrition.* The changes in cardiac output are mirrored by changes in basal metabolic rate (BMR). The increase is proportional to the size of the burn and the presence of infection; it peaks at 7–10 days. There is an increase in core temperature by 1–2°C. Ambient temperature is important as the warmer the critical care environment the less the increase in BMR due to decreased heat and water loss. The ideal ambient temperature is 28–32°C with high humidity.

Nutritional assessment of calorific requirements is guided by formulae that take into account BSA, age, burn size and pre-existing nutritional state. Protein losses are large and difficult to assess due to wound loss but urinary nitrogen loss is a guide. Protein needs are calculated in relation to caloric needs; 20% of total calories are administered as protein with non-protein calorie to nitrogen ratio of 100:1.

Gut protection is essential due to risk of gastric ulceration (Curling's ulcers) and is best provided for by early enteral feeding (within 4 hours of injury).

4. *Infection control.* Down regulation of immune responses and loss of the skin barrier render patients highly susceptible to infection. The major cause of death in severely burned patients is pulmonary sepsis, especially in the presence of smoke inhalation. Wound infection with streptococci and *Pseudomonas* sp. may be decreased by early surgical excision, improved wound dressings and topical anti-microbials. Bacterial colonization is not preventable but controlling superficial infection is important so healing is not impaired and systemic spread is limited.

Diagnosis of sepsis is difficult as leukocytosis, erythema, fever and a hyper-dynamic state are all normal findings in a severely burned patient. Ongoing sepsis should be suspected if there is any change in mental status, new glucose intoler-ance, increasing base deficit or hypothermia. Regular inspection, surveillance cultures and wound biopsy may be required to confirm diagnosis.

5. *Pharmacology.* The changes in metabolism, cardiac output and fluid shifts will effect, volume of distribution, protein binding and clearance of drugs over time and make careful plasma and clinical monitoring essential. Blood flow (usually increased) and hepatic enzyme activity (decreased) affect hepatic elimination of agents. In the kidney there is increased glomerular filtration but decreased tubular secretion of drugs.

6. *Analgesia.* In the early phases, incremental i.v. boluses of an opioid such as morphine are titrated to effect and later given either by PCA or continuous infusion, depending on the patient's functional state. Ketamine can be used in con-junction with a benzodiazepine for wound dressing changes after the acute phase of injury.

7. *Psychological/rehabilitation.* The long-term effects of severe illness, pain, disfigurement and loss of independence have profound effects on the survivors of severe burns. Post-traumatic stress disorder may contribute to low mood, agitation and sleep disturbance. A compassionate approach with the early involvement of a multi-disciplinary team containing physiotherapists, psychologists, nurses, coun-cillors and occupational therapists is vital to help reduce long term impairment.

Surgical management

Early tangential surgical excision and grafting removes the source of the inflam-matory response and provides a barrier to infection. Early excision of burned tissue decreases pain, the number of operations required, blood loss, length of hospital stay, and mortality rate as well as achieving a better functional result. After a period of stabilization (up to 48 hours) excision and grafting of up to 20–25% BSA per operation can take place. With the use of multiple teams, tourniquets to limit blood loss and aggressive temperature control larger areas may be excised. Scalds should be treated more conservatively as they are associated with less severe second degree burns that may heal well without scarring.

Massive burns (> 60% BSA) provide difficulty with suitable donor sites. This can be overcome by:

- Use of widely expanded meshed autologous skin graft, which can be overlaid with unmeshed cadaver skin.
- Biosynthetic materials have a non-cellular matrix material which mimics the 3D structure of the dermis and is overlaid with a silastic covering membrane to mimic the physical properties of the epidermis. Such material is as effective as autologous skin grafting but is extremely expensive.

- Cultured epithelial autograft is very expensive and has an unacceptably high failure rate.
- In the future, artificial skin may be available in the form of cultured allograft epidermal cells. If successful, this would have the advantage of being pathogen free, universally available, and produce growth factors enhancing the healing process.

Further reading

MacLennan, N, Heimbach, DM, Cullen, BF. Anaesthesia for major thermal injury. *Anaesthesiology* 1998; **89** (3): 749–770.

Nguyen, TT, Gilpin, DA, Meyer, NA, Herndon, DA. Current treatment of severely burned patients. *Annals of Surgery* 1996; **233** (1): 14–25.

Related topic of interest

Fluid therapy, p. 122

CALCIUM, MAGNESIUM AND PHOSPHATE

Calcium

Over 98% of body calcium is in bone, of which about 1% is freely exchangeable with extracellular fluid (ECF). Ionized calcium is crucial to many excitatory processes including nerve and neuromuscular conduction/contraction and coagulation. Normal daily intake is 10–20 mmol and the normal total serum calcium is in the range 2.25–2.7 mmol l^{-1}. Intestinal calcium absorption is enhanced by 1,25-dihydroxyvitamin D_3 ($1,25(OH)_2D_3$). Around 40% is bound to albumin and total serum calcium falls 0.02 mmol l^{-1} for each 1g l^{-1} fall in albumin. Ionized calcium is the physiologically important form and the normal level is 1.15 mmol l^{-1}. The ionized calcium should be used whenever possible to guide therapy. Measurement of total serum calcium corrected for albumin is a poor substitute for ionized calcium.

Hypocalcaemia

1. Causes. Hypocalcaemia occurs when calcium is lost from the ECF (most commonly through renal mechanisms) in greater quantities than can be replaced by bone or the intestine. Common causes of hypocalcaemia are:

- Renal failure.
- Hypoparathyroidism.
- Sepsis.
- Burns.
- Hypomagnesaemia.
- Pancreatitis.
- Malnutrition.
- Osteomalacia.
- Citrate toxicity (massive transfusion).

As a result of reduced absorption of dietary divalent cations or poor dietary intake, hypocalcaemia and hypomagnesaemia often coexist.

2. Clinical features. The symptoms of hypocalcaemia correlate with the magnitude and rapidity of the fall in serum calcium. The main features include neuromuscular irritability evidenced by paraesthesiae of the distal extremities and circumoral area, Chvostek and Trousseau signs, muscle cramps, laryngospasm, tetany, and seizures. Cardiac manifestations comprise a prolonged QT interval, which may progress to VT/VF, and hypotension.

3. Treatment. Appropriate therapy depends on the severity of the hypocalcaemia and its cause. The serum magnesium and potassium should be checked and, if low, corrected. Chronic, asymptomatic mild hypocalcaemia can be treated with oral calcium supplements. If metabolic acidosis accompanies hypocalcaemia calcium must be replaced before the acidosis is corrected. Calcium and hydrogen ions compete for protein-binding sites so an increase in pH will lead to a rapid fall in ionized calcium. In the presence of acute symptomatic hypocalcaemia an intra-venous bolus of calcium (100–200 mg or 2.5–5 mmol) should be given over 5 min. This can be followed by a maintenance infusion of 1–2 mg kg^{-1} h^{-1}. Calcium chloride 10% contains 27.2 mg Ca ml^{-1} (0.68 mmol ml^{-1}) and calcium gluconate 10% contains 9 mg Ca ml^{-1} (0.225 mmol ml^{-1}). Calcium gluconate is more appropriate for prolonged infusion because it causes less venous irritation than calcium chloride.

Hypercalcaemia

1. Causes. Hypercalcaemia occurs generally when the influx of calcium from bone or the intestine exceeds renal calcium excretory capacity. Thus, common causes include:

- Hyperparathyroidism (the commonest cause of hypercalcaemia, accounting for more than 50% of patients).
- Neoplasms [primary with ectopic parathyroid hormone (PTH) secretion, secondary with bone metastases] are the second commonest cause of hyper-calcaemia.
- Sarcoidosis (increased production of 1,25(OH)$_2$D$_3$ by granulomatous tissue).
- Drugs (e.g., thiazides increase renal calcium reabsorption).
- Immobilization.
- Vitamin D intoxication.
- Thyrotoxicosis.
- Milk-alkali syndrome (consumption of large amounts of calcium-containing antacids).

2. Clinical features. The symptoms associated with hypercalcaemia depend on the rate of rise as well as the absolute level. Mild hypercalcaemia is usually asymptomatic. Severe hypercalcaemia causes neurological, gastrointestinal, and renal symptoms. Neurological features range from mild weakness, depression, and psychosis, and may progress to coma. Gastrointestinal symptoms may include nausea, vomiting, abdominal pain, constipation, and peptic ulceration. Hypercalcaemia may induce nephrogenic diabetes insipidus (DI), nephrolithiasis, and nephrocalcinosis.

3. Treatment. The underlying cause of the hypercalcaemia must be treated. The measures taken to lower the serum calcium depend on its level. Most cases of mild hypercalcaemia are caused by primary hyperparathyroidism and many of these patients will require parathyroidectomy. Patients with symptomatic moderate (serum total calcium > 3.0 mmol l^{-1}) or severe (> 3.4 mmol l^{-1}) hypercalcaemia require intravenous saline to restore intravascular volume and enhance renal calcium excretion. Thiazide diuretics should be avoided but a loop diuretic such as frusemide will enhance calcium excretion. Patients with severe hypercalcaemia associated with raised PTH should be referred for urgent parathyroidectomy. Bisphosphonates (e.g., etidronate, sodium pamidronate) have become the main therapy for the management of hypercalcaemia due to enhanced osteoclastic bone reabsorption. Steroids are effective in hypercalcaemia associated with haemato-logical malignancy and in diseases related to 1,25(OH)$_2$D$_3$ excess (e.g., sarcoidosis and vitamin D toxicity).

Magnesium

Magnesium is essential for normal cellular and enzyme function. The total body magnesium store is around 1000 mmol, of which 50–60% is in bone. The normal plasma range is 0.7–1.0 mmol l^{-1} but because it is primarily an intracellular ion the plasma level does not reflect total body stores. The normal daily intake is 10–20 mmol, which is balanced by urine and faecal losses. The kidney is the primary organ involved in magnesium regulation.

Hypomagnesaemia

Hypomagnesaemia occurs in up to 65% of critically ill patients. It is often associated with hypokalaemia.

1. **Causes.** The usual reason is loss of magnesium from the gastrointestinal tract or the kidney.

- Gastrointestinal causes include prolonged nasogastric suction, diarrhoea, extensive bowel resection, severe malnutrition, and acute pancreatitis.
- Renal losses occur with volume expanded states, hypercalcaemia, with diuretics, and during the diuretic phase of acute tubular necrosis. Other drugs such as alcohol, aminoglycosides, and cisplatin are associated with renal loss of magnesium.
- Other causes of hypomagnesaemia include phosphate depletion, hyperparathyroidism, and diabetes mellitus.

2. **Clinical features.** Most of the symptoms of hypomagnesaemia are rather non-specific. The accompanying ion abnormalities such as hypocalcaemia, hypokalaemia, and metabolic alkalosis account for many of the clinical features. Neurological signs include confusion, weakness, ataxia, tremors, carpopedal spasms, and seizures. Cardiological features are: wide QRS, long PR, inverted T, U wave on ECG, arrhythmias including severe ventricular arrhythmias (torsade de pointes), and an increased potential for cardiac glycoside toxicity.

3. **Treatment.** The underlying cause of the hypomagnesaemia must be addressed. Symptomatic moderate-to-severe hypomagnesaemia will require parenteral therapy. In the event of an acute arrhythmia or seizures, 8 mmol of magnesium sulphate can be given over 5 min followed by 25 mmol over 12 hours. This rate can be titrated against serum magnesium levels. Potassium should be replaced at the same time. Oral magnesium sulphate is a laxative and may cause diarrhoea.

Hypermagnesaemia

Hypermagnesaemia is usually iatrogenic (e.g., excessive intravenous administration). High magnesium levels antagonize the entry of calcium into cells and prevent excitation.

1. **Clinical features.** Clinical manifestations of hypermagnesaemia include hypotension, bradycardia, drowsiness, hyperreflexia (knee jerk is a useful clinical test and is lost > 4 mmol l^{-1}). Levels in excess of 6 mmol l^{-1} will cause coma and respiratory depression.

2. Treatment. The administration of magnesium should be stopped. Calcium chloride will antagonize the effect of magnesium. Diuretics will increase renal loss. In severe cases dialysis will be required.

Phosphate

The total body phosphate in normal adults is about 700 g. Approximately 85% is found in bone, the remaining 15% is in the extracellular fluid and soft tissues. Phosphate is found in adenosine triphosphate (ATP), 2,3-diphosphoglycerate (2,3 DPG) in red blood cells, phospholipids and phosphoproteins. Phosphate is essential for many cellular actions and also acts as a buffer. The normal serum level is $0.85–1.4 \text{ mmol l}^{-1}$.

Hypophosphataemia

1. Causes. Hypophosphataemia results from internal redistribution, increased urinary excretion, and decreased intestinal absorption.

- Internal redistribution of phosphate may result from respiratory alkalosis, re-feeding after malnutrition, recovery from diabetic ketoacidosis, and the effects of hormones and other agents (insulin, glucagon, adrenaline, cortisol, glucose).
- Increased urinary excretion of phosphate occurs in hyperparathyroidism, vitamin-D deficiency, malabsorption, volume expansion, renal tubular acidosis, and alcohol abuse.
- Decreased intestinal absorption of phosphate occurs in antacid abuse, vitamin-D deficiency, and chronic diarrhoea.

2. Clinical features. The clinical features of hypophosphataemia are usually seen when the plasma phosphate falls below 0.3 mmol l^{-1}. They are often non-specific but may include muscle weakness (which may contribute to respiratory failure and cause problems with weaning from mechanical ventilation), cardiac dysfunction, paraesthesiae, coma, and seizures.

3. Treatment. The underlying cause of hypophosphataemia should be corrected. Oral phosphate can be given in tablets of sodium or potassium phosphate in doses of 2–3 g daily. Where necessary, 10 mmol of intravenous potassium phosphate can be given over 60 min and repeated depending on measured levels (sodium phosphate preparation is available). There is a high risk of hypocalcaemia associated with intravenous phosphate replacement and serum calcium must be maintained.

Hyperphosphataemia

1. Causes. Renal failure is the commonest cause of hyperphosphataemia. The causes of hyperphosphataemia can be divided into:

- Reduced urinary excretion: renal failure, hypoparathyroidism, acromegaly, biphosphonate therapy, and magnesium deficiency.
- Increased exogenous load: intravenous infusion, excessive oral therapy, and phosphate-containing enemas.

- Increased endogenous load: tumour-lysis syndrome, rhabdomyolysis, bowel infarction, malignant hyperthermia, haemolysis, and acidosis
- Pseudohyperphosphataemia: multiple myeloma.

2. Clinical features. Hypocalcaemia and tetany may occur with rapid rises in plasma phosphate. A large rise in the calcium × phosphate product with cause ectopic calcification in soft tissues and may cause renal stones.

3. Treatment. Aluminium hydroxide is used as a binding agent. Magnesium and calcium salts are also effective and are preferred in renal failure when aluminium accumulation is a risk. Dialysis may be required

Further reading

Bushinsky DA, Monk RD. Calcium. *Lancet* 1998; **352**: 306–311.
Weisinger JR, Bellorin-Font E. Magnesium and phosphorus. *Lancet* 1998; **352**: 391–396.

Related topics of interest

Fluid therapy, p. 122; Potassium, p. 180; Sodium, p. 231

CANCER THERAPY
Cynthia Uy

Several malignancies are curable with aggressive treatments including chemotherapy, radio-therapy and bone marrow transplant. The commonest cause of death in such patients is failure of the malignant process to respond to treatment. The second commonest is infection. Patients being treated for malignancy may require admission to a critical care unit for management of:

- Specific cancer therapy (usually performed in specialist units).
- Complications associated with the disease and treatment.
- Infection.

Admission of such patients to critical care facilities requires careful assessment by both critical care and oncology specialists and a realistic view of long term prognosis by all involved (including the patient and their relatives).

Complications of cancer therapy
Side effects of chemotherapy:

- Nausea and vomiting is associated with most cytotoxic agents.
- Bone marrow suppression of haematopoietic progenitor cells leading to leuco-paenia and thrombocytopaenia after 10–14 days. The lowest blood counts are called the nadir. Recovery occurs over 3–4 weeks.
- Oral mucositis which may reflect damage to the whole of the gastrointestinal epithelium. Mucositis is due to the effect of chemotherapy on the GI tract (GIT) mucosa, which like marrow is a rapidly dividing cell population. The result is inflammation, necrosis and subsequent regeneration.
- Diarrhoea and constipation are frequent and rarely a paralytic ileus may be present (vinca alkaloids).
- Peripheral and autonomic neuropathies (platinum drugs, taxanes and vinca alkaloids). Cerebellar toxicity (5-fluoruracil).
- Ototoxicity may be irreversible (cisplatin).
- Nephrotoxicity is seen with platinum agents (particularly cisplatin).
- Haemorrhagic cystitis (cyclophosphamide and ifosfamide).
- Cardiomyopathy with arrhythmias and fibrosis (doxorubicin).
- Acute myocardial necrosis (cyclophosphamide).
- Coronary artery spasm and ischaemia (5-fluorouracil).
- Many cytotoxics are vesicants and extravasation is associated with severe damage.
- Pulmonary fibrosis (bleomycin and busulphan). Most alkylating agents can cause fibrosis or pneumonitis.

Metabolic complications
- Hyperuricaemia (treatment includes hydration, alkalinization of urine, allo-purinol).
- Hypercalcaemia (due to bony metastases or ectopic PTH secretion).
- Tumour lysis syndrome (hyperkalaemia, hyperphosphataemia, hypocal-caemia, lactic acidosis).

- Hyperviscosity (particularly seen in multiple myeloma and may be an indication for plasmaphoresis).
- Hyponatraemia due to SIADH (vincristine, cyclophosphamide) (see page 232).

Bone marrow failure

(a) Anaemia. Blood transfusion is used to maintain Hb of approximately 10 g dl^{-1}.

(b) Bleeding (due to thrombocytopaenia but DIC may also be a feature) Platelets are transfused to maintain a count > 10–15×10^9 l^{-1}, in the presence of fever and evidence of blood loss this level may need to be higher ($> 20 \times 10^9$ l^{-1}).

(c) Infection (neutropenia). Neutropenia is a neutrophil count $< 1.0 \times 10^9$ l^{-1}. Infection is not usually a problem until counts fall below this level. At 0.5×10^9 l^{-1} the risk becomes significant. In general, neutropenia for less than 10 days is well tolerated. Sepsis should be assumed in any patient presenting with a fever (temperature $> 38°C$) and neutropenia, and should be managed accordingly (septic screen and empirical antibiotics). Because of low neutrophil counts and continued immunosuppression (steroids), patients often do not show the usual signs of infection. Granulocyte transfusion is rarely used to increase the granulocyte count since the introduction of granulocyte colony stimulating factor (GCSF). GCSF is used to stimulate stem cells after chemotherapy and before stem cell harvest. Treatment reduces the duration and severity of neutropenia. Patients at high risk of infection include those with:

- Prolonged persistent neutropenia.
- Pneumonitis.
- Severe mucositis.
- Invasive catheters (i.v., urethral, tracheal).
- Local sepsis.

Prevention of infection

Infection arises from endogenous spread (e.g., oropharynx, GI tract, i.v. lines) and exogenous spread (from staff, other patients, food, parenteral drugs and nutrition and blood products). Methods used to reduce infection include:

- Hand washing.
- Protective isolation and reverse barrier nursing.
- Sterile technique for all procedures.
- Minimizing invasive procedures.
- Prophylactic antibiotics.
- Screening all blood products.

Respiratory complications

ARDS is the most common reason for admission of patients receiving chemotherapy to a general critical care unit. On clinical grounds it may be difficult to differentiate infection from pneumonitis. There may also be pulmonary haemorrhage in the presence of very low platelet counts. Management is empirical and supportive. Confirmatory tests to consider include CT scan, bronchoalveolar lavage, bronchial brushings and biopsies.

Nutritional failure

This is common because of poor nutritional status, disease of the GI tract that limits enteral nutrition, and a high metabolic nutritional requirement. Whenever possible enteral nutrition is preferred but some patients with prolonged, severe mucositis will require parenteral nutrition. The use of parenteral nutrition is a recognized risk factor for infection in these patients.

Bone marrow transplantation complications

Respiratory failure secondary to infection remains the most common cause of death. Organisms implicated include cytomegalovirus, *Pneumocystis carinii*, varicella zoster, toxoplasmosis, Gram-positive and Gram-negative bacteria and *Candida* and *Aspergillus* species. Antimicrobial therapy requires multiple drugs and close microbiological collaboration. Such patients are often treated with a third generation cephalosporin (to cover common Gram-positive and -negative organisms), an aminoglycoside, vancomycin, fluconazole, an antiviral, and co-trimoxazole.

Veno-occlusive liver disease may occur early after transplantation and is associated particularly with busulphan regimens.

Graft versus host disease (GvHD)

A common, potentially fatal complication of allogeneic BMT. There is frequently a rash associated with variable degrees of hepatic abnormalities and gastrointestinal failure. Therapy includes steroids, cyclosporin, antithymocyte globulin, methotrexate, thalidomide, azathioprine and psoralen plus ultraviolet A (PUVA).

Empirical antibiotic therapy

Best bet antimicrobial therapy for suspected infection in immunocompromised patients must cover Gram-negative (including *Pseudomonas aeruginosa*) and Gram-positive organisms (including streptococci and staphylococci). Two drug therapy with a third generation cephalosporin (e.g., ceftriaxone of cefotaxime) is initiated. There should be a low threshold for adding a glycopeptide (e.g., vancomycin or teicoplanin) if there is suspicion of infection with coagulase negative staphylococci, MRSA and resistant streptococci. Antifungal treatment is given if there is evidence of fungal infection. Antimicrobials should be reviewed on a daily basis in the light of culture results and microbiologist advice.

Further reading

Rubenfeld GD, Crawford SW. Withdrawing life support from mechanically ventilated recipients of bone marrow transplants: A case for evidence-based guidelines. *Annals of Internal Medicine* 1996; 125: 625–633.
Sculier JP. Intensive care and oncology. *Support Care Cancer* 1995; 3: 93–105.

Related topics of interest

Infection control, p. 140; Infection in critical care, p. 143

CARDIAC ARRHYTHMIAS

Arrhythmias in critically ill patients are common. Arrhythmias arise from either abnormal generation or conduction of cardiac impulses. Abnormal impulse generation results from either increased automaticity (e.g., sinus tachycardia, sinus bradycardia, atrial tachycardia, junctional rhythm, idioventricular rhythm) or triggered activity (e.g., long QT syndrome, digoxin toxicity).

Disorders of impulse conduction include AV and AV nodal re-entry tachycardias, atrial flutter, atrial fibrillation, ventricular tachycardia, VF, SA and AV heart block, bundle branch block.

Assessment

The extent of haemodynamic compromise will dictate the urgency of intervention. The arrhythmia and any cardiac pathology should be identified. Management is directed at correcting any underlying abnormalities and specific therapy that includes drugs cardioversion/defibrillation and cardiac pacing.

The history and examination may reveal correctable causes of arrhythmias. These include:

- Myocardial ischaemia.
- Respiratory compromise (hypoxia, hypercarbia).
- Circulatory compromise (hypovolaemia, hypotension, hypertension, low haemoglobin, reduced cardiac output).
- Electrolyte abnormalities (especially of potassium, magnesium and calcium).
- Metabolic abnormalities (acidosis, alkalosis).
- Presence of drugs (tricyclics, MAOIs, cocaine, amphetamine, antiarrhythmic overdose/toxicity).
- Endogenous catecholamines (inadequate sedation, pain, phaeochromocytoma).
- Exogenous catecholamines (catecholamine infusions, direct and indirect vasopressors, theophylline toxicity).
- Mechanical stimulation (pacing wire, CVP line, pulmonary artery catheter).
- Mechanical cardiac abnormalities (cardiomyopathy, valvular heart disease, pulmonary embolism, tamponade).
- Raised intracranial pressure (ICP).
- Thyrotoxicosis.
- Hypothermia or hyperthermia.
- Vagal stimulation.

Management of specific arrhythmias

For arrhythmias associated with cardiac arrest see page 214.

There are three treatment options available for the management of cardiac arrhythmias not associated with cardiac arrest. They are:

- Cardioversion. Relatively reliable way of converting a tachycardia to sinus rhythm. It may, unusually, precipitate VF. It is thus reserved for those patients with adverse signs or in whom drug therapy has failed.

- Antiarrhythmic drugs. Although less likely to produce life-threatening consequences than cardioversion, antiarrhythmic drugs are also less likely to be successful in converting a tachycardia to sinus rhythm.
- Cardiac pacing. This is a reliable way of treating most bradycardias and some tachycardias. Transvenous pacing requires expertise to establish. External pacing and fist or percussion pacing are easier techniques that may be used as temporizing manoeuvres. In percussion pacing gentle blows are delivered rhythmically to the chest overlying the heart.

The following are the treatment algorithms of the European Resuscitation Council. In all circumstances it is assumed that the patient is being given additional oxygen to breathe and intravenous access has been established.

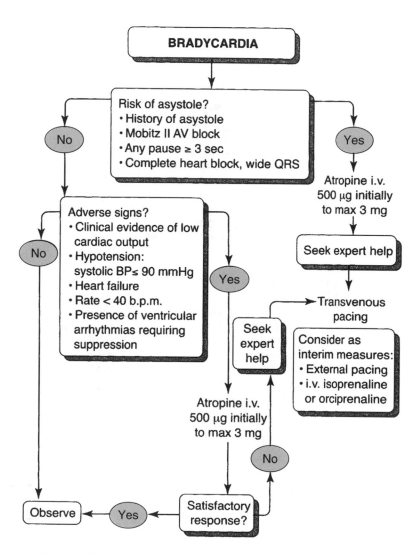

Reprinted from *Resuscitation*, Volume 37, 1998 with permission from Elsevier Science.

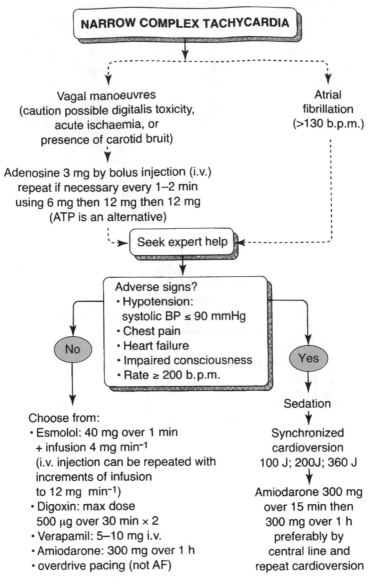

NARROW COMPLEX TACHYCARDIA

Vagal manoeuvres
(caution possible digitalis toxicity,
acute ischaemia, or
presence of carotid bruit)

Atrial
fibrillation
(>130 b.p.m.)

Adenosine 3 mg by bolus injection (i.v.)
repeat if necessary every 1–2 min
using 6 mg then 12 mg then 12 mg
(ATP is an alternative)

Seek expert help

Adverse signs?
• Hypotension:
  systolic BP ≤ 90 mmHg
• Chest pain
• Heart failure
• Impaired consciousness
• Rate ≥ 200 b.p.m.

No

Yes

Choose from:
• Esmolol: 40 mg over 1 min
  + infusion 4 mg min⁻¹
  (i.v. injection can be repeated with
  increments of infusion
  to 12 mg min⁻¹)
• Digoxin: max dose
  500 µg over 30 min × 2
• Verapamil: 5–10 mg i.v.
• Amiodarone: 300 mg over 1 h
• overdrive pacing (not AF)

Sedation

Synchronized
cardioversion
100 J; 200J; 360 J

Amiodarone 300 mg
over 15 min then
300 mg over 1 h
preferably by
central line and
repeat cardioversion

Notes: *Vagal manoeuvres include the Valsalva manoeuvre, and
carotid sinus massage (performed unilaterally and only after a
carotid bruit has been excluded).
β-blockade after verapamil may result in AV node standstill.*

Reprinted from *Resuscitation*, Volume 37, 1998 with permission from Elsevier Science.

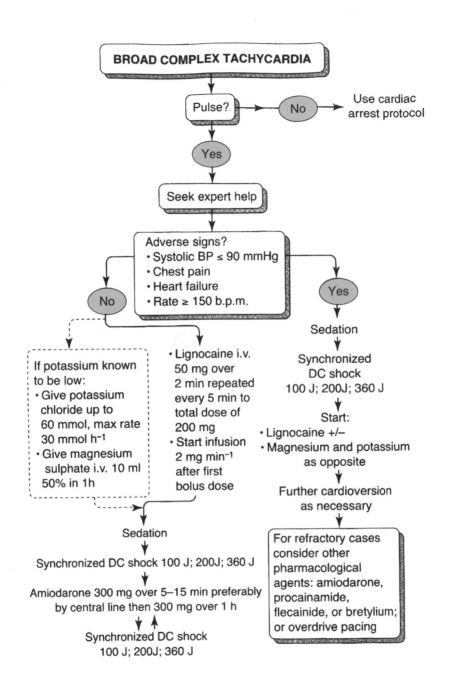

BROAD COMPLEX TACHYCARDIA

Pulse? → No → Use cardiac arrest protocol

Yes

Seek expert help

Adverse signs?
- Systolic BP ≤ 90 mmHg
- Chest pain
- Heart failure
- Rate ≥ 150 b.p.m.

No

Yes

If potassium known to be low:
- Give potassium chloride up to 60 mmol, max rate 30 mmol h^{-1}
- Give magnesium sulphate i.v. 10 ml 50% in 1h

- Lignocaine i.v. 50 mg over 2 min repeated every 5 min to total dose of 200 mg
- Start infusion 2 mg min^{-1} after first bolus dose

Sedation

Synchronized DC shock 100 J; 200J; 360 J

Amiodarone 300 mg over 5–15 min preferably by central line then 300 mg over 1 h

Synchronized DC shock 100 J; 200J; 360 J

Sedation

Synchronized DC shock 100 J; 200J; 360 J

Start:
- Lignocaine +/–
- Magnesium and potassium as opposite

Further cardioversion as necessary

For refractory cases consider other pharmacological agents: amiodarone, procainamide, flecainide, or bretylium; or overdrive pacing

Reprinted from *Resuscitation*, Volume 37, 1998 with permission from Elsevier Science.

Further reading

Bossaert L (ed). Periarrest arrhythmias: management of arrhythmias associated with cardiac arrest. In: *European Resuscitation Council Guidelines for Resuscitation*. Amsterdam; Elsevier, 1998, pp. 159–168.

Parr MJ and Craft TM. *Resuscitation; Key Data Third Edition*. Oxford; BIOS Scientific Publishers, 1998.

Related topic of interest

Resuscitation – cardiopulmonary, p. 213

CARDIAC CHEST PAIN

Cardiac chest pain is one of the most common reasons for emergency admission to hospital. Acute myocardial infarction is seen in approximately 30% of these admissions. The mortality of acute myocardial infarction can be markedly reduced with the early administration of thrombolytic agents. Patients presenting with chest pain thus require a rapid assessment of their condition to determine whether or not urgent thrombolysis is indicated. At the same time, their symptoms need controlling and physical condition stabilizing.

Angina

Angina is defined as unstable when attacks are increasingly frequent and/or prolonged, occur at rest, or are brought on with minor provocation. The vast majority of such patients have atheromatous obstructive coronary disease. Unstable angina may be precipitated by an atheromatous plaque fissuring or rupturing leading platelets to form an overlying mural thrombus.

1. Treatment aims
- Pain relief.
- Reduction of platelet activity and thus thrombus formation.
- Prevention of progression to myocardial infarction (MI).

2. Immediate actions
- **Oxygen** by face mask or nasal cannulae.
- **Intravenous access.**
- **Pain control.** Give diamorphine 2.5–5 mg i.v. by slow injection (1 mg min^{-1}) repeated as required together with an antiemetic, e.g., metoclopramide 10 mg or cyclizine 25–50 mg i.v. The equivalent dose of morphine is 5–10mg i.v by slow injection (2 mg min^{-1}).
- **Aspirin** 75 mg orally or 300 mg chewed then swallowed.
- **12 lead ECG** and continuous ECG monitoring (CXR later).
- **Blood tests.** FBC, U&Es, glucose, cardiac enzymes, cholesterol.

The patient should then be admitted to a critical care unit for bedrest, monitoring, and continued management.

3. Anti-anginal therapy
- **Nitrates.** Nitrates reduce the pain of unstable angina. Sublingual glyceryl trinitrate (GTN) provides rapid but transient relief. A continuous intravenous infusion of isosorbide dinitrate ($2–10 \text{ mg h}^{-1}$) or GTN ($10–200 \text{ μg min}^{-1}$) should be titrated against the clinical response. Headache, nausea, or hypotension may limit the use of nitrates. It is not known whether the use of intravenous nitrates will prevent progression to infarction.
- **β-blockade.** Treatment usually relieves symptoms and may prevent progression to infarction. Early (within 12 hours) intravenous therapy followed by oral treatment reduces the risk of progressing to infarction from 32% to 28%.

4. _Antiplatelet therapy._ Thromboxane A_2 promotes the aggregation of platelets. Aspirin inhibits its synthesis, reduces the incidence of MI, and improves the survival of patients with unstable angina. Following the initial, immediate, dose of aspirin it should be continued indefinitely.

5. _Anticoagulants_

- **Unfractionated heparin.** When given by intravenous infusion, unfractionated heparin (UFH) reduces symptomatic and silent ischaemic episodes in patients with unstable angina. It has been difficult to see this translated into a difference in outcome, however. In a meta-analysis of studies comparing groups treated with UFH and aspirin in combination or aspirin alone the incidence of death or infarction was 7.9% in the combined therapy groups versus 10.4% with aspirin alone. There is thus probably a small but clinically significant benefit in combined therapy.
- **Low molecular weight heparins.** The anticoagulant effect of LMWH is more predictable than UFH. It can thus be given by s.c. injection in a fixed dose adjusted for body weight. Anticoagulation monitoring is not required. Double blind studies have found LMWHs to be more effective in combination with aspirin at reducing the incidence of MI or death than aspirin alone and at reducing the need for early revascularization procedures than UFH.

6. _Revascularization._ Revascularization comprises either coronary artery bypass grafting (CABG) or percutaneous transluminal coronary angioplasty (PTCA). Acute complications, procedure-related death and MI are all more common in patients with unstable angina, regardless of the procedure, than in patients having the same procedure for stable angina. Where it is suitable on angiographic grounds, PTCA will, over a 5 year period, avoid the need for CABG in most patients. Outcome following CABG performed on patients with unstable angina is as good as that performed on those with stable angina once they survive the early complications (90% survival at 5 years, 80% at 10 years, and relief of angina).

Patients with angina resistant to medical therapy or which persists after 48 hours of inpatient treatment require urgent angiography to determine suitability for revascularization. Patients whose symptoms settle should be investigated non-invasively for severe residual ischaemia (exercise ECG, thallium screening, stress echocardiography).

Acute myocardial infarction

Given early enough, aspirin will save 20–30 lives per 1000 infarcts. Giving thrombolytic agents early enough will save 30 lives per 1000 infarcts. The difference between thrombolysis during the first hour following the onset of symptoms compared with the second to third hour is 10–12 lives saved per 1000 infarcts.

1. _Thrombolysis_

- **Indications.** Patients within 24 hours of the onset of major symptoms suggestive of acute MI. Supporting ECG changes are ST elevation > 0.2 mV in more than two adjacent chest leads or > 0.1 mV in limb leads.
- **Absolute contraindications.** Active haemorrhage. Recent CNS infarction, haemorrhage, or surgery. Trauma or malignancy.

- **Relative contraindications.** Recent non-CNS surgery ($<$ 10 days). Recent trauma ($<$ 10 days). Recent gastrointestinal haemorrhage. Recent protracted chest compressions (cardiac massage). Coagulation disorders. Pregnancy or $<$ 10 days post partum. Severe hypertension (diastolic $>$ 130 mmHg).

2. Thrombolytic agents
DO NOT WAIT FOR CONFIRMATORY LAB RESULTS OF MI

1. **Streptokinase** (for almost all patients). Streptokinase is a fibrin non-specific plasminogen activator. It causes widespread activation of circulating plasminogen resulting in a systemic lytic state. It is antigenic.
   Dose: 1.5 million units in 0.9% sodium chloride given over 60 min.
2. **t-PA (tissue plasminogen activator) with intravenous heparin.** t-PA is a fibrin specific plasminogen activator which produces direct activation at the site of the fibrin clot occluding the coronary artery. It is indicated if:
- Streptokinase given within 5 days–12 months previously.
- Patient aged $<$ 75 years, with a large anterior MI, and within 4 hours of onset of symptoms (large infarcts are defined by ST segment elevation in more than six of the 12 ECG leads).
- Severe persistent hypotension, especially if aggravated by streptokinase.
   Dose: 15 mg bolus i.v., then infusion of 0.75 mg kg^{-1} over 30 min (max 50 mg), then 0.5 mg kg^{-1} over 60 min (max. 35 mg).
   The dose of i.v. heparin is 5000 unit bolus then 1000 units h^{-1} for 48 hours. Heparin is commenced simultaneously with t-PA.

3. Alternatives to thrombolysis.
Emergency coronary angiography with angioplasty, placement of intraluminal stents, intracoronary thrombolysis or emergency coronary artery bypass surgery are the subject of current investigation and should be considered if available. At present emergency angiography is not widely available in many countries.

4. Other drugs
- **β-blockade** should be started as soon as possible by either the oral or intravenous route unless contraindicated (e.g. asthma, bradycardia). Agents in common use include metoprolol and atenolol. β-blockade probably reduces mortality, arrhythmias (including VF), cardiac rupture and reinfarction rate.
- **ACE inhibitor.** After 48 hours an ACE inhibitor should be started. Captopril 12.5 mg bd increasing to 50 mg has been shown to be effective. Captopril given in this way will save an extra five lives per 1000 patients with MI. The benefit continues for at least 1 year. Evidence from the SAVE study suggests that patients with poor left ventricular function following an MI treated with captopril 50 mg tds had a reduced mortality (over 40 lives per 1000 patients), fewer recurrent MIs and reduced need for hospitalization for heart failure over a 3.5 year period.
- **Aspirin.** Aspirin administration should be continued after thrombolysis because it reduces the chances of reocclusion.

Consider

- **Heparin.** Intravenous heparin is commenced in conjunction with t-PA and continued for at least 24 hours. While there is no convincing evidence that heparin infusions are beneficial after streptokinase they are often initiated within 6–12 hours of thrombolysis. After intravenous heparin has been stopped subcutaneous heparin (5000 units bd) should be continued for all patients at risk from DVT. Compression stockings should be worn.
- **Warfarin.** Oral anticoagulation is commenced for those patients with large anterior MI.

5. Rehabilitation. Patients who survive require a sympathetic explanation of their condition and its implications. They should then commence a cardiac rehabilitation programme and receive advice about their risk factors (family history, smoking, hyperlipidaemias, hypertension, and diabetes mellitus).

Cholesterol-lowering drugs. Three recent large clinical trials have all confirmed that cholesterol lowering is a safe and effective means of preventing initial or recurrent coronary events in at risk patients. In the CARE trial pravastatin (a competitive inhibitor of cholesterol biosynthesis) saved 150 fatal and non-fatal CVS events per 1000 patients treated for 5 years when it was given to post MI patients with average cholesterol levels. Patients aged > 60 years and women showed the greatest benefit. Pravastatin does not interact with warfarin.

Further reading

Louie EK, Edwards L. Reynertson, SI. Acute myocardial infarction and guidelines for treatment. *Current Opinion in Critical Care* 1998; **4**: 304–316.
Owen A. Intravenous β-blockade in acute myocardial infarction. *British Medical Journal* 1998; **317**: 226–227.

Related topics of interest

Cardiac pacing, p. 80; Resuscitation – cardiopulmonary, p. 213; Resuscitation – post-resuscitation care, p. 216

CARDIAC FAILURE

Manivannan Gopalkrishnan

Cardiac failure occurs when the heart fails to maintain an adequate circulation despite adequate filling pressures. This results in failure to meet tissue oxygen and metabolic requirements. Cardiogenic shock is severe acute cardiac failure and defined by a systolic BP <90 mmHg with evidence of impaired tissue perfusion. This condition has a poor prognosis.

Factors affecting cardiac output

Cardiac output is the product of stroke volume and heart rate. Stroke volume is determined by preload, contractility and afterload. Cardiac output maybe optimized by manipulation of these factors.

1. Preload. This refers to the diastolic myocardial tension or left ventricular (LV) end diastolic volume. Increasing preload increases cardiac output by the Frank–Starling mechanism when LV function is normal. In patients with poor LV function, decreasing preload may improve cardiac output if left atrial pressures are high. Preload may be increased by volume loading and decreased by diuresis and venodilation.

In cardiac failure with normal LV systolic function, reducing preload may be deleterious. Such hearts are preload dependent (e.g., pericardial constriction, high output failure).

2. Contractility. This is the force of LV contraction independent of preload and afterload. Contractility is increased by inotropic drugs and relief of ischaemia and hypoxia. It is decreased by ischaemia, hypoxia and negatively inotropic drugs (e.g. thiopentone, calcium channel blockers).

3. Afterload. This refers to the systolic myocardial wall tension. It is increased with high intraventricular pressures, increased aortic impedance/systemic vascular resistance (SVR), increased ventricular radius and negative intrathoracic pressure. Afterload is decreased by reduced aortic impedance/SVR, reduced intraventricular pressure, positive intrathoracic pressure and increased ventricular wall thickness.

The failing heart is generally more afterload dependant (compared to the heart with normal LV function which is preload dependant).

Heart rate

Heart rate is increased in most patients with cardiac failure as an acute compensatory mechanism. However, increased heart rate results in reduced diastolic filling time, reduced time for coronary perfusion and increasing cardiac work.

Rhythm

Arrhythmias with loss of coordinated atrial activity (atrial fibrillation, atrial flutter, and heart block) can impair LV diastolic filling resulting in lowered stroke volumes which may trigger cardiac failure in susceptible patients.

Manipulation of these factors to improve cardiac output must be performed without increasing myocardial work or oxygen demand.

Clinical features

The main symptoms of cardiac failure are dyspnoea, orthopnoea, paroxysmal nocturnal dyspnoea (PND) due to pulmonary congestion, and fatigue (due to low cardiac output).

The main signs are due to:

- Sympathetic stimulation: tachycardia, sweating, peripheral vasoconstriction.
- Myocardial dysfunction: cardiomegaly, added heart sounds (gallop rhythm), functional tricuspid and mitral regurgitation.
- Sodium and water retention: elevated venous pressure, pulmonary and peripheral oedema, pleural effusions, hepatomegaly and ascites.

Similar symptoms may be caused by non-cardiogenic pulmonary oedema, pulmonary pathology and non-pulmonary causes (e.g. obesity, psychogenic). Gallop rhythms may occur normally in the aged and in pregnancy. Oedema may be caused by renal and liver disease and venous insufficiency. Patients in cardiac failure with normal LV systolic function often have normal sized hearts.

Sudden deterioration in well compensated chronic cardiac failure may be caused by ischaemia/infarct, arrhythmias, pulmonary embolism, hypertension, and increased cardiac work e.g. due to asthma, infection and poor compliance with medical therapy.

In patients difficult to wean from ventilation, occult cardiac failure must be considered.

Investigations

(a) Investigations for coexisting and precipitating conditions.
(b) Full blood count, urea, electrolytes, creatinine, cardiac enzymes and thyroid function tests.
(c) ECG for diagnosis of myocardial ischaemia/ infarct and arrhythmias.
(d) CXR for assessment of cardiac size and shape and pulmonary oedema.
(e) Arterial blood gas and lactate for assessment of severity of decompensation.
(f) Echocardiogram for confirmation of diagnosis, assessment of cause and severity.
(g) Pulmonary artery catheterization will usually demonstrate high PAOP and CVP with a low cardiac output and low mixed venous oxygen saturation.
(h) Other investigations:

- For coronary artery disease: stress testing and coronary angiography.
- Electrophysiogical studies and radiofrequency ablation for arrhythmias.
- Endomyocardial biopsy for diagnosis of infiltrative diseases.

Management

1. Aims

- To reduce cardiac work and optimize coronary O_2 supply.
- To improve cardiac output to meet tissue needs.
- To treat precipitating event and underlying cause.

2. General treatment

(a) Rest will reduce metabolic requirements.
(b) O_2 by mask or nasal prongs. In acute pulmonary oedema, mask CPAP is useful. It helps to correct hypoxia and hypercapnoea, reduces work of breathing by

improved alveolar stability and by increased lung volume and thus lung compliance, and reduces LV afterload and thus cardiac work. Intubation and ventilation may be required in fulminant pulmonary oedema and ventilatory compromise.

(c) Drugs

- Nitrates produce venodilatation and reduction of preload, provided that the patient is not hypotensive. In comparison with high dose frusemide, first line therapy with nitrates will improve outcome from heart failure.
- Diuretics: In acute heart failure frusemide produces rapid venodilatation followed by diuresis. However, in chronic congestive heart failure (CHF) frusemide stimulates the renin–angiotensin aldosterone system and causes an initial increase of afterload with reduction of stroke volume and cardiac output and increased pulmonary capillary pressure. In chronic CHF, if large doses of diuretic are needed, thiazides or metalozone may be considered.
- Vasodilators: In acute heart failure with evidence of increased afterload, a short acting vasodilator such as GTN or sodium nitroprusside can be titrated rapidly. Both systolic and diastolic function may be improved. Angiotensin converting enzyme (ACE) inhibitors improve exercise tolerance and signs and symptoms of heart failure and reduce mortality. To prevent hypotension they should be introduced cautiously in severe heart failure e.g., captopril 6.25 mg tds or less. Calcium channel blockers also produce reduction of afterload. However, they make heart failure worse and may increase the risk of death.

(d) Inotropes: Inotropes improve cardiac output and tissue perfusion.

- Dobutamine has both inotropic and vasodilatory actions and may be the drug of choice in heart failure. However, it may occasionally cause severe hypotension and tachycardia.
- Adrenaline produces good improvement of cardiac output but often at the cost of tachycardia and increased cardiac work.
- Noradrenaline causes less tachycardia but may be inappropriate in vasoconstricted states.
- Phosphodiesterase inhibitors have independent lusitropic effects in addition to inotropic effects. They are useful in diastolic failure. Because of their different site of action, they may also be useful in down-regulated states.
- Digoxin: In the critically ill the role of digoxin is restricted to the treatment of supraventricular tachycardia and AF. It has a narrow therapeutic index with increased risk of toxicity in renal failure. It is a poor inotrope especially in the presence of high sympathetic activity and may actually reduce cardiac output in cardiogenic shock by increasing SVR.
- Beta-blockers: Have been shown to improve survival in severe heart failure after acute myocardial infarction.

3. Specific treatment

- Treatment of arrhythmias: Anti-arrhythmic agents, radiofrequency ablation, pacemakers, implantable cardiodefibrillators.
- Treatment of coronary artery disease: Coronary angioplasty +/- stent, CABG.
- Other surgical treatment: Cardiomyoplasty, cardiomyomectomy, cardiac transplantation.

4. **Outcome.** Cardiac failure has a high mortality. More than 30% of patients will die within a year of diagnosis. Cardiogenic shock is associated with an initial mortality of >50%.

Further reading

Calvin JE. Use of clinical practice guidelines in congestive cardiac failure. *Current Opinion in Critical Care* 1999; **5**: 317–321.

Teo KK. Recent advances. Cardiology. *BMJ* 1998; **316**: 911–915.

Related topics of interest

Cardiac arrhythmias, p. 64; Cardiac chest pain, p. 69; Cardiac output – measurement of, p. 77; Resuscitation – cardiopulmonary, p. 213

CARDIAC OUTPUT – MEASUREMENT OF

Martin Schuster-Bruce

The maintenance of adequate tissue perfusion is one of the primary goals in the management of the critically ill. Cardiac output is the major determinant of oxygen delivery and the variable that can be most effectively manipulated therapeutically. Preload, afterload, cardiac contractility and compliance affect cardiac output. The monitoring and manipulation of cardiac filling and cardiac output form the basis of much of critical care practice.

Clinical

Clinical assessment, vital signs, urine output and core/peripheral temperature gradients can provide valuable information about the cardiac output and circulation. In all forms of shock there is evidence of poor end organ perfusion (oliguria, altered mental state, lactic acidosis). In low cardiac output states the peripheries are cool and the pulse volume low, whereas in septic shock the peripheries are warm and the pulse volume high. However, in critically ill patients with multisystem failure, clinical assessment alone may be inadequate and the accuracy of estimation of volume status compared to invasive techniques may be as low as 30%.

Invasive

1. **Pulmonary artery catheter.** Pulmonary artery catheterization without the need for X-ray can be achieved via a percutaneous sheath, placed in a central vein. The waveform and pressure are monitored continually. The balloon is inflated and the catheter 'floated' through tricuspid valve into the right heart and finally 'wedged' in a pulmonary artery. It allows direct measurement of CVP, pulmonary artery pressure and PAOP.

   (a) **Preload.** Inflation of the balloon isolates a pulmonary vascular segment and flow in that segment ceases. The PAOP is equivalent to left ventricular end diastolic pressure (LVEDP). PAOP is measured at end-expiration to minimize the effect of intrathoracic pressure. LVEDP is used as an indicator of the preload of the left ventricle (i.e. LVEDV). The relationship between LVEDP and LVEDV depends on the compliance of the ventricle, which is often altered and may be difficult to predict in many critically ill patients.

   (b) **Cardiac output.** The addition of a thermistor near the tip of the catheter allows determination of cardiac output by the thermodilution technique. A known volume of liquid at a known temperature is injected as a bolus into the right atrium. This mixes with and cools the blood, causing a drop in temperature at the thermistor in the pulmonary artery. The dilution curve is analysed by computer to calculate the cardiac output. The mean of three consecutive measurements, taken randomly through the respiratory cycle, is calculated. The precision of the measurements is at best 4–9%. The results will be inaccurate in the presence of intracardiac shunts or pulmonary/tricuspid regurgitation.

   Complications of pulmonary artery catheterization include all those of central venous catheterization plus trauma to the atria, ventricles and valves, arrhythmias, pulmonary infarction and haemorrhage, catheter knotting and infection (particularly after 72 hours).

(c) **Derived variables.** Measurement of cardiac output, intravascular pressures and heart rate allows the calculation of a number of haemodynamic and oxygen transport variables.

Body surface area is used to index the variables and compensate for differences in patient size.

Pulmonary and sytemic vascular resistance can be useful in diagnosis of the type of shock and estimate the afterload of the right and left ventricles respectively.

(d) **Semi-continous cardiac output and mixed venous oxygen saturation.** A thermal filament is attached to the catheter so that it is located in the right ventricle after insertion. Pulses of heat emitted by the filament are detected by the thermistor at the tip of the catheter to produce a thermodilution washout curve. Values are updated every 30 s and the average over the last 5 min displayed. It appears as accurate and reproducible as intermittent thermodilution in routine practice. However, the response time is too slow for immediate detection of acute changes in cardiac output and rapid infusion of cold solutions can interfere with measurements.

The addition of a fibreoptic oximeter at the tip provides continuous mixed venous oxygen saturation. Based on the Fick principle, when oxygen consumption is constant, changes in mixed venous oxygen saturation are directly proportional to cardiac output.

(e) **Right ventricular ejection fraction catheter.** A rapid-response thermistor allows temperature changes in the pulmonary artery on a beat-to-beat basis to be measured after right atrial injection of a cold fluid bolus. Right ventricular end diastolic volume (RVEDV) can be calculated (RVEDV=SV/RVEF) and has been suggested to be a better indicator of preload than CVP and PAOP, particularly in sepsis, ARDS and when high levels of PEEP are applied.

(f) **Indications for pulmonary artery catheterization:**
- Assessment of intravascular volume, cardiac output, SvO_2, DO_2 and VO_2.
- Rational use of volume, inotropes and vasoactive drugs.
- Manipulation of PAOP and PAP in ARDS.

As yet, there are no unambiguous data showing that pulmonary artery catherization reduces mortality.

Normal values (CO, cardiac output)

Variable	Calculation	Normal range
Cardiac index (CI)	CO/BSA	$2.8–4.2 \, l \, min^{-1} \, m^{-2}$
Stroke volume	CO/HR	80 ml
Left ventricular stroke work index	$CI \times (MAP–PAOP) \times 0.0136$	$44–64 \, g \, m \, m^{-2}$ per beat
Right ventricular stroke work index	$CI \times (MPAP–CVP) \times 0.0136$	$7–12 \, g \, m \, m^{-2}$ per beat
Systemic vascular resistance	$(MAP–CVP) \times 80/CO$	$1000–1200 \, dyn \, s \, cm^{-5} \, m^{-2}$
Pulmonary vascular resistance	$(MPAP–PAOP) \times 80/CO$	$60–120 \, dyn \, s \, cm^{-5} \, m^{-2}$
Oxygen delivery	$CO \times CaO_2$	$850–1050 \, ml \, min^{-1}$
Oxygen consumption	$CO \times (CaO_2 - CvO_2)$	$180–300 \, ml \, min^{-1}$

2. **Direct Fick method.** The Fick principle can be applied to the consumption of oxygen by the body (cardiac output = $VO_2/[CaO_2-CvO_2]$). A metabolic cart is used to measure VO_2. Current technology allows measurement of breath by breath VO_2 and in conjunction with continuous SvO_2 and SpO_2, this technique can be used to calculate continuous cardiac output.

Non-invasive

1. **Aortic Doppler flow probes.** When a sound wave is reflected off a moving object the frequency is shifted by an amount proportional to the relative velocity of the object. This is the Doppler principle. Reflected signals from a probe placed in either the oesophagus or suprasternal notch are analysed to produce a velocity–time curve for blood flow in the aorta. From analysis of the area under the curve, cardiac output and SV can be calculated. There is reasonable correlation between Doppler and thermodilution estimates of cardiac output, though relative rather than absolute values are obtained. The major advantage of this technique is that the probes are relatively non-invasive and easy to place, although in some patients signal strength can be poor.

2. **Echocardiography.** Echocardiography utilizes an ultrasound beam to generate intermittent real-time images of the heart. It has been traditionally performed via the transthoracic approach, but up to 30% of mechanically ventilated patients have poor transthoracic windows, particularly in those who have undergone cardio-thoracic surgery. Transoesophageal echocardiography (TOE) uses a transducer mounted on the tip of an endoscope. The image obtained is more refined since the transducer within the oesphagus is juxtaposed against the heart and it is easier to maintain a stable transducer position. Cardiac performance can be estimated by the calculation of ejection fractions and from Doppler velocity traces of aortic flow. The chief advantage of echocardiography is its ability to detect other pathologies. TOE is sensitive enough to detect ischaemia by regional wall motion abnormalities prior to any ECG changes. Other diagnostic uses include the detection of aortic dissection or trauma, cardiac tamponade, valvular lesions and intracardiac thrombus.

3. **Others**
- Impedence cardiography.
- Radionucleotide techniques.
- MUGA scans.

These have limited use in bedside assessment of cardiac output in the ICU.

Further reading

Gomez CMH, Palazzo MGA. Pulmonary artery catheterization in anaesthesia and intensive care. *British Journal of Anaesthesia* 1998; **81**: 945–956.

Shephard JN, Brecker SJ, Evans TW. Bedside assessment of myocardial performance in the critically ill. *Intensive Care Medicine* 1994; **20**: 513–521.

Related topics of interest

Arterial cannulation, p. 29; Central venous pressure monitoring, p. 87

CARDIAC PACING

Jas Soar

Cardiac pacing is necessary when normal impulse formation fails (bradyarrhythmias) or conduction fails (heart block) and there is a decrease in cardiac output with associated hypotension or syncope. Pacing can also be used to override tachyarrhythmias.

Permanent pacemakers

Assessment of patients with a permanent pacemaker should include the following key points

1. Why was the patient paced? Indications include symptomatic heart block, sinus node disease, carotid sinus or malignant vasovagal syndromes. The underlying cause may be idiopathic or include congenital abnormalities, ischaemic heart disease, valve disorders, connective tissue diseases, and problems associated with antiarrhythmic drug therapy. An ECG rhythm strip will indicate the underlying rhythm or if the patient is pacemaker dependent.

2. What type of pacemaker is fitted? Pacemakers are classified using the North American Society of Pacing and Electrophysiology/British Pacing and Electrophysiology Group five-letter code. The first letter refers to the paced chamber and the second to the sensed chamber. The chamber codes are A (atrium), V (ventricle), D (dual), O (none) or S (atrium or ventricle). The third letter refers to the sensing mode and may be T (triggering), I (inhibition), D (dual, inhibition and triggering) or O (none, pacemaker in asynchronous mode). The fourth letter indicates programmability and rate response functions (adjustments in heart rate according to patient activity). The fifth letter refers to overdrive pacing, and implantable defibrillator functions.

Temporary pacemakers

1. Indications include:
- Life threatening bradyarrhythmia until a permanent pacemaker is implanted.
- Temporary bradyarrhythmia. Transient atrioventricular block may occur after myocardial infarction, cardiac surgery, especially valve surgery, or with drug therapy e.g., amiodarone toxicity.
- Pacemaker dependent patients who develop pacemaker malfunction. Temporary pacing allows the permanent pacemaker to be changed.
- Patients undergoing surgical procedures at risk of life threatening bradyarrhythmia.

2. Methods of temporary pacing
- **Transvenous pacing** is the commonest temporary mode. A single bipolar right ventricular lead is placed with fluoroscopy. Temporary dual chamber pacing is also possible. The lead is connected to a pacing box. The commonest modes are VOO or VVI. Leads can stay in place for 1–2 weeks although puncture site infection and septicaemia is a risk.

- **Transcutaneous pacing** is rapid, safe and easy to initiate. Adhesive electrodes with a large surface area are used. The negative electrode is placed anteriorly (cardiac apex) and the second electrode posteriorly (below the tip of the scapula). Multifunction electrodes (pacing and defibrillation) are placed in the usual positions for defibrillation. A high threshold is required for pacing causing chest muscle stimulation and pain. In an emergency, transcutaneous pacing buys time for transvenous pacing to be initiated.
- **Epicardial pacing** is common after cardiac surgery. Wires are positioned on the atrial and ventricular surfaces at the end of surgery and passed out through the chest wall.
- **Transoesophageal pacing.** The posterior left atrium comes into close proximity with the oesophagus. Ventricular capture is difficult to achieve and use of this method is limited.
- **Percussion pacing** by gentle blows over the precordium may produce a cardiac output in patients with ventricular standstill where P waves are seen. This temporizing manoeuvre may buy time to institute other therapies and avoid the need for CPR.

Pacemaker problems

It is important to ensure that electrical activity on the ECG is accompanied by a palpable pulse. A CXR will show position of leads and may indicate misplacement, dislodgement or damage.

1. Failure to capture. The ECG show pacing spikes with no following P or QRS waves. Myocardial ischaemia at the site of electrode attachment or of conducting pathways can cause loss of capture. There may be scarring at the contact site. Increasing the generator output may correct this. Potassium abnormalities also cause failure to capture. These affects are amplified in critically ill patients who may have hypoxia acidosis and other metabolic abnormalities.

2. Failure to pace. There are no pacing spikes when they should occur. Battery failure, loose connections and lead damage should be excluded.

3. Failure to sense. Pacing spikes occur inappropriately. May precipitate ventricular arrhythmias.

4. Oversensing. Pacemaker is inhibited by non-cardiac stimuli. Electro-magnetic interference from diathermy, MRI scanners, and mobile phones can interfere with pacemakers. Patient shivering can also interfere with pacemaker function.

5. Defibrillation. Paddles should be placed at least 12–15 cm from the pacing unit.

Permanent pacemakers may be converted to a VOO (asynchronous) mode by placing a magnet over the pacemaker box but specialist help should be sought if time permits as the magnet may set the unit to a reprogrammable mode. For modern pacemakers it is thus preferable to use the programming transceiver for any adjustment.

Automatic implantable cardioverter-defibrillators (AICDs)

AICDs may be of benefit in patients who suffer recurrent ventricular tachyarrhythmias. They deliver small energy shocks (less than 30 J). AICDs may be disabled by applying a magnet over the unit, but specialist help should be sought if time permits as the unit may be set in a reprogrammable mode by the use of a magnet. They should be disabled if patients undergo surgery (diathermy) or the AICD malfunctions and discharges inappropriately. These patients can have external defibrillation in the same way as patients with pacemakers.

Further reading

ACC/AHA guidelines for implantation of cardiac pacemakers and antiarrhythmia devices: Executive Summary. A report of the American College of Cardiology/American Heart Association task force on Practice guidelines (Committee on pacemaker implantation). *Circulation* 1998; **97**: 1325–1335.

Cardiac Pacing. *Resuscitation Council (UK) Advanced Life Support Course Provider Manual* (3rd edition) 1998 London, Resuscitation Council.

Related topics of interest

Cardiac arrhythmias, p. 44; Cardiac chest pain p. 69; Resuscitation – cardiopulmonary, p. 213

CARDIAC VALVE DISEASE

Cathal Nolan

Life expectancy of patients with valvular heart lesions has improved dramatically over the past 15 years. This coincides with a reduction in rheumatic fever in the developed world, better non-invasive monitoring of cardiac function, improved prostheses and surgical techniques. There has also been a greater understanding of valvular pathology and timing of surgical intervention.

Surgery on stenotic lesions may be deferred until symptoms appear. Regurgitant lesions however may cause severe left ventricular dysfunction before symptoms occur. Conservation of the native valve structure is preferable to mechanical replacement where possible.

Aortic stenosis

Aortic stenosis may be congenital (bicuspid valve) or acquired (calcification, rheumatic fever). Symptoms include, dyspnoea, angina and syncope. Signs include, slow rising anacrotic pulse and an ejection-systolic murmur that is loudest at the 2nd right intercostal space and radiating to the neck. There may be an associated thrill if there is severe stenosis, when the murmur occurs late, the S_2 is soft and there may be reversed splitting of the second sound.

1. Investigations
- ECG findings may be those of left ventricular hypertrophy.
- CXR. The heart is of normal size unless there is left ventricular dilatation. There may be aortic calcification or post-stenotic dilatation of the aorta.
- Doppler echocardiography allows estimation of the valve area, the trans-valvular gradient, ventricular hypertrophy and ejection fraction.
- Cardiac catheterization will add to the echocardiographic findings as well as define the anatomy of the coronary arteries.

2. Management
- The cardiac output is 'fixed'. The blood pressure is thus directly related to SVR.
- Tachycardia resulting in a reduced time for diastolic myocardial perfusion should be avoided.
- The presence of symptoms and a documented stenotic valve should prompt immediate valve replacement
- 75% of patients with symptomatic aortic stenosis die within 3 years of the onset of symptoms unless the valve is replaced.
- A gradient of $>$ 50 mmHg or a valve area $<$ 0.8 cm^2 represent severe stenosis.
- Balloon aortic valvotomy is a palliative procedure only and is associated with serious complications (death, stroke, aortic rupture and aortic regurgitation in 10% of cases). Mortality with this procedure is 60% at 18 months, which is similar to no treatment.
- Prophylaxis against infective endocarditis.

Mitral stenosis (MS)

The vast majority of MS is due to rheumatic fever but other causes include left atrial myxoma, calcification of the annulus and SLE.

1. **Symptoms.** Dyspnoea, recurrent bronchitis, palpitations (atrial fibrillation), haemoptysis (due to pulmonary oedema), acute neurological events (due to embolism).

2. **Signs.** Mitral facies, small volume pulse (+/− atrial fibrillation), tapping apex beat (palpable S_1), parasternal heave (RVH), loud S_1, opening snap (if non-calcified). A diastolic murmur with or without presystolic accentuation may be present if the patient is in sinus rhythm.

3. **Investigations**
- ECG may show p mitrale, atrial fibrillation, or right ventricular hypertrophy.
- CXR. There may be an enlarged left atrium, calcification of the valve, and pulmonary venous congestion
- Echocardiography allows an accurate calculation of the valve area (MS is severe if the area is $< 1 \text{ cm}^2$)

4. **Management**
- Digoxin or β-blockers to increase diastolic-filling time and to reduce the heart rate.
- Anticoagulation is needed in the presence of atrial fibrillation to prevent neurological complications.
- Prophylaxis against infective endocarditis.
- Preload should be maintained to optimize filling, avoid tachycardia, hypoxia will increase pulmonary vasoconstriction, putting further strain on the right ventricle.
- MS eventually leads to pulmonary hypertension through the increase in left atrial pressure. Balloon valvotomy or valve replacement should be performed before irreversible pulmonary hypertension results.

Mitral regurgitation

The causes include infective endocarditis, myxomatous degeneration of the mitral valve (including mitral valve prolapse), collagen vascular disease, rheumatic fever and spontaneous rupture of the chordae. Regurgitation may be acute or chronic. In acute mitral regurgitation there is sudden volume overload on the left atrium and pulmonary veins leading to pulmonary oedema.

In chronic mitral regurgitation the volume overload is compensated for by the development of cardiac hypertrophy.

1. **Symptoms** are those of left and right heart failure.

2. **Signs.** Cardiac enlargement, the apex beat is displaced and there may be a parasternal heave. The S_1 is followed by a pansystolic murmur which radiates to the axilla. A third heart sound signifies reduced compliance.

3. **ECG signs** include left ventricular hypertrophy, p mitrale, and possible atrial fibrillation.

4. *Echocardiography or cardiac catheterization* may show the enlarged cardiac chambers and permit estimation of severity of regurgitation.

5. *Management*
- Prophylaxis against infective endocarditis.
- The amount of blood regurgitated will depend on the gradient across the valve, the heart rate and SVR (a slow heart rate and raised SVR favour regurgitation).
- Vasodilators and maintenance of mild tachycardia will reduce regurgitation.

Aortic regurgitation (AR)

Chronic AR is due to disease of the aortic leaflets (infective endocarditis, rheumatic fever or the seronegative arthropathies), or disease affecting the aortic root (Marfan's syndrome, aortic dissection, syphilis or idiopathic associated with aging and hypertension).

1. *Symptoms.* Fatigue, dyspnoea, orthopnoea (signs of left heart failure), or angina.

2. *Signs.* The increased stroke volume produces a large pulse pressure with a waterhammer (collapsing) pulse. Corrigan's sign (visible carotid pulses) and head nodding may be apparent. Quincke's sign (nail bed capillary pulsation) and pistol-shot femoral pulses are also a feature. The apex beat is displaced. The murmur of AR is typically high-pitched and early in diastole. The Austin Flint murmur (due to the aortic jet impinging on the mitral valve apparatus) may contribute to a physiological mitral stenosis (due to early closure of the mitral valve).

3. *ECG* may show left ventricular hypertrophy with or without strain.

4. *CXR.* Cardiomegaly.
Echocardiography or cardiac catheterization allow measurement of the aortic valve gradient and the extent of regurgitation. Left ventricular size and function may also be assessed.

5. *Management*
- Prophylaxis against infective endocarditis.
- Vasodilators such as nifedipine or ACE inhibitors are used to reduce the afterload. If the patient is asymptomatic these can delay the need for surgery for 2–3 years.
- Surgery should be performed on the valve before the LV end-systolic dimension exceeds 55 mm or the ejection fraction falls below 55%.
- Acute AR (or MR) is a surgical emergency. The left ventricle does not have time to adapt in the face of increased volume load and cardiogenic shock with pulmonary oedema result. The coronary blood vessels are affected both by the reduction in perfusion and the increase in left ventricular end-diastolic pressure so worsening myocardial ischaemia. Infective endocarditis is the usual cause. Concerns of valve replacement in infected patients are offset by the life threatening nature of the insult. (The risk of prosthetic valve infection is 10%.)

Further reading

Anonymous. ACC/AHA guidelines for the management of patients with valvular heart disease. A report of the American College of Cardiology/American Heart Association. Task Force on Practice Guidelines (Committee on Management of Patients with Valvular Heart Disease). *Journal of the American College of Cardiology* 1998; **32**: 1486–1588.

Roldan CA. Valvular disease associated with systemic illness. *Cardiology Clinics* 1998; **16**: 531–550.

Related topics of interest

Cardiac arrhythmias, p. 64; Cardiac chest pain, p. 69; Cardiac failure, p. 73; Cardiac output – measurement of, p. 77

CENTRAL VENOUS PRESSURE MONITORING

Central venous pressure (CVP) measurement is one of the most commonly used monitors in critically ill patients. The CVP is not a measure of blood volume but allows assessment of the ability of the right heart to accept and deliver blood. The CVP is influenced by several factors: venous return, right heart compliance, intrathoracic pressure and patient position. Venous blood returning to the right atrium is delivered via the superior vena cava (SVC), the inferior vena cava, and the coronary veins. Right ventricular compliance is the change in end-diastolic pressure with change in ventricular volume. In a healthy heart, volume administration does not cause a dramatic rise in end-diastolic pressure; the ventricle is compliant. Certain disease states cause the ventricle to be less compliant or stiff e.g., pericardial effusion, cardio-myopathies, or cardiac failure.

The correct catheter position for valid CVP monitoring is in the superior vena cava. The zero point is level with the mid-axillary line in the fourth intercostal space.

A normal CVP is 0–8 mmHg. The absolute value is not as important as the response to therapy. Serial measurements and the resulting trend provide valuable information.

Catheter insertion sites

1. ### Internal jugular vein
   - **Advantages.** Large vessel. Easy to locate/access. Short straight path to SVC. Low rate of complications.
   - **Disadvantages.** Uncomfortable for patient. Difficult to dress/nurse. Close to carotid artery.

2. ### Subclavian vein
   - **Advantages.** Large vessel. High flow rates possible. Low infection rate. Easy to dress. Less restricting for patient.
   - **Disadvantages.** Risk of pneumothorax. Close to subclavian artery. Difficult to control bleeding (non-compressible vessel).

3. ### Basilic vein
   - **Advantages.** Accessible during resuscitation.
   - **Disadvantages.** Increased risk of phlebitis. Catheter movement with arm movement. Greater distance to SVC. High rate of misplacement.

4. ### Femoral vein
   - **Advantages.** Easy access. Large vessel. High flow rates possible. Accessible during resuscitation.
   - **Disadvantages.** Decreased patient mobility. Increased risk of thrombosis. Risk of femoral artery puncture. Dressing problematic.

Insertion guidelines

All CVP insertion sites risk air entrainment and consequent embolism as well as infection. Thus, the patient should be positioned with head down tilt (Trendelenburg). This produces venous engorgement as well as reducing the risk of air entrainment. Femoral venous cannulation does not require the patient to be head down. Strict aseptic procedures should be followed. Continuous ECG monitoring should be used as insertion of wires or catheters into the right ventricle may trigger cardiac arrhythmias. A CXR should be performed after insertion of the CVP to check for catheter position and exclude complications.

The normal waveform

- The **a wave**. This occurs during atrial contraction. Some blood regurgitates into the vena cavae during atrial systole. In addition, venous inflow stops and the rise in venous pressure contributes to the a wave. A large a wave occurs in tricuspid stenosis, pulmonary stenosis, in complete heart block (cannon wave) and in severe pulmonary hypertension. There is no a wave in atrial fibrillation.
- The **c wave**. This is the transmitted manifestation of the rise in atrial pressure produced by the bulging of the tricuspid valve into the right atrium during ventricular contraction.
- The **v wave** mirrors the rise in atrial pressure during atrial filling before the tricuspid valve opens. A large v wave occurs in tricuspid incompetence and is known as a giant v wave.

CVP is often not a reflection of left atrial pressure in the seriously ill.

Further reading

Randolf AG, *et al*. Ultrasound guidance for placement of central venous catheter: a meta-analysis of the literature. *Critical Care Medicine* 1996; **24**: 2053–2058.

Related topics of interest

Arterial cannulation, p. 29; Cardiac failure, p.73; Cardiac output – measurement of, p. 77

CHEST TUBE THORACOSTOMY

Indications

The indications for insertion of a chest drain include the drainage of established or threatened collections of air, blood, fluid, or pus from the pleural cavity. According to the guidelines produced by the British Thoracic Society, simple, spontaneous pneumothoraces can be aspirated without the need for a chest drain. However, any patient developing a pneumothorax while receiving positive pressure ventilation should have a chest drain inserted. Without chest drainage, 50% of these will develop into a tension pneumothorax. A tension pneumothorax requires immediate decompression by inserting a cannula in the 2nd intercostal space in the mid-clavicular line of the affected side. This will reverse the life threatening mediastinal compression while preparations are made for chest drainage. A patient with fractured ribs who requires intubation and positive pressure ventilation should have a chest tube inserted prophylactically. This is indicated particularly before inter-hospital transfer or prolonged anaesthesia for associated injuries; under these circumstances a developing tension pneumothorax is likely to be discovered late. Pleural effusions that cannot be drained by repeated thoracocentesis may require the insertion of a chest drain. Many of these may be managed more appropriately, and less traumatically, with the insertion of a pig-tailed catheter.

Equipment

In adults, drainage of blood requires at least a 32F chest drain; smaller drains will tend to become blocked. Sharp trocars should never be used for chest drain insertion – they may lacerate the lung or pulmonary vessels. The chest drain is usually attached to an underwater seal bottle. Some chest drainage systems (e.g., PleurEvac) will allow the re-infusion of blood collected from a massive haemothorax. A purpose-designed bag with a built-in flutter valve can be used instead of an underwater seal. This is particularly useful in the pre-hospital environment or if the patient requires inter-hospital transfer.

Technique

Ideally, the patient is placed in a semi-recumbent position with their upper trunk at 75° to the horizontal. The patient is given additional oxygen to breath. Local anaesthesia is infiltrated into the skin and along the proposed incision line. Under aseptic conditions the drain is inserted in the 5th intercostal space just anterior to the mid-axillary line. The track is defined down to parietal pleura using blunt dissection and staying close to the upper border of the rib. The pleura is punctured with the blunt tip of a clamp. The clamp is then removed and a finger used to perform a 'sweep' of the pleural cavity to exclude adhesions or abdominal viscera prior to insertion of the drain.

The drain is connected to an underwater seal or flutter valve. Mattress sutures are inserted across the skin incision. These can be tightened after drain removal. Traditional 'purse' string sutures produce very poor cosmetic results and are now less often used.

A clean dressing is applied and a check CXR taken.

Bronchopleural fistulae will cause large air leaks. A bronchoscopy will rule out the presence of a ruptured bronchus. If the lung is non-compliant or the air leak is large, and a major airway injury has been excluded, continuous, high-flow suction (20–30 cm H_2O) may be applied to the drainage system. This may help to bring the visceral and parietal pleural surfaces together.

Complications

Intercostal vessels or nerves may be inadvertently damaged during chest tube insertion. It is possible to lacerate the lung or pulmonary vessels, particularly if a sharp introducer is used. A common error committed by the inexperienced is to place the tube outside the pleural cavity (extrapleural or intra-abdominal). Inadequately tied drains will fall out. A persistent air leak will occur if the proximal side-hole of the chest tube is outside the pleural cavity. Empyema occurs in about 2% of patients having chest tubes inserted. It is particularly likely after blunt trauma.

Removal of chest drains

Whilst the indications for chest drain insertion are relatively clear cut, explicit guidance on removal of chest drains is hard to find. Chest tubes inserted to drain a pneumothorax are removed on resolution of the pneumothorax. Assuming there is no air leak or excessive drainage of fluid (> 100 ml day^{-1}), chest tubes inserted prophylactically into patients with rib fractures can probably be removed after the patient has been stabilized and any early, prolonged surgery has been completed.

Further reading

Feliciano DV. Tube thoracostomy. In: Benumoff JL (ed). *Clinical Procedures in Anesthesia and Intensive Care*. Philadelphia: J.B. Lippincott Company, 1992.

Related topics of interest

Trauma – primary survey and resuscitation, p. 257; Trauma – secondary survey, p. 260; Trauma – anaesthesia and critical care, p. 263

CHRONIC OBSTRUCTIVE PULMONARY DISEASE

Chronic obstructive pulmonary disease (COPD)is a slowly progressive disorder and in the developed world is one of the most common causes of death. Up to 20% of cigarette smokers develop clinically significant COPD. It is a disease almost entirely confined to smokers. Other less common causes include occupational exposure to pulmonary toxins and hereditary α1-antitrypsin deficiency.

There is no agreed definition of COPD. The main feature of the disease is slowly progressive chronic airflow limitation with a reduced FEV_1 and FEV_1/VC ratio. There is usually underlying chronic bronchitis and emphysema. Wall fibrosis follows airway inflammatory processes. There may be an element of reversibility to the airflow obstruction but most of the obstruction is fixed. Chronic bronchitis is defined by sputum production on most days for 3 months of 2 consecutive years. There are features of mucosal hypertrophy, increased mucous secretion, increased bronchial reactivity and reduced pulmonary compliance. Emphysema is a histological diagnosis (although the CXR is often suggestive). Elastic tissue destruction results in dilatation of the terminal airways and reduced elastance.

Diagnosis of COPD

This requires both:

- A history of chronic progressive symptoms (cough and/or wheeze with or without breathlessness).
- Objective evidence of airway obstruction (spirometry) that does not return to normal with treatment.

Severe COPD is associated with marked reductions in forced inspiratory and expiratory flows. This results in early airway closure and air trapping with patients breathing at abnormally high lung volumes. This in turn results in smaller tidal volumes and a more rapid respiratory rate to maintain a normal minute ventilation, especially during an acute exacerbation. The efficiency of respiratory muscles is impaired at these high volumes and rapid rates and eventually fatigue will precipitate further respiratory failure.

Acute exacerbation of COPD

This is a new respiratory event or complication superimposed on established COPD. They occur on average 1–2 times per year. It is manifest by:

- Increased sputum purulence.
- Increased sputum volume.
- Increased dyspnoea.
- Increased wheeze.
- Increased chest tightness.
- Increased fluid retention.
- Worsened gas exchange.

The differential diagnosis of acute exacerbation of COPD includes

- Infection/pneumonia.
- Segmental pulmonary collapse due to secretions (particularly associated with surgery, chest trauma and depressed level of consciousness which result in hypoventilation and ineffective cough).
- Pneumothorax (NB. do not confuse lung bulla with pneumothorax).
- Heart failure (pulmonary oedema may be difficult to diagnose because of the abnormal pulmonary pathology).
- Pulmonary embolus.
- Lung cancer.
- Airway obstruction.

Clinical features

1. Symptoms. Cough, sputum production, dyspnoea, smoker.

2. Signs. Pyrexia, hyperinflation, respiratory distress, accessory muscle use, decreased breath sounds, wheeze, cyanosis, signs of cor pulmonale.

Investigations

1. CXR. Hyperinflation with flat diaphragms, >6 anterior ribs visible, bulla, areas of consolidation due to infection. Malignancy. Heart failure may be difficult to diagnose because of the abnormal pulmonary pathology. Pulmonary hypertension results in large proximal pulmonary artery shadows with peripheral attenuation of vessel markings.

2. Lung function tests. Demonstrate an obstructive pattern with FEV_1/FVC <70%, high residual volume and total lung capacity, transfer factor for carbon monoxide is low. The pattern is mainly irreversible.

3. Arterial blood gas analysis. Patients with an acute exacerbation of COPD frequently exhibit severe hypoxaemia. Increased resistance and hyperinflation will increase ventilation-perfusion (V/Q) mismatch, which often causes significant hypercarbia.

4. Blood count. To assess polycythaemia and neutrophilia.

5. ECG. Is often normal but may progress to show signs of right atrial and ventricular enlargement associated with pulmonary hypertension.

Treatment

1. Controlled oxygen therapy. COPD patients with acute respiratory failure are often profoundly hypoxaemic. Restoration of an adequate PaO_2 is a priority. These patients are chronically hypoxaemic and will have developed compensatory mechanisms such as an increased haematocrit and a high oxygen extraction ratio. The aim of oxygen therapy should be to increase the PaO_2 to approximately 8 kPa. This marks the end of the steep portion of the oxygen dissociation curve and will result in an acceptable arterial oxygen saturation. Increased airway resistance reduces ventilation in some zones of the lungs (low V/Q) and hyperinflation reduces blood flow in distended alveoli (high V/Q). These alterations in V/Q mismatch are the main reason for an increase in $PaCO_2$ despite maintenance of minute ventilation. The degree of V/Q mismatch is limited by hypoxic vasoconstriction. Administration of high concentration oxygen will abolish the hypoxic vasoconstriction reflex and exacerbate the V/Q mismatch. This may cause a profound rise in $PaCO_2$ with the onset of CO_2 narcosis and respiratory arrest. It is this mechanism and not the elimination of 'hypoxic drive' that dictates the need for carefully titrated oxygen therapy. Oxygen is provided using a Venturi mask and is increased in increments of 0.04 from an initial level of 0.24 or 0.28. Arterial blood gases should be checked every 30 min. If the PaO_2 remains < 8.0 kPa and the $PaCO_2$ has not increased by more than 2 kPa, the FIO_2 can be increased to the next level. If it is not possible to achieve adequate arterial oxygenation without a steep increase in $PaCO_2$, ventilatory assistance will be required.

2. *Bronchodilators*. β_2 agonists (salbutamol or terbutaline) are best given by nebulizer (salbutamol is also available as an intravenous preparation). They act as bronchodilators and enhance mucociliary clearance. They may cause hypokalaemia, tachycardia and tremor.

The anticholinergic ipratropium is used in conjunction with β_2 agonists for its bronchodilator action. It has a slower onset of action with a peak effect at 60–90 min. Dry mouth and urinary retention are side effects.

Aminophylline by continuous infusion is used as an adjunct to β_2 agonists but is of unproven efficacy. Loading doses should be avoided in patients already taking theophylline preparations. Levels must be monitored because of narrow therapeutic limits.

3. *Antibiotics*. Most exacerbations are treated as infections although it is common that no particular organism is identified as the cause. The most common organisms responsible for infective exacerbations are *Haemophilus influenzae*, *Streptococcus pneumoniae* and *Moraxella catarrhalis*. In patients with very severe COPD ($FEV_1 < 35\%$ predicted) Gram-negative organisms (particularly enterbacteriaceae and *Pseudomonas*) also appear to be important. Antibiotic prescribing should follow local protocols that are governed by organism sensitivities. Amoxycillin and tetracycline are common first line treatments for out of hospital exacerbations. In-hospital acquired and life threatening infection should be managed with more aggressive intravenous therapy.

4. *Steroids*. Although fewer than 25% of patients with COPD are steroid responsive they are commonly given during an acute exacerbation. Courses of steroid should be tapered rapidly. Commonly, hydrocortisone 200 mg every 6 h is commenced, converted to oral prednisolone after improvement and withdrawn over 7–14 days.

5. *Secretion clearance*. Sputum retention is common in COPD. Mucolytics are of unproven benefit. Physiotherapy and tracheal suction are crucial in intubated patients with extensive sputum production, though may be detrimental in the absence of sputum production. Bronchoscopy and tracheal suction may be beneficial in the presence of large airway obstruction due to mucous plugging and may be required to aid the diagnosis of infection or malignancy. Tracheostomy aids weaning and pulmonary toilet for those with ineffective coughs. A mini-tracheostomy (size 4.0) may be useful in selected patients but plugging with tenacious secretions may limit its efficacy.

6. *Diuretics/vasodilators.* Hypoxia and acidosis increase pulmonary artery pressure (which may be chronically raised) and precipitate right heart failure. In this situation oxygen, diuretics and vasodilators may improve heart function. Electrolyte abnormalities (hypokalaemia, hypomagnesaemia, hypophosphataemia) secondary to diuresis should be prevented or corrected.

7. *Nutrition.* Avoid excessive carbohydrate loads in those patients with CO_2 retention.

8. *Ventilatory support.* Non-invasive ventilatory support may be achieved with non-invasive intermittent positive pressure ventilation, bilevel positive airway pressure (BiPAP) or CPAP by nasal or face mask. Invasive positive pressure ventilation following intubation may be required for patients who fail to improve with a non-invasive strategy. Respiratory muscle activity will account for up to 50% of oxygen consumption in patients with severe COPD. Resting these muscles by mechanical ventilation allows correction of hypoxia, oxygen utilization by other tissues, and the correction of acidosis. Where possible, spontaneous ventilation is preserved, excessive inflation pressures avoided ($<$ 35 mmHg), and a degree of respiratory acidosis is accepted. Relative hypoxia is acceptable provided sufficient oxygen is available to meet the metabolic requirements of the tissues. Patients with severe COPD may have auto-PEEP due to early airway closure and gas trapping which results in volume trauma and barotrauma. Adequate time for expiration must be allowed.

The potential difficulties in weaning patients with COPD from ventilatory support does not exclude this therapy for selected cases. The decision to admit these patients to a critical care environment and the decision to embark on invasive ventilation must be made by senior clinicians. Many patients with COPD progress to end respiratory failure where aggressive intensive care management is futile. Where prolonged intubation is probable, early tracheostomy is likely to provide better conditions for weaning from ventilation.

Criteria supporting the use of mechanical ventilation include:

- A reversible reason for the current decline (e.g., pneumonia).
- A quality of life/level of activity prior to this exacerbation that is acceptable to the patient.

Factors against aggressive ventilation include:

- Where aggressive management is likely to be futile.
- Previous severe COPD unresponsive to optimal therapy.
- Poor quality of life, with an expected outcome that would be unacceptable to the patient.
- Severe comorbidity (e.g., heart failure, neoplasia).
- The need for continuous home oxygen.

Doxapram

Doxapram is a respiratory stimulant that acts principally on peripheral chemoreceptors. It may be helpful if the pH is $<$ 7.26 and/or the $PaCO_2$ is elevated in avoiding the need for ventilation and allowing time for other therapies to take effect.

Outcome

The outcome from the management of an acute exacerbation of COPD is not related to the patient's age or the $PaCO_2$. Hospital survival of an acute exacerbation exceeds 80% but long-term survival is poor and dependent on the respiratory reserve and comorbidity.

Prevention of exacerbations of COPD requires the following:

- Stop smoking.
- Weight loss if obese.
- Avoidance of sedatives (including excess alcohol).
- Avoiding infection (influenza and pneumococcal vaccination).
- Control of cardiovascular disease and fluid overload.
- Venesection for polycythaemia (decreases the risk of thrombosis and cardiac work).

Cor pulmonale

Chronic lung disease that results in hypoxic pulmonary vasoconstriction eventually leads to chronic pulmonary hypertension and right heart failure.

The features include a raised venous pressure, peripheral oedema, hepatomegaly and ascites. Tricuspid regurgitation may be present. A left parasternal heave and loud pulmonary component of the second heart sound are features. The CXR demonstrates cardiomegaly and large pulmonary arteries. The ECG shows a p pulmonale, right axis deviation, right ventricular hypertrophy with strain pattern or right bundle branch block.

Pulmonary vasodilators

- The best and easiest to give is oxygen (continuous therapy for more than 15 hours per day improves survival from cor pulmonale due to COPD).
- Systemic vasodilators (calcium antagonists).
- Pulmonary vasodilators (inhaled nitric oxide, intravenous prostacyclin).

Further Reading

Madison JM. Chronic obstructive pulmonary disease. *Lancet* 1998; **52**: 467–473.
British Thoracic Society Guidelines for the management of chronic obstructive pulmonary disease. *Thorax* 1997; **52**(suppl 5).

Related topics of interest

Asthma, p. 31; Pneumonia – community acquired, p. 173; Respiratory support – weaning from ventilation, p. 210

COMA

Coma is the manifestation of a depressed level of consciousness. Coma is usually defined as a GCS (see page 219) of 8 or less. Coma reflects pathology in the reticular activating system of the brain stem or the cerebral cortex. The principles of critical care management of coma include:

- Protecting the patient from further injury.
- Diagnosing the underlying cause.
- Managing the patient to ensure an optimal outcome.

Causes of coma

- **Primary cerebral lesion.** Head injury, intracranial haemorrhage, meningitis/encephalitis, abscess, tumour, hydrocephalus, cerebral oedema, and epilepsy.
- **Secondary to systemic illness.** Any cause of hypoxia and hypotension (e.g. cardiac arrest and shock), liver failure, renal failure, CO_2 narcosis, hypoglycaemia, ketoacidosis, electrolyte abnormalities, hyper- and hypo-osmolar states, myxoedema, hypothermia, sepsis (including tropical diseases).
- **Drug induced.** Therapeutic drugs, drugs in overdose or non-therapeutic drugs and poisons. Anaesthetic agents, benzodiazepines, opioids, antidepressants, alcohol.

Assessment

- **A rapid assessment** with simultaneous resuscitation following the ABC format is required.
- **The history will often provide the likely diagnosis.**
- **Exclude hypoxia and hypotension.** Assess respiration (absent in brain stem death and following overdosage of certain drugs)
- **Assess external signs of head injury** (if suspicious immobilize cervical spine). NB. Blood in external auditory meatus or from the nose or over the mastoid area are signs of base of skull fracture.
- **Assess and record the GCS.**
- **Localizing neurological signs** suggest intracranial pathology.
- **Examine the pupils** for asymmetry, size and reactions. Bilateral unreactive pupils suggest brain stem pathology. A unilateral dilated and unreactive pupil suggests ipsilateral III nerve palsy. Meiosis suggests opioids or brain stem disease. Dysconjugate gaze suggests cranial nerve lesion (III, IV, VI) or internuclear opthalmoplegia. Conjugate gaze deviation suggests an ipsilateral frontal lesion. Fundoscopy for retinopathy (hypertensive, diabetic) and papilloedema.
- **Consider assessment of other cranial nerves.**
- **Meningism** suggests meningitis or subarachnoid haemorrhage.
- **Assess temperature.** Pyrexia suggests sepsis, meningitis. Exclude hypothermia.
- **Look for venepuncture marks** (opioid overdose, other illicit drugs, septicaemia, and intracerebral abscess).
- **Examine the abdomen** for signs of liver and renal disease.

Investigations

- Blood sugar on finger prick test.
- Laboratory blood sugar, urea, creatinine, electrolytes, liver function tests and FBC.
- Drug screen for suspected agents and hold urine for toxicology.
- Blood alcohol level.
- CT / MRI scan.
- Lumbar puncture is rarely required as an urgent procedure and should never be performed in the presence of signs of raised intracranial pressure.
- EEG is useful to demonstrate abnormal activity.

Management

- Specific therapy is directed at the underlying pathology.
- Hypoxia and hypotension must be rapidly corrected.
- GCS <10 will require intubation to protect the airway, prevent secondary brain injury and facilitate investigation (e.g., CT scan).
- Ventilate the patient's lungs to achieve a normal PaO_2 and $PaCO_2$ if there is any ventilatory failure.
- Hypoglycaemia is corrected with 50 ml intravenous glucose 50%.
- Give thiamine, 100 mg, if suspicion of history of alcohol abuse.
- Correct electrolyte abnormalities and ensure adequate hydration.
- Commence early enteral nutrition.
- Commence DVT prophylaxis.
- Consider the use of anticonvulsants.
- Consider insertion of ICP monitor.
- Initiate therapy to reduced a raised ICP.
- Consider cerebral protective therapy (hypothermia, reduce $CMRO_2$).

Specific antagonists

- Naloxone for opioid overdose.
- Flumazenil for benzodiazepine overdose.

Extradural haemorrhage

Usually caused by a head injury. There may be an initial lucid period followed by a rapid deterioration in GCS progressing to coma often with focal signs (lateralizing weakness or pupillary signs). This is consistent with a minor brain injury with a rapid accumulation of blood from a middle meningeal artery rupture. Surgical drainage following CT scan localization has a relatively good prognosis, provided the time period to surgery is short and the initial GCS immediately after injury was high.

Subdural haemorrhage

Acute presentations following trauma are associated with, severe underlying brain injury, initial low GCS post-injury and a poor prognosis. In acute head injury subdural haemorrhage is more common than extradural haemorrhage and the onset of coma is immediate.

Chronic subdural haematoma presents days to weeks after head trauma which is often described as trivial. Presentation may be vague with a fluctuating level of consciousness, agitation, confusion, seizures, localizing signs, or a slowly evolving stroke. Diagnosis is made by CT or MRI scan. Treatment is by surgical drainage.

Intracerebral haemorrhage

Intracerebral haemorrhage is associated with hypertension, haemorrhage into a neoplasm, haemorrhage into an infarct, AV malformations, vasculitis, coagulopathy (including post-thrombolysis) and mycotic aneurysms associated with bacterial endocarditis.

Clinical features are governed by the area of involvement. Extensive haemorrhage presents as sudden onset of coma, drowsiness and/or neurological deficit. The rate of evolution depends on the site and size of the bleed.

Intracerebral infarction

Cerebral infarction follows thrombosis or embolism. Few of these patients benefit from intensive care management. Those that may benefit include those with embolic strokes where the source of the embolism is amenable to therapy, those with thrombosis secondary to medical intervention (e.g. post carotid or neurosurgery) or where surgery, invasive radiology or thrombolysis may be of use. Management is largely supportive.

Brain stem death (see p.48)

Vegetative state

Refers to an uncommon state where there is severe cortical damage but with preservation of some brain stem activity. Vegetative states usually follow severe hypoxic brain injury or severe head injury. Consciousness is impaired, although there may be eye opening, and there is no voluntary movement. It is a diagnosis that can be made only after a prolonged period of observation (months), at which stage it is usually permanent.

Locked-in syndrome

Refers to a state of normal consciousness but with impaired movement due to lower cranial nerve damage and brain stem/spinal cord damage that results in paralysis. Careful assessment of responsiveness is required and the EEG will demonstrate awake rhythms.

Pseudo-coma/psychogenic coma

Is a diagnosis of exclusion. Signs are usually not consistent with accepted neurological damage. Cranial nerve reflexes will remain intact and the EEG will demonstrate awake rhythms.

Global ischaemia

Global cerebral ischaemia is the usual result of a prolonged period of circulatory arrest but will also result from prolonged periods of severe hypoxia and/or hypotension of any cause. Prognosis is related to the duration of the ischaemic/hypoxic period and the presence of comorbidity. Fewer than 10% of patients demonstrating severe global ischaemic injury will regain independent activity. Recovery can be delayed and prolonged which leads to guarded prognosis. After 6 months the potential for major improvement in patients with severe brain injury is small. Those patients that have the potential for significant recovery will demonstrate improvements within the first 72 hours. If there is improvement in cranial nerve activity and motor activity during this period continued aggressive intensive care may be indicated. Seizures in the initial post resuscitation period do not correlate with outcome but myoclonic activity carries a poor prognosis. EEG and evoked potentials may provide some aid to judging prognosis.

Further reading

Chiappa KH, Hill RA. Evaluation and prognostication in coma. *Electroencephalography and Clinical Neurophysiology* 1998; **106**: 149–155.

Giacino JT. Disorders of consciousness: differential diagnosis and neuropathological features. *Seminars in Neurology* 1997; **17**: 105–111.

Related topics of interest

Brain stem death and organ donation, p. 48; Convulsions, p. 100; Scoring systems, p. 219

CONVULSIONS

Status epilepticus describes prolonged or repetitive convulsive or non-convulsive seizures which continue without a period of recovery between attacks and last for longer than 30 min. Status epilepticus may arise in known epileptics (epilepsy has a prevalence of 1:200) or in non-epileptic individuals. Status epilepticus is an emergency during which the brain is at risk of secondary injury from hypoxia, hypotension, cerebral oedema and direct neuronal injury. The risk of permanent brain damage is proportional to the duration of seizures.

Status epilepticus may present as

- Generalized tonic/clonic seizures without full neurological recovery between attacks.
- Focal epileptic seizures without impaired consciousness.
- Non-convulsive seizures with impaired consciousness.

Causes of status epilepticus

- Idiopathic epilepsy (particularly associated with non-compliance with medication, changes in medication).
- Infection (meningitis, abscess, encephalitis, HIV).
- Head injury.
- Intracranial tumour (primary, secondary).
- Cerebrovascular disease (haemorrhage, thrombosis, embolism, eclampsia, cerebral vasculitis).
- Drug induced/overdose (local anaesthetics, tricyclic antidepressants, theophylline, amphetamines, cocaine, LSD, insulin).
- Drug withdrawal (benzodiazepines, alcohol).
- Metabolic (hypoglycaemia, hyponatraemia, hypocalcaemia, hyperpyrexia, uraemia, hepatic failure, pyridoxine deficiency, porphyria).
- Pseudoepilepsy.

Investigations

- Blood biochemistry (glucose, sodium, calcium, magnesium, phosphate).
- Arterial blood gas.
- Drug screen for suspected drugs.
- Urinalysis.
- Anticonvulsant drug levels.
- Brain CT or MRI to identify structural brain lesions.
- Lumbar puncture (contraindicated if raised ICP or space occupying lesion suspected).
- ECG and echocardiography to exclude cardiac embolism.
- EEG is required in all patients presenting with epilepsy. It will differentiate secondary generalized (focal seizures) from primary generalized seizures. It will occasionally detect subclinical epileptic activity in the absence of external signs of convulsions.

Clinical features

1. *Airway compromise.* During seizures the airway is compromised and there is risk of aspiration. Hypoxia is common because of inadequate ventilation combined with high oxygen requirements of continuous muscle activity. Hypercarbia occurs due to increased CO_2 production and reduced ventilation.

2. *Metabolic changes.* Hyperthermia, dehydration, acidosis, rhabdomyolysis, hyperkalaemia and possible renal impairment result from the excessive muscle activity. Hypoglycaemia or hyperglycaemia can occur, both of which may result in secondary brain injury.

3. *Cerebral consequences.* Brain oedema may occur due to increased cerebral blood flow, hypercapnia, impaired venous drainage (position and raised venous pressure). Hypertension is common and may further add to cerebral oedema. Hypotension will usually signify hypovolaemia.

Management

Management follows the ABC priorities. Specific therapy should be directed to the underlying problem.

- Intubation should be performed to protect the airway in those who do not rapidly recover an adequate level of consciousness with intact airway reflexes.
- Adequate ventilation should be ensured. Excessive hyperventilation should be avoided.
- Adequate circulating volume is maintained. Hypotonic solutions that will increase cerebral oedema should be avoided.
- Hypoglycaemia is corrected with 50 ml of 50% glucose i.v.
- If alcoholism is suspected give thiamine 100 mg i.v.

Choice of anticonvulsant:

1. *Status epilepticus (grand mal).* Diazepam [given i.v. or rectally (rectal doses are effective within about 10 min)], phenytoin, phenobarbitone or thiopentone, magnesium sulphate, propofol.

2. *Tonic-clonic (grand mal).* Sodium valproate, carbamazepine, phenytoin, and phenobarbital.

3. *Partial (focal).*

(a) Psychomotor: carbamazepine, phenytoin
(b) Absence (petit mal): sodium valproate, ethosuxamide
(c) Myoclonic: clonazepam, sodium valproate

- Anticonvulsant levels should be checked and corrected in known epileptics.
- Cerebral oedema should be managed with sedation, controlled hyperventilation and osmotic diuretics.
- Steroids should be considered for those with a known tumour, arteritis or parasitic infections.
- Surgery should be considered for space occupying lesions (e.g., haemorrhage, abscess, tumour).
- Hyperthermia should be corrected.

- A brisk diuresis should be maintained if there is any evidence of rhabdomyolysis.

There is no role for the use of long acting muscle relaxants purely to control seizures. Continuing seizure activity implies inadequate anticonvulsant levels. Occasionally paralysis may be required to facilitate ventilation if there is associated severe lung injury or for the control of ICP. If neuromuscular blockade is used continuous EEG monitoring is mandatory to assess seizure activity.

Pseudoepilepsy

Pseudoepilepsy is a diagnosis of exclusion. Simulated seizures may be differentiated from true epilepsy by features such as atypical movements (e.g., asynchronous limb and rolling movements), the presence of eye lash reflexes, resistance to eye opening, normal pupillary responses during convulsion, retained awareness or vocalization and normal tendon reflexes and plantar responses immediately after convulsion. They may be brought on by approaching the patient, are often recurrent, and seen in individuals who have some knowledge of what epilepsy looks like (health care workers or relatives of epileptics). Pseudoepilepsy is more common in females with a history of psychological disturbance. Occasionally the diagnosis will only become clear on EEG monitoring.

Outcome

Outcome from status epilepticus is directly related to the duration of seizures, the incidence of secondary brain injury and the underlying pathology.

Further reading

Delanty N, Vaughan CJ, French JA. Medical causes of seizures. *Lancet* 1998; **352**: 383–390.
Feely M. Fortnightly review: drug treatment of epilepsy. *BMJ* 1999; **318**: 106–109.

Related topics of interest

Coma, p. 96; Head injury, p. 128

DEATH CERTIFICATION

The medical certificates which are completed for transmission to the Registrar of Births and Deaths serve both legal and statistical purposes. A death must be registered before a funeral director can proceed with the final arrangements for the body. There are three types of death certificate:

- Stillborn certificate (after 24 weeks of pregnancy).
- Neonatal Death Certificate (any death up to 28 days of age).
- Medical Certificate of Death (any other death).

The certificate should only be completed by a medical practitioner who attended the deceased during their final illness.

Cause of death statement

The cause of death on a death certificate should refer to the state or condition directly leading to death. The mode of dying should not be stated (e.g., heart failure, cardiac arrest, renal failure, coma, old age). The addition of acute or chronic to any of these terms does not make them acceptable as a cause of death. Abbreviations or medical symbols should be avoided. Registrars of Births and Deaths are instructed to refer Medical Certificates to the Coroner for further enquiry if only a mode of death (and not a cause) has been recorded. This will almost certainly result in unnecessary delay and distress to the deceased's family.

The coroner

A death should be referred to the Coroner if:

- The cause of death is unknown.
- The deceased was not seen by the certifying doctor either after death or within the 14 days before death.
- The death was violent or unnatural or there are suspicious circumstances.
- The death may be due to an accident (whenever it occurred).
- The death may be due to self-neglect or neglect by others.
- The death may be due to an industrial disease or may be related to the deceased's employment.
- The death may be due to an abortion.
- The death occurred during an operation or before recovery from anaesthesia was complete.
- The death may be a suicide.
- The death occurred during or shortly after detention in police or prison custody.

Death related to employment

Categories of death which may be of industrial origin:

	Causes include
Malignant diseases	
Skin	Radiation and sunlight pitch or tar, mineral oils
Lung	Asbestos, nickel, radiation
Nasal	Wood or leather work, nickel
Pleura	Asbestos
Urinary tract	Benzidine, dye, chemicals in rubber
Liver	PVC manufacture
Bone	Radiation
Infectious diseases	
Anthrax	Imported bone, bonemeal, hide or fur
Brucellosis	Farming or veterinary
Leptospirosis	Farming, sewer or underground workers
Rabies	Animal handling
Pneumoconiosis	Mining and quarrying, potteries, asbestos

A more complete list is found on the reverse of each death certificate.

If there is any doubt as to whether a death should be reported the advice of the local Coroner's officer should be sought.

Where the death has been reported to the Coroner, the death certificate will be issued by the Coroner and sent directly to the Registrar of Births and Deaths. This normally takes approximately 2 working days to complete. In some cases when the death has been discussed with the Coroner's officer, a doctor will be given permission to issue a death certificate without further enquiry.

What happens next?

The death certificate is taken to the Registrar's office, usually by a close relative, and the deceased's death recorded. The Registrar will issue two certificates. A white certificate which is for Department of Social Services purposes and will ensure that any benefits (such as a widow's pension) that are due from the state can be claimed for. The green certificate is for the funeral director and authorizes burial or the application for cremation.

The Registrar is also able to issue certified copies of the death certificate which will be required for probate or insurance purposes. Such certificates are needed to access bank accounts, pension policies, or investments for example.

Further reading

Completion of Medical Certificates of Cause of Death, May 1990. Office of Population Censuses & Surveys, St Catherine's House, 10 Kingsway, London WC2B 6JP.

Related topic of interest

Brain stem death and organ donation, p. 48

DIABETES MELLITUS

Diabetes in the critical care setting presents with end organ damage secondary to long-standing diabetes and the problems of acute diabetic emergencies.

Most cases of insulin dependent diabetes mellitus (IDDM) are associated with autoimmune destruction of pancreatic cells producing insulin deficiency, but it may also follow pancreatitis or pancreatectomy. With non-insulin dependent diabetes mellitus (NIDDM) there is insulin resistance; insulin levels are initially high but later in the disease process they are reduced and overt hyperglycaemia develops. In the critical care setting, hyperglycaemia in IDDM is best managed by infusions of a short acting insulin and frequent blood sugar estimation. The same is often true for NIDDM patients who can usually return to non-insulin control after resolution of any intercurrent illness. Hyperglycaemia also occurs in normal individuals secondary to administration of glucose containing solutions, corticosteroids, catecholamines and the stress response. In this non-diabetic group the hyperglycaemia resolves with the clinical illness and long term anti-diabetes treatment is rarely required.

Long standing diabetes results in end organ damage producing severe morbidity and an increased mortality.

- Vascular disease (15–60%), coronary artery disease, cerebrovascular disease.
- Hypertension (30–60%).
- Cardiomyopathy.
- Nephropathy.
- Retinopathy.
- Autonomic neuropathy (at risk of arrhythmias, cardiac arrest, respiratory arrest and hypoglycaemia).
- Infection.
- Increased respiratory disease.
- Neuropathy.

Management is directed at maintaining normoglycaemia (blood glucose 6–10 mmol l^{-1}) and at associated disorders.

Specific diabetic emergencies

1. Diabetic ketoacidosis (DKA). DKA accounts for the majority of diabetic emergencies admitted to critical care units. It is usually seen in patients with IDDM and evolves over a period of days. Lack of insulin combined with increases in glucagon, catecholamines and cortisol stimulate lipolysis, free fatty acid production and ketogenesis. Accumulation of keto-acids (β-hydroxybutyrate and acetoacetate) results in metabolic acidosis. Increased gluconeogenesis and glycolysis result in hyperglycaemia which is not taken up peripherally because of the lack of insulin. The renal retention threshold for glucose is exceeded and glycosuria and ketonuria results in the loss of large amounts of water and electrolytes. Hypovolaemia ensues and impaired tissue perfusion result in anaerobic metabolism which adds to the metabolic acidosis.

(a) **Clinical features.** Thirst, polyuria, nausea, abdominal pain, vomiting, weight loss. Confusion progressing to coma. Hyperventilation (Kussmaul respiration) due to acidosis, ketone breath. Dehydration and hypovolaemia

(b) **Precipitants.** Infection and sepsis, surgery, MI, non-compliance with drug therapy.

(c) **Investigations.** Blood sugar, urea, creatinine and electrolytes (potassium should be measured frequently as deficits are often large and only become obvious once treatment has been commenced). Serum bicarbonate < 16 mmol l^{-1} signifies a severe acidosis and is an indication for ABG analysis. Serum lactate, ketone levels (serum levels rarely needed, confirmed on urine stick testing). Serum osmolality and calculation of anion gap. Amylase (which may be raised in the absence of pancreatitis). Full blood count. ECG. Septic screen: blood culture, urine for microscopy and culture, CXR and sputum culture if signs of infection.

(d) **Management**

- Severe DKA has a mortality rate of around 5%.
- Follow the ABC principles.
- Intubation is required if the patient's consciouness is significantly obtunded. There is the risk of aspiration from both the depressed level of consciousness and gastric dilatation. When assisted ventilation is employed the minute ventilation must take into account the large respiratory compensation of the spontaneously ventilating patient; an inadequate minute volume at this stage may precipitate profound acidosis and cardiovascular decompensation.

(e) **Fluid resuscitation.** Hypovolaemia must be reversed rapidly to ensure adequate tissue perfusion; the overall fluid deficit can then be replaced over a longer period. The volumes infused must be assessed repeatedly against resuscitative end points (HR, BP, peripheral perfusion, CVP).

Average fluid losses are around 6 l of water and 350 mmol of sodium. Hypotension is corrected initially with 0.9% sodium chloride. Half-normal saline can be substituted later as it contains more free water and approximates more closely to the urinary sodium and water losses.

In general, the fluid and electrolyte deficits should be corrected over a 48–72 hour period. Regular measurement of urine output and blood electrolytes allows the fluid replacement to be tailored individually.

Potassium, magnesium and phosphate require regular measurement and replacement. Acidosis and excess potassium administration may cause hyperkalaemia, while fluid and insulin will cause hypokalaemia.

Potassium requirements range from 5–40 mmol h^{-1}; some should be given as potassium phosphate to replace lost phosphate.

The magnesium deficit mirrors that of potassium. Initial replacement is started at 10–20 mmol h^{-1}. Hypomagnesaemia may contribute to insulin resistance and increase the risk of arrhythmias.

Once the blood sugar is approaching normal levels (< 15 mmol^{-1}) it is appropriate to change to 5% glucose.

During fluid and electrolyte replacement these patients are at risk of volume overload, hypernatraemia and hyperchloraemic acidosis from excess sodium chloride infusion, hypokalaemia, hypophosphataemia and hypomagnesaemia from inadequate replacement, hypoglycaemia from excess insulin, and cerebral oedema from excess fluid and too rapid replacement.

(f) **Insulin infusion.** A low dose insulin infusion ($1-2$ U h^{-1}) is commenced and titrated against frequent blood glucose measurements. Insulin resistance is seen in around 10% of IDDM. The blood glucose level should be corrected over 48–72 hours (at a rate of 2–3 mmol h^{-1}), as rapid correction is likely to result in osmotic shifts and serious complications.

(g) **Correction of acidosis.** The metabolic acidosis will improve with restoration of tissue perfusion and reduction in ketosis. The use of sodium bicarbonate is controversial because of numerous side effects including: adverse effects on tissue oxygenation because of increased haemoglobin oxygen affinity, increased carbon dioxide production, which will require increased minute ventilation, paradoxical intracellular and cerebrospinal acidosis, a high osmotic and sodium load with the risk of volume overload, hypokalaemia; hypocalcaemia.

Bicarbonate may be indicated in the presence of profound acidosis and cardio-vascular depression. Bicarbonate is not generally indicated if the pH is $>$ 6.9. If bicarbonate is administered, small boluses (50 mmol) should be titrated against frequent blood gas estimations.

A nasogastric tube should be inserted Stress ulcer prophylaxis should be initiated and early enteral feeding commenced.

(h) **DVT prophylaxis.** Compression stockings, mechanical compression devices and subcutaneous heparin.

2. *Hyperosmolar non-ketotic coma (HNKC).* HNKC occurs much less frequently than DKA. The mortality of hyperosmolar coma is much greater than for DKA and can be as high as 50%. In HNKC, severe hyperglycaemia develops over a period of days or weeks without significant ketosis. It is usually seen in elderly uncontrolled NIDDM but may also be the first presentation of late onset diabetes. Precipitants include infection, steroid and diuretic use, an excessive glucose intake and inter-current surgery or illness. The characteristic presentation is of non-specific anorexia, malaise and weakness which progresses to coma, severe dehydration and renal impairment. The severe dehydration and renal impairment will result in a metabolic acidosis but ketosis is not a feature. Coma will necessitate intubation, confusion, agitation and drowsiness may persist for weeks. The principles of fluid replacement are the same as for DKA but the dehydration is often more severe and replacement should be more gradual as the risk of cerebral oedema is higher. Saline is used to correct hypotension, and half-normal saline is used to replace the water and sodium losses. The fluid deficits should be corrected over a period of days. Despite the levels of hyperglycaemia often exceeding those seen in DKA the insulin requirements are lower than for DKA. Thrombotic events appear to be more common in HNKC and are a major cause of morbidity and mortality.

3. *Hypoglycaemia.* Life-threatening hypoglycaemia may be seen in diabetics and non-diabetics. Coma in diabetics is most commonly due to hypoglycaemia. Hypoglycaemia (BS $<$ 2.5 mmol l^{-1}) may be precipitated by:

- Inadequate diet carbohydrate, missed meals.
- Excess glucose uptake (exercise, insulin overdose).

- Change in therapy/commencement of insulin therapy.
- Liver failure.
- Alcohol (inhibition of gluconeogenesis).
- Hypoadrenalism (including Addison's disease), hypopituitarism.

The threshold for symptoms and clinical features of hypoglycaemia vary widely:

- Nausea, vomiting.
- Sweating, tachycardia, tremor (may be absent if autonomic neuropathy).
- Altered behaviour, confusion, agitation and depressed level of consciousness.
- Seizures, coma and focal neurological signs, permanent neurological damage occurs rapidly because of the brain's dependence on glucose for metabolism and the lack of any significant brain stores of glycogen.

(a) **Management.** Sufficient glucose must be given to rapidly reverse hypoglycaemia. High concentration glucose (e.g., 50 ml 20% glucose) must be given without delay and repeated if necessary while blood sugar levels by stick test are measured.

A continuous infusion of glucose may be required to maintain normal blood sugar levels. Injection of glucagon 1 mg (IM/SC) can be used if there is no venous access or glucose solution immediately available. Its use will have to be followed by glucose administration.

(b) **Outcome.** Insulin dependent diabetes is associated with an increased morbidity and mortality with the risk of death being up to eight times greater than non-diabetics. The main increased risk is from cardiovascular complications.

Diabetic ketoacidosis has a mortality rate of up to 10%, while in hyperosmolar non-ketotic hyperosmolar coma the risk of death may be as high as 50%. The main causes of death are the underlying diseases that precipitate DKA or HNKC with cardiovascular complications being common.

Further reading

Lebovitz HE. Diabetic ketoacidosis. *Lancet* 1995; **346:** 767–772.
Genuth SM. Diabetic ketoacidosis and hyperglycemic hyperosmolar coma. *Current Therapy in Endocrinology and Metabolism* 1997; **6:** 438–447.

Related topics of interest

Calcium, magnesium and phosphate, p. 56; Fluid therapy, p. 122; Potassium, p. 180; Sodium, p. 231

DRUG OVERDOSE

Minh Tran

Drug overdose may be accidental or intentional as seen in suicidal or parasuicidal patients. The number of drugs available is enormous and clinical presentations vary greatly. However, BLS and ALS measures remain the mainstay of treatment and the majority of patients will recover without the need for specific measures. A systematic approach to assessment and management comprises resuscitation, substance identification, drug elimination, and specific treatment.

Resuscitation

Resuscitation should follow the well established ABC principles. However, there are a few specific problems:

- Hypothermia is common especially at the extremes of age. Core temperature should be measured (see page 136).
- Hyperthermia is relatively uncommon but is seen with salicylates, amphetamine, cocaine and anticholinergic drugs. Neuroleptic malignant syndrome and malignant hyperthermia are rare causes. Sepsis may be the cause, particularly in obtunded patients.
- Rhabdomyolysis should be excluded in hypothermic, comatose or traumatized patients. It may also occur in narcotic and cocaine abuse without coma, or it may complicate prolonged seizures.

Substance identification

The history is often unreliable but important information includes:

- Drug: drug name(s), dosage, when taken, route taken.
- Circumstance: intention, witnesses, empty bottles, packets, syringes, associated trauma.
- Background: previous attempt(s), past medical history, allergy.
- Symptoms and signs: description and first aid prior to presentation. A full physical examination is essential.

Investigations. Identify the drug (blood, urine, or gastric aspirate) and decide on the need for a specific treatment. It is often routine practice to check for paracetamol, aspirin and alcohol. Other helpful investigations might include:

- Blood count and coagulation.
- Urea, creatinine and electrolytes, liver function tests and CPK.
- Serum osmolality (ethanol, methanol and ethylene glycol).
- Arterial blood gas analysis.
- CXR in obtunded or intubated patients.
- 12-lead ECG.

Drug elimination

There are a number of strategies for drug elimination:

1. **External decontamination** is indicated for toxins which can be absorbed transdermally e.g. organophosphates and hydrocarbons.

2. **Induced emesis** with syrup of ipecacuanha is not indicated when time of ingestion is more than 1 hour. Less than 40% of ingested substance is usually recovered. It is contraindicated in children less than 6 months old, when there is coma or a depressed level of consciousness, following ingestion of caustic agents, alkalis and hydrocarbons. Potential complications include aspiration, Mallory–Weiss tears, protracted vomiting, and gastric rupture.

3. **Gastric lavage** is generally only useful within 1 hour of ingestion but worthwhile recovery of some drugs (e.g., salicylate, theophylline) may occur later. It is not effective against alcohol ingestion and is potentially harmful following petroleum product and caustic ingestion. It should be performed only when the airway is protected. Complications include aspiration and inhalation of gastric contents, oropharyngeal trauma and oesophageal perforation.

4. **Activated charcoal** (AC) is an effective adsorbent for many drugs. It is superior to emesis or lavage. Activated charcoal does not bind elemental metal (e.g., iron, lithium), alcohol (e.g., ethanol, methanol), cyanide or some pesticides (malathion, DDT). Commercially available AC is in an aqueous slurry with added cathartic and flavoring. AC promotes active elimination of aspirin, carbamazepine, dapsone, phenobarbitone, quinine and theophylline.

5. **Cathartics** cause diarrhoea and are used in combination with AC. Fluid and electrolyte losses may be excessive.

6. **Endoscopy** may be used for iron, alkali or acid ingestion, where gastric lavage and AC may cause further harm.

7. **Surgical removal** is rarely indicated (e.g., iron overdose, body packers).

8. **Diuresis** relies on bulk flow to decrease drug concentrations in blood. Intravenous fluid with or without a diuretic is used to produce a urine output of 2–5 ml kg^{-1} h^{-1}. Electrolyte and volume status must be closely monitored. There is a major risk of fluid overload. Alkalinization with sodium bicarbonate may enhance barbiturate and salicylate elimination but is generally no longer recommended.

9. **Haemodialysis** is effective for low molecular weight compounds with small volume of distribution, low protein binding, low lipid solubility and low spontaneous clearance. Examples include methanol, ethanol, ethylene glycol, salicylates, lithium and chloral hydrate.

10. **Haemoperfusion** using either charcoal or resin columns may be useful for lipid soluble drugs such as theophylline and barbiturates.

Specific treatment

1. **Tricyclic antidepressants.** Toxicity is due to anticholinergic effects and post-ganglionic noradrenaline reuptake blockade (increased sympathetic stimulation). They also cause quinidine-like effects on cardiac conduction (rhythm and conduction disturbances). There is no specific antidote and rapid metabolism results

in recovery within 24 hours. Gastric elimination and AC are effective up to 24 hours after ingestion. Ventricular arrhythmias usually respond to correction of acidosis and hypoxia.

2. *Paracetamol.* Ingestion of > 150 mg kg^{-1} by a child or > 7.5 g by an adult is considered toxic. In the early phase (< 20 hours) there are relatively few symptoms apart from some abdominal pain, and nausea and vomiting. In the 2nd phase (> 20 hours), clinical (pain and tenderness) and biochemical signs of hepatocellular necrosis are present. In the 3rd phase (Day 3–4) liver damage is maximal. The recovery phase lasts for 7–8 days.

Initial management includes gastric lavage and AC up to 2 hours after ingestion. Intravenous acetylcysteine is most effective within 10–12 hours of ingestion but may be worthwhile beyond this period. Methionine is an oral alternative if used within 10–12 hours. Acetylcysteine is indicated if more than 10 g has been ingested, if there is doubt about the amount taken, or if the paracetamol level is above the line on the treatment graph. Acetylcysteine may cause urticaria, bronchospasm and anaphylaxis, especially with rapid administration. Liver transplantation is indicated for severe established liver failure.

3. *Aspirin.* Absorption may be delayed (enteric formulations) and blood concentrations within 6 hours may be misleadingly low. Aspirin toxicity causes hyperventilation, tinnitus, vasodilatation, and an initial respiratory alkalosis that progresses to metabolic acidosis if severe. There is no specific antidote. Gastric emptying may be useful up to 4 hours after ingestion. If the plasma salicylate concentration is > 350 mg l^{-1} in children or > 500 mg l^{-1} in adults, sodium bicarbonate may enhance urine excretion. Severe overdose (plasma level > 700 mg l^{-1}) is an indication for haemodialysis.

4. *Anticholinergic drugs.* Atropine and other belladonna alkaloids, antihistamines, phenothiazines and tricyclic antidepressants have anticholinergic activity. This results in hyperthermia, dilated pupils, loss of sweating, delirium, visual hallucination, ataxia, dystonic reactions, seizures, coma, respiratory depression, labile blood pressure, arrhythmias, urinary retention, and ileus.

Management comprises resuscitation, GI elimination and supportive care. Physostigmine, an anticholinesterase, crosses the blood brain barrier and may be useful in severe cases but is not widely available.

5. *Amphetamines and ecstasy (MDMA).* These drugs cause sympathomimetic effects including arrhythmias, hypertension, seizures, coma, hyperthermia, rhabdomyolysis, renal and hepatic failure, intracerebral haemorrhage and infarction and hyponatraemia. There are no specific antidotes but beta-blockers can be used to treat arrhythmias.

6. *Benzodiazepines.* Supportive care alone will usually result in a good recovery. The antagonist flumazenil may be used but its short half-life dictates the need for an infusion and it may precipitate seizures, particularly in chronic benzodiazepine users.

7. *Beta-blockers.* Beta-blockers will cause bradyarrhythmias, atrioventricular block, and hypotension. They may cause an altered mental state, delirium, coma and seizures. Sotalol may cause VT (sometimes torsade de pointes). Bradycardia is treated with atropine. Isoprenaline and cardiac pacing may also be useful in refractory cases. Glucagon is used a beta-receptor independent inotrope and chronotrope in refractory bradycardia and hypotension.

8. Calcium channel blockers. In overdose, calcium channel blockers will cause hyperglycaemia, nausea and vomiting, coma, seizures, bradycardia, varying degrees of AV block, hypotension, and cardiac arrest. Gastric lavage may precipitate arrhythmias. Hypotension and bradycardia may respond to 10% calcium chloride. Glucagon, vasopressors, and inotropes may be required.

9. Digoxin. Nausea, vomiting, drowsiness and confusion are prominent. The ECG may show many types of rhythm and conduction abnormality. Management includes gastric elimination and correction of electrolytes, particularly potassium and magnesium. Digoxin-specific antibody fragments (Fab) are indicated in arrhythmias associated with haemodynamic instability. Ventricular tachyarrhythmias may respond to phenytoin, lignocaine or amiodarone. Atropine may be effective for bradycardia but temporary pacing may be required.

10. Ethanol. Very high doses of ethanol will cause severe cortical and brain-stem depression (coma and hypoventilation) with obvious risk of aspiration of vomit. Depressed gluconeogenesis may cause hypoglycaemia and there may be a high anion gap metabolic acidosis. Management comprises correction of fluid, electrolyte and acid-base disturbance.

11. Methanol. The metabolites of methanol (formaldehyde and formic acid) are toxic. The lethal dose is 1–2 ml kg^{-1} or 80 mg dl^{-1}. A latent period of 2–18 hours may occur before the onset of a triad of GI symptoms (nausea, vomiting, pain, bleeding), eye signs (blurred, cloudy vision, central scotoma, yellow spots or blindness) and metabolic acidosis. There is an elevated serum osmolality and increased anion gap. Ethanol is a competitive inhibitor for metabolism and is used as an antidote to methanol. Aim to maintain a serum ethanol level at 1 g l^{-1} or 20 mmol l^{-1}). Haemodialysis should be considered if:

- Peak methanol levels > 15 mmol l^{-1} (> 50 mg dl^{-1}).
- Renal failure.
- Visual impairment.
- Mental disturbance.
- Acidosis not corrected with bicarbonate therapy.

12. Ethylene glycol. Ethylene glycol causes an odourless intoxication with high serum osmolality, severe metabolic acidosis, and oxalate crystalluria. It is associated with hyperthermia, hypoglycaemia and hypocalcaemia. Toxicity is due due to hepatic metabolites (glycoaldehyde, glycolic acid, glycoxylate and oxalate). Management is as for methanol toxicity.

13. Opioids. An opioid overdose will cause respiratory depression, pin-point pupils, and coma. Seizures are usually due to hypoxia but can be caused by nor-pethidine, the neurotoxic metabolite of pethidine. Rhabdomyolysis, endocarditis and pulmonary complications are common. Naloxone is a specific antagonist that can be given i.v. and/or i.m. Its short half-life dictates the need for repeated injections or an infusion. Titration will avoid precipitating withdrawal in habitual users.

14. Lithium. Polyuria, thirst, vomiting, diarrhoea and agitation are common presentations of lithium overdose. Coma, seizures and nephrogenic diabetes insipidus also occur. Serum lithium levels > 1.5 mmol l^{-1} are toxic. Fluid and electrolyte disturbances should be corrected. Consider haemodialysis when concentrations reach 2 mmol l^{-1}.

15. Organophosphates and carbonates. Toxicity is due to cholinergic over-activity and symptoms appear within 2 hours of exposure. The symptoms can be memorized with the following mnemonics:

- **DUMBELS:** diarrhoea, urination, miosis, bronchospasm, emesis, lacrimation, salivation.
- **SLUDGE:** salivation and sweating, lacrimation, urination, diarrhoea, gastro-intestinal pain and emesis.

Observe strict isolation and avoid contact exposure. Gastric elimination is appropriate. Atropine is used treat bradycardia and pulmonary secretions. Pralidoxime is a specific reactivator of cholinesterase but is only effective if given within 24 hours of exposure. Plasma cholinesterase levels require monitoring until recovery.

Further reading

Sporer KA. Acute heroin overdose. *Annals of Internal Medicine* 1999; **130:** 584–590.
Trujillo MH, Guerrero J, Fragachan C, Fernandey MA. Pharmacologic antidotes in critical care medicine: a practical guide for drug administration. *Critical Care Medicine* 1998; **26:** 377–391.

Related topics of interest

Hyperthermia, p. 133; Hypothermia, p. 136; Liver dysfunction, p. 147; Renal replacement therapy, p. 197; Resuscitation-cardiopulmonary, p.213

ENDOCARDITIS

Antony Stewart

Infective endocarditis results in the formation of infective vegetations on the endocardium. The cardiac valves are most commonly involved but other areas of endocardium may also be affected e.g., VSD, ASD, PDA, coarctation. Endocarditis is seen in one of three groups of patients: native valve endocarditis, prosthetic valve endocarditis and endocarditis in i.v. drug users.

Causative organisms

1. Native valve endocarditis

- *Streptococcus viridans* (30–40%).
- Other streptococci. (15–25%) *Strep. bovis* is frequently associated with colonic polyps or malignancy.
- Staphylococci (30) (90% of which are *Staphylococcus aureus*). This is often hospital acquired.
- Enterococci (5–18%) and fungi (candida) are more rarely hospital acquired.
- Very rare: rickettsia (Q fever), brucella, mycoplasma, legionella, histoplasma.

2. Organisms in intravenous injecting drug addicts

- Staphylococci (60%).
- Gram-negative organisms (10%).
- Streptococci and fungi (6–12%).

5% of patients will have more than one organism.

3. Prosthetic valve endocarditis

Early (within 60 days):

- *Staph. aureus* and *Staph. epidermidis* (50%).
- Gram-negative organisms (20%).
- Fungi (10–12%).

Late onset (after 60 days):

- Staphylococci (30–40%).
- Streptococci (25–30%).
- Gram-negative (10–12%).

Pathogenesis

Endocarditis most commonly involves the left side of the heart with the mitral valve most frequently affected. Drug addicts often have right sided involvement most commonly of the tricuspid valve. Vegetations consisting of fibrin, platelets and infecting organisms form in areas with high velocity and abnormal blood flow, flow from high to low pressure chambers, and flow through a narrow orifice.

The risk of endocarditis is increased in patients with structural heart disease, rheumatic valve disease, and mitral valve prolapse with regurgitation. However, 40–50% of cases occur in patients with no abnormalities. Usually these cases are due to virulent organisms such as *Staph. aureus*.

Clinical features

Low virulence organisms such as *Strep. viridans* tend to have insidious clinical courses. High virulence organisms such as *Staph. aureus* and fungi result in more dramatic presentations. Fever is present in up to 90% of patients as are new murmurs or changing murmurs (may not be detected in tricuspid involvement). Myalgia, arthralgia, fatigue, anorexia and anaemia are common presenting features. Embolic phenomena are common, especially if vegetations are larger than 10 mm. Splenomegaly (40%) and clubbing are both late signs. Neurological signs occur in 20–40% due to embolism, encephalopathy, and haemorrhage from mycotic aneurysms. Heart failure due to fulminant valvular regurgitation and cardiac conduction abnormalities also occur.

Immune complex deposition results in vasculitis, splinter haemorrhages, Osler's nodes in the finger pulp, Roth spots in retina and microscopic haematuria (due to either proliferative glomerulonephritis or focal embolic glomerulonephritis).

In severe cases shock and MOF are features.

Diagnosis

1. Definite infective endocarditis
(a) Pathological criteria

- Micro-organisms: on culture or histology in a vegetation, an embolus or in an intracardiac abscess.
- Pathological lesions: histology confirming endocarditis.

(b) Clinical diagnosis based on major and minor criteria

- 2 major criteria, or
- 1 major and 3 minor criteria, or
- 5 minor criteria

2. Possible infective endocarditis.
Clinical findings fall short of a definite diagnosis, but endocarditis is not rejected.

3. Rejected.
Firm alternative diagnosis, or resolution of clinical manifestations with 4 or less days of antibiotics, or no evidence of endocarditis at autopsy or surgery

4. Definitions
(a) Major criteria.
Positive blood culture with typical micro-organism for infective endocarditis from:

- Blood cultures more than 12 hours apart, or
- all three or a majority of four or more blood cultures with first and last at least 1 hour apart.

Evidence of endocardial involvement. Positive echocardiogram for endocarditis

- Oscillating intracardiac mass on a valve or supporting structures, in the path of regurgitant jets or on implanted material in the absence of an alternative explanation.
- Abscess.
- New partial dehiscence of prosthetic valve or new valvular regurgitation.

(b) Minor criteria

- Predisposing heart lesion or i.v. drug use.
- Fever > 38.0°C.
- Vascular phenomena.
- Immunological phenomena: e.g., glomerulonephritis, Osler's nodes.
- Microbiological evidence; positive blood cultures not meeting major criteria or serological evidence of active infection with organisms consistent with infective endocarditis.
- Echo consistent with endocarditis but not meeting major criteria.

Investigations

- Blood count may show neutrophilia and anaemia.
- Urinalysis for haematuria and casts.
- Blood cultures, at least three, from different sites an hour apart before antibiotics are given. Cultures are positive in up to 90% of patients. Culture may be negative because of prior antibiotic exposure, fastidious organism e.g., *Coxiella burnetii* (Q fever), HACEK organisms (*Haemophilus* spp., *Actinobacillus actinomycetemcomitans*, *Cardiobacterium hominis*, *Eikenella corrodens*, and *Kingella* sp.), fungi, anaerobes, right sided endocarditis, or non-infective endocarditis e.g., Libman-Sacks disease in systemic lupus erythematosus (SLE) or marantic endocarditis.
- Echocardiography: transthoracic echo detects vegetations larger than 2–3 mm. Transoesophageal echocardiography (TOE) is more sensitive.

Management

- General resuscitative, management following the ABC priorities.
- Aggressive antimicrobial therapy.
- Repeated assessment for worsening valvular function, heart failure, abscess formation, embolic phenomena (especially cerebral) and MOF.
- Cardiac surgery may be required for acute valvular regurgitation, myocardial abscess, prosthetic valve dysfunction and replacement, high risk of emboli (vegetations > 10 mm), persistent positive blood cultures despite treatment and fungal endocarditis.

Principles of antimicrobial therapy:

- Empirical therapy (e.g., benzylpenicillin, flucloxacillin, and gentamicin) is commenced in fulminant endocarditis and then modified depending on organisms isolated from blood cultures. Rifampicin may be added if prosthetic valve endocarditis is suspected.
- Prolonged treatment is required (4–6 weeks) because the high density of micro-organisms protected in vegetations is associated with a high relapse rate.
- If treatment is effective the fever should decrease in 3–7 days. A persistent fever may reflect ineffective treatment, abscess formation, septic emboli or antibiotic fever.

Prognosis

Streptococcal and tricuspid endocarditis carry a 10% mortality. The prognosis is poor (> 20% mortality) in non-streptococcal disease, severe heart failure, aortic and prosthetic valve involvement, age > 65, valve ring or myocardial abscess, and large vegetations. Death is usually due to heart failure and embolic events. Prognosis is worst (60% mortality) in early prosthetic valve endocarditis. Recurrent or second episodes are seen in 6% of patients.

Prophylaxis

Although there is little evidence of the efficacy of antibiotic prophylaxis it is common practice to administer antibiotics to high risk patients who are having procedures associated with the risk of bacteraemia.

The recommendations for prophylaxis vary depending on the procedure, from country to country and depending on local factors. Expert microbiologist advice should be sought.

Further reading

Bayer AS *et al*. Diagnosis and management of infective endocarditis and its complications. *Circulation* 1998; **98**: 2936–2948.

Dajani AS, Taubert KA, Wilson W, *et al*. Prevention of bacterial endocarditis. Recommendations by the American Heart Association. *Circulation* 1997; **96**(1): 358–366.

Related topics of interest

Cardiac failure, p. 73; Infection control, p. 140; Infection in critical care, p. 143

EPIGLOTTITIS

Acute epiglottitis is an uncommon but dangerous bacterial infection of the throat. It is usually seen in children aged less than 8 years with a peak incidence between 2 and 5 years. It may also occur in adults. The usual causative organism is *Haemophilus influenzae* type B but this is not invariable and β-haemolytic streptococci, staphylococci, or pneumococci may also be isolated, especially in adult cases. The differential diagnosis in children is acute laryngotracheo-bronchitis (croup) which is a viral infection occurring principally in those under 3. The mortality in adults is quoted to be as high as 6–7% but this is usually due to misdiagnosis and inappropriate treatment.

Problems
- Upper airway obstruction.
- Lethargy and exhaustion.
- Potential difficulty with intubation.

Diagnosis
The provisional diagnosis is made on the history and examination. Typically the history is short with a rapid deterioration. The patient presents with a sore throat, fever, muffled voice and dysphagia. Pain may exceed that expected from the brevity of the history. Inspiratory stridor develops rapidly and progression to complete respiratory obstruction may occur within 12 hours.

Children prefer to sit up and drool saliva from the mouth. Swallowing is avoided because of the extremely sore throat.

Indirect laryngoscopy should not be undertaken to confirm the diagnosis as this frequently precipitates airway obstruction, especially in children. Lateral neck X-rays may confirm a swollen epiglottis but are not essential. A sick child should not be sent to the X-ray department without the continual presence of someone skilled in paediatric intubation. A child with suspected epiglottitis will invariably require an examination of their upper airway under anaesthesia and X-rays are frequently unnecessary. The airway can then be secured with a tracheal tube.

Management
The child is moved to a quiet induction area where all the necessary aids to a difficult paediatric intubation are readily to hand. The child is allowed to remain in an upright posture as sudden changes in position, especially lying down, may result in complete airway obstruction.

An inhalational induction of anaesthesia is usually preferred. Venous access can be obtained once the child is unconscious. Atropine may then be administered if required. In the presence of airway obstruction it may take more than 15 minutes before anaesthesia is deep enough to permit safe laryngoscopy.

Laryngoscopy will show a swollen 'cherry red' epiglottis. There is often associated swelling of the aryepiglottic folds. In severe cases the only clue to the glottic opening may be bubbles issuing from behind the epiglottis during expiration.

Once intubated the child should then be transferred to a critical care area. Blood cultures and throat swabs are taken for microbiological examination. Therapy is continued with intravenous rehydration, humidified inspired gases, airway toilet, and antibiotics.

The management of adult cases follows a similar course, although observation of the unintubated patient in a critical care environment has been recommended by some. The risk in this strategy is the possibility of death from sudden complete respiratory obstruction.

Antibiotics

Ampicillin and chloramphenicol are the usual 'best bet' antibiotics until the organism's sensitivities are known. Cefuroxime is an alternative.

Progress

Epiglottic oedema settles rapidly following commencement of the antibiotics and an increasing leak around the tracheal tube is expected. Once the patient is afebrile and appears well, extubation may be considered. This is usually within 24–48 hours. It is not necessary to re-examine the larynx prior to extubation.

Related topic of interest

Infection in critical care, p. 143

FIBREOPTIC BRONCHOSCOPY

Diagnostic uses

Fibreoptic bronchoscopy (FOB) allows the direct inspection and instrumentation of the upper and lower airway. Aspiration, bronchoalveolar lavage, bronchial brushings, transbronchial biopsy and protected specimen brushings can obtain diagnostic material. Indications for FOB include:

- Investigation of atelectasis. Areas of atelectasis may require bronchoscopy to exclude an obstruction.
- Evaluation of haemoptysis.
- Evaluation of radiological abnormalities. Lesions can be biopsied but the incidence of complications, particularly pneumothorax, is highest with this technique especially in those mechanically ventilated (as high as 20%).
- Diagnosis of pneumonia. Indicated particularly in those immunocompromised and in those with suspected nosocomial pneumonia. Protected specimen brushes or bronchoalveolar lavage affords better correlation with the infective cause of infection by reducing contamination from a colonized upper airway (see Pneumonia – hospital acquired p. 177).
- Localization of the tracheal tube tip.
- Determination of the site of barotrauma.
- Evaluation of major airway trauma and thermal injury.

Therapeutic uses

- Aspiration of mucous plugs. Chest physiotherapy and suctioning are usually successful in treating mucous plugs and resultant atelectasis. If these techniques fail, bronchoscopy with bronchoalveolar lavage can be used to remove the plugs and re-expand the atelectatic lung. The relatively narrow suction channel in the FOB will limit its efficacy in the presence of very thick mucous.
- Local treatment of haemoptysis. A fibreoptic bronchoscope can be used to instil adrenaline solution onto a bleeding endobronchial site or to assist the placement of a Fogarty catheter into that segment to tamponade the bleeding focus.
- Removal of aspirated foreign bodies. Although the rigid bronchoscope traditionally is the preferred instrument for the removal of foreign bodies, the FOB used with a variety of forceps and baskets, has been shown to be safe and effective.
- Treatment of bronchopulmonary fistula. Proximally located fistulae may be directly visualized, whereas more distal fistulae may be localized by systematically passing an occluding balloon into each bronchial segment. When the correct segment is located inflation of the balloon will result in reduction of the air leak.

Airway management

Indications for bronchoscopic airway management include:

- Tracheal intubation. Especially in the setting of difficult intubation, anatomical deformity, head and neck immobility and upper airway obstruction.
- Percutaneous tracheostomy. The FOB is used to confirm correct position of the Seldinger wire within the lumen of the trachea.
- Bronchial intubation (double lumen tube).
- Changing tracheal tube.
- Placement of a nasogastric tube.

Complications

FOB is a safe procedure when performed on critically ill patients. The most common complications are oxygen desaturation, hypotension, frequent premature ventricular beats, fever and pulmonary haemorrhage. These are generally transient and rarely life threatening. Relative contraindications include: difficult ventilation or oxygenation, severe coagulopathy, acute myocardial infarction or ischaemia; status asthmaticus.

Further reading

Ovassapian A, Randel GI. The role of the fibrescope in the critically ill. *Resp. Proc. Monitoring* 1995; 11(1): 29–50.

Silver MR, Balk RA. Bronchoscopic procedures in the intensive care unit. *Resp. Proc. Monitoring* 1995; 11(1): 97–109.

Related topics of interest

Chest tube thoracostomy, p. 89; Tracheostomy, p. 250

FLUID THERAPY

Total body water (TBW) is approximately 60% of body weight in young adult males (42 1 for 70 kg male). Adult females comprise slightly less water and slightly more fat per kilogram body weight. TBW is distributed between two compartments; extracellular fluid (ECF) and intracellular fluid (ICF). ECF itself comprises two compartments; interstitial fluid (ISF) (that part of the ECF which is outside the vascular system bathing the body's cells) and plasma (the non-cellular component of blood).

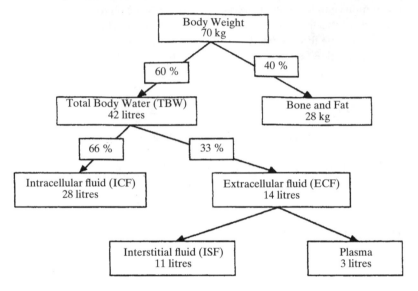

Physiology

ICF is separated from ECF by a cell membrane that is highly permeable to water but not to most electrolytes. Intracellular volume is maintained by the membrane sodium–potassium pump, which moves sodium out of the cell (carrying water with it) in exchange for potassium. Thus, there are significant differences in the electrolytic composition of intracellular and extracellular fluid

The intravascular space and the ISF are separated by the endothelial cells of the capillary wall (the capillary membrane). This wall is permeable to water and small molecules including ions. It is impermeable to larger molecules such as proteins. The higher hydrostatic pressure inside capillaries (compared with that in the ISF) tends to force fluid out of the vessel into the ISF.

The osmotic pressure of a solution is related directly to the number of osmotically active particles it contains. The total osmolarity of each of the fluid compartments is approximately 280 mOsm l^{-1}. Oncotic pressure is that component of osmotic pressure provided by proteins. The higher osmotic pressure inside capillaries tends to pull fluid back in to the vessels.

Electrolyte concentrations differ markedly between the various fluid compartments. Notably, sodium and chloride are chiefly extracellular whilst the majority of total body potassium is within the intracellular compartment. There is also a relatively low content of protein anions in interstitial fluid compared to intracellular fluid and plasma.

Crystalloids

Crystalloids are fluids comprised of water to which solutes (e.g., sodium chloride) have been added. Their distribution following intravenous administration is determined chiefly by their sodium concentration. Since sodium is confined mainly to the ECF, fluids with high sodium concentrations (e.g., 0.9% sodium chloride) will be distributed mainly through the ECF. Solutions with lower sodium concentrations (e.g., 5% glucose) will be distributed throughout both ECF and the intracellular compartment.

Colloids

Colloidal solutions are fluids containing large molecules that exert an oncotic pressure at the capillary membrane. Natural colloids include blood and albumin. Artificial colloids contain large molecules such as gelatin, dextran, starch, and haemoglobin solutions. Intravenous administration of colloids results chiefly in expansion of the intravascular compartment, at least in the first instance. The duration of intravascular persistence depends on molecular size, shape, and ionic charge. Albumin is a negatively charged substance and as such is repelled by the negatively charged endothelial glycocalyx, thus extending its intravascular duration. Colloid solutions that have an oncotic pressure greater than that of plasma are also able to draw fluid from the interstitial space back into the circulating compartment.

1. Blood. Blood is an appropriate replacement fluid following severe haemorrhage. It will increase the haemoglobin concentration in the circulating compartment and thus improve oxygen carriage in the blood. Intravenous administration of blood results in expansion of the intravascular compartment with little or no increase in interstitial fluid.

2. Albumin. Human albumin is a single polypeptide with a molecular weight of around 68 kDa. It has transport functions, is able to scavenge free radicals, and has anticoagulant properties. In health, it contributes about 80% of oncotic pressure but in the critically ill serum albumin correlates poorly with colloid oncotic pressure. Albumin is prepared in two concentrations (4–5% and 20%) from many thousands of pooled donors. There is a theoretical risk of transmission of the prion causing New Variant Creutzfeld–Jakob disease. The half-life of exogenous albumin in the circulating compartment is 5–10 days assuming an intact capillary wall membrane. It is expensive to prepare but has a long shelf-life.

3. Gelatins. Gelatins are produced by modifying bovine collagens and suspending them in ionic solutions. They have long shelf-lives and do not transmit infection. Gelatin solutions contain molecules of widely varying size that are excreted by the kidney chiefly unchanged. Gelatin solutions remain in the circulating compartment for a short period, only 15% being found in the intravascular space 24 hours after administration.

4. Dextrans. Dextrans are polysaccharide products of sucrose. The polysaccharides themselves are of varying molecular weight and their classification is based upon this. Dextran 70 (average molecular weight 70 000) has an intravascular half-life of about 12 hours. Dextrans cause a mild alteration in platelet stickiness and function and thus have an antithrombotic effect. They have been shown to reduce the incidence of fatal pulmonary embolism in susceptible patients.

5. Hydroxyethyl starch. Hydroxyethyl starch (HES) is manufactured by polymerizing cornstarch. A number of HES solutions are produced, each with a different average molecular weight. Most HES solutions have a longer intravascular half-life than other synthetic colloids. The higher molecular weight starch solutions will impair factor VII and von Willebrand factor function, thus altering haemostatic function. There is a theoretical concern about accumulation of higher molecular weight HES in the reticular activating system. Some starch solutions (e.g., Haes 10%) have a higher oncotic pressure than plasma.

6. Haemoglobin solutions. Blood is the only fluid in clinical use that has significant oxygen carrying capability. While this property makes it indispensable during resuscitation of haemorrhagic shock, it is expensive, in short supply, antigenic, requires cross-matching, has a limited shelf-life, requires a storage facility and carries a risk of disease transmission. Free haemoglobin causes severe renal injury. Polymerization of the haemoglobin overcomes this problem and improves intravascular persistence. Haemoglobin solutions under development are derived from one of three sources; bovine blood, out of date human blood (5–13% of blood donated in the United States is discarded), and recombinant haemoglobin. The products currently under investigation do not require cross-matching, have similar oxygen dissociation curves to blood, and are apparently free from risk of transmitting viral or bacterial infections. They have an intravascular half-life of about 24 hours. Diaspirin cross-linked haemoglobin and bovine haemoglobin solution have a significant vasopressor effect which is thought to result from scavenging endothelial nitric oxide.

Fluid therapy

Fluid therapy is based on an assessment of the water and electrolyte deficiency and anticipated needs of the physiological fluid compartments. Resuscitation of the intravascular space is the most important aspect of fluid therapy in the hypovolaemic patient. The status of the intravascular space can be assessed clinically using heart rate, blood pressure, urine output, CVP and PAOP for guidance. The interstitial and intracellular fluid spaces are more difficult to assess but remain in dynamic equilibrium with the intravascular space. Serial body weight measurements offer an indicator of total body fluid balance. Hidden 'losses' (e.g., ileus, pleural effusion) will not be accounted for by weight measurements.

In patients with continuing blood loss haemorrhage control must be achieved. Thereafter, the goals of fluid resuscitation are to optimize oxygen delivery and improve microcirculatory perfusion.

Crystalloids vs. colloids

A lack of quality outcome data to allow evidence-based decisions over the choice of crystalloid or colloidal solutions for resuscitation has allowed a debate to simmer for many years. Crystalloid containing isotonic concentrations of sodium or colloids can be used to expand the intravascular space. Crystalloid solutions are readily available, cheap, and associated with fewer adverse reactions. However, a greater fluid and sodium load is required to resuscitate a volume depleted intravascular space using crystalloids than colloids. Crystalloids offer no oxygen carrying capacity. Loss of more than 40% of the total blood volume is likely to require replacement with red cells. However, acute anaemia is far better tolerated than hypovolaemia. Thus, initial resuscitation is acheived with non-blood solutions, and, where appropriate, blood is given at a later stage. Patients with SIRS are more likely to loose fluid from the intravascular space through endothelial leakage (e.g., burns, sepsis, and critical illness). Fluid resuscitation of such patients may be better achieved with colloids than with crystalloid solutions although this remains controversial. Crystalloids may worsen tissue oxygenation in such patients, especially if leakage occurs into the lungs.

Fluid warming

All intravenous fluids given to critically ill patients should be warmed. Hypothermia has a number of adverse effects including: shifting the oxygen-dissociation curve to the left (impairing tissue oxygen unloading), decreasing haemostatic function, increasing oxygen demand and lactic acidosis if shivering is induced, and increasing the chance of an adverse cardiac event.

Further reading

Haljamae H, Dahlqvist M, Walentin F. Artificial colloids in clinical practice: pros and cons. *Bailliere's Clinical Anasthaesiology* 1997; **11**: 49–79.

Hillman K, Bishop G, Bristow P. The crystalloid versus colloid controversy: present status *Bailliere's Clinical Anasthaesiology* 1997; **11**: 1–13.

Related topics of interest

Burns, p. 51; Calcium, magnesium and phosphate, p. 56; Potassium, p. 180; Sodium, p. 231; Trauma-primary survey and resuscitation, p. 257

GUILLAIN–BARRÉ SYNDROME

Guillain–Barré syndrome (GBS) is an acute inflammatory demyelinating polyradiculo-neuropathy. It is the commonest cause of acute generalized flaccid paralysis and has an incidence of ~2 per 100000 population per anum. It is commoner in men. Around 70% of cases occur after a viral infection that usually comprises a short-lived flu-like illness. It may occur following recently acquired HIV, after infection with CMV, Epstein–Barr virus, hepatitis or infectious mononucleosis. It may also occur after *Campylobacter jejuni* enteritis, a feature that carries a worse prognosis. It is likely that immune responses directed towards the infecting organisms cross-react with ganglioside surface components of peripheral nerves.

Occasionally it occurs as a complication of an underlying systemic condition such as SLE, sarcoidosis, or Hodgkin's lymphoma. GBS should be differentiated from neuropathy of the critically ill and that associated with porphyria. It may also be confused with poisoning by neurotoxic fish or following exposure to certain heavy metals.

Approximately one third of patients with GBS require admission to a critical care unit and subsequent ventilatory support.

Clinical features

Typically, the first symptoms of GBS are paraesthesiae in the toes or fingers. This may progress over a few days to be weakness of the legs, arms, face, and oropharynx. Examination may show bilateral, symmetrical, flaccid tetraparesis. There may also be facial weakness, reduced deep tendon reflexes, but only minimal sensory signs. In more severe cases progression is more rapid. There may also be respiratory muscle weakness and involvement of the extraocular muscles and dysphagia.

Two clinical variants have been described:

- The axonal form, which has a more rapid onset, a higher incidence of preceding *C. jejuni* infection, anti-GM$_1$ ganglioside antibodies as a frequent finding, and a generally worse prognosis.
- The Miller Fisher syndrome is, strictly, a separate condition but shares some overlap features with GBS, especially those involving the eye muscles. It comprises an acute ophthalmoparesis, areflexia without weakness, and ataxia.

Autonomic dysfunction is common in severe cases. This may manifest as cardiovascular signs with both brady- and tachyarrhythmias. There may also be constipation, especially if the patient is profoundly weak.

Some patients with GBS suffer considerable pain and acutely inflamed nerves may be unusually prone to pressure palsies.

Investigation

1. Electrophysiology. Nerve conduction studies show evidence of demyelination. This may manifest as a slowed motor nerve conduction velocity or a conduction block.

2. Lumbar puncture. A normal CSF opening pressure and white cell count but raised protein concentration (> 0.45 g l^{-1}) after the first week of the illness are typical.

3. *Immunology* may show antibodies to *C. jejuni*, especially in patients with the axonal form. Some patients have antibodies to myelin protein.

Management

1. *General measures*

- Careful assessment and monitoring of patients with GBS will determine those that need admission to a critical care unit. Frequent measurement of the vital capacity will allow semi-elective ventilation to be established in those becoming progressively weaker.
- Continuous ECG and direct arterial blood pressure monitoring are advised to detect those with autonomic involvement. Autonomic disturbances should be minimized by ensuring an adequate circulating volume. Sedation may be required, especially during tracheal suction of the intubated patient. Beta-blockade may be required to control episodes of hypertension and/or tachy-cardia. Since hypotension and bradycardia are also likely in those with autonomic involvement, esmolol, a drug with a short half-life, given by continuous infusion may be the best beta-blocker to use. Significant bradycardia may necessitate the insertion of a pacemaker.
- Active measures to prevent DVT should be taken.
- Attention to nutrition is important and those with dysphagia may require nasogastric or percutaneous enterostomy feeding.
- Limb pains are common, especially during passive physiotherapy. Anti-prostanoid analgesics may control the pain but opioids are frequently required.

2. *Specific measures.* Both plasma exchange and intravenous immunoglobulin have been shown to be beneficial in GBS. Since the latter is simpler to administer and less invasive, it is now the treatment of choice. Immunoglobulin is given for 5 days at $0.4 \, \text{g} \, \text{kg}^{-1} \, \text{day}^{-1}$.

Prognosis

The prognosis for complete recovery is good, though 10% are left with a long term disability whilst 10% die in the acute illness from complications. A poor prognosis is suggested by: older age, preceding *C. jejuni* infection, evidence of axonal damage and a rapid onset of weakness.

Some suggest avoiding vaccinations in the future unless essential.

Further reading

Hahn, AF. Guillain–Barré Syndrome. *Lancet* 1998; **352**: 635–641.
Plasma Exchange/Sandoglobulin Guillain–Barré Syndrome Trial Group. Randomised trial of plasma exchange, intravenous immunoglobulin, and combined treatments in Guillain–Barré syndrome. *Lancet* 1997; **349**: 225–230.

Related topics of Interest

Respiratory support-weaning from ventilation, p. 210; Stroke, p. 243

Head injury accounts for approximately a third of all trauma deaths and is the leading cause of death and disability in young adults. However, severe head injury may still be compatible with a good outcome. Only preventative measures will help to address the primary brain injury. The role of critical care is to assess and resuscitate, identify intracranial pathology that can be improved by surgery, prevent secondary brain injury through monitoring and intervention and prevent other complications that will reduce the chances of the best possible recovery.

Causes of secondary brain injury and therapeutic aims

Cause	Aim
Hypotension	systolic blood pressure (SBP) $>$ 120 mmHg (maintain cerebral perfusion pressure $>$ 70 mmHg)
Hypoxia	$SpO_2 > 95\%$
Hypo/hypercapnia	$PaCO_2$ 4.5 kPa
Raised intracranial pressure (ICP)	ICP $<$ 20–25 mmHg
Seizures	treat convulsions with diazepam and phenytoin
Hyperthermia	core temperature 35–37°C
Hyperglycaemia	blood sugar 4–7 mmol l^{-1}

Assessment and resuscitation

Initial resuscitation of patients with severe head injury should follow the ABCDE format. Hypoxia ($SpO_2 < 95\%$) and hypotension (SBP $<$ 90 mmHg) independently increase mortality after severe head injury and must be treated aggressively. A rapid neurological assessment, including response to commands and any focal signs should be made before any sedative/paralysing drugs are given.

Management of intubation

Patients with head injuries should be sedated, paralysed, intubated and ventilated if there is airway compromise, ventilatory failure, a GCS $\leq$ 8 or if warranted because of another injury. The airway should also be secured if there is any doubt that there may be airway compromise, or agitation requiring sedation for a CT scan. It is appropriate to sedate and intubate patients with GCS scores of $>$ 8 to ensure optimal conditions for CT scanning and prevention of secondary brain injury. No head-injured adult or child should be sedated for a CT scan without control of the airway, even if this is to be reversed immediately afterwards.

An unstable cervical spine injury should be assumed until excluded. Oral tracheal intubation should follow a rapid sequence induction of anaesthesia and neuromuscular blockade with in-line stabilization of the cervical spine and cricoid pressure. Care should be taken to avoid hypotension during induction of anaesthesia as all intravenous anaesthetic agents are cardiovascular depressants.

Once intubated, sedation (+/−paralysis) should be maintained and an oro-gastric tube inserted. The oral route is preferred because of the risk of intracranial passage of a nasogastric tube in the presence of a base of skull fracture.

Breathing

All head injured patients requiring intubation will need ventilatory support. Ventilation should be monitored by arterial blood gas analysis and capnography. In most cases the patient should be ventilated to normocapnia. In the early stages after head injury the patient should not be hyperventilated excessively because it induces vasoconstriction which results in a reduced cerebral blood flow (CBF). Long-term outcome has been shown to be worse following prolonged hyper-ventilation ($PaCO_2$ < 3.4 kPa) in adults with severe head injuries. If used, hyper-ventilation should be titrated against the ICP and jugular bulb oxygen saturation (SjO_2).

Circulation

Haemorrhage should be controlled by whatever means is required. Large-bore intravenous cannulae are inserted and the blood pressure maintained with i.v. fluid. Hypotonic solutions should be avoided. In the adult, BP should be maintained above 120 mmHg systolic (children > 90 mmHg systolic). A vaso-pressor may be needed to counteract the vasodilatory effects of anaesthetic drugs, once hypovolaemia has been excluded. In the multi-trauma patient persistent hypotension and tachycardia implies blood loss from extracranial injuries. The haemoglobin should be maintained at > 10 g dl^{-1} in an attempt to ensure adequate cerebral oxygen delivery. Circulatory monitoring should include ECG, pulse oximetry, invasive blood pressure measurement, and urinary output. Severely head injured patients should not be moved or transferred until life threatening injuries are stable and an adequate mean arterial pressure has been achieved.

Disability

A rapid assessment of the GCS should be undertaken before anaesthesia is induced. An accurate assessment of the GCS and pupillary abnormalities takes a few seconds and has therapeutic and prognostic implications. See Scoring systems (p. 219).

Exposure

All patients should be fully exposed. Head injuries are often associated with other injuries. This exposure should include a log-roll. Life threatening extracranial injuries should be assessed fully and treated. X-rays of the chest and pelvis should be obtained and a urinary catheter inserted. Spinal X-rays should be obtained during the secondary survey.

Management of critically raised ICP

Critically raised ICP secondary to a CT proven or clinically suspected intracranial haematoma may be treated with a mannitol bolus (0.25–0.5 g kg^{-1}) and short-term hyperventilation. Mannitol is effective in lowering an acute rise in ICP but the hyperosmolality and dehydration may cause hypotension. Mannitol should be given as a bolus and not as an infusion. The use of hyperventilation or mannitol before ICP monitoring or CT scanning must be based on evidence of intracranial hypertension (pupillary dilation, motor posturing or progressive neurological deficit). Adequate sedation is essential. Serum osmolality may be used as a guide to mannitol therapy. The osmolality should not be allowed to rise above 310 mosmol kg^{-1}. Frusemide may be given instead of or in conjunction with mannitol.

Patients with severe head injury should be nursed approximately 30° head-up. This allows for adequate venous drainage and also reduces the risk of nosocomial pneumonia. A semi-rigid collar (if in place) should not be allowed to impede venous return and increase ICP.

Steroids

There is currently no evidence to support the use of steroids to lower ICP or improve outcome in patients with a severe head injury. Given the high incidence of side effects, their use in the management of severe head injury is not supported at this time.

Management of seizures

Seizures should be treated aggressively as they increase the cerebral metabolic rate and may lead to a critically raised ICP. The ABC sequence should be rechecked followed by a bolus of diazepam (0.1–0.2 mg kg^{-1}), thiopentone or propofol. This is usually followed by a loading dose of phenytoin (15–20 mg kg^{-1}).

Identifying head-injured patients who require immediate life-saving neurosurgery

Patients who have an expanding intracranial haematoma and a critically rising ICP, as shown by a deteriorating level of consciousness and/or progressive focal signs, require immediate neurosurgery. If it is necessary to transfer the patient to another centre for neurosurgery, CT scan should not delay transfer if it can be performed more rapidly at the neurosurgical centre. Surgery may also be required for hydrocephalus and elevation of a depressed skull fracture.

Reducing cerebral metabolic requirements

If conventional therapy fails to control intracranial pressure adequately, an infusion of thiopentone or propofol will reduce cerebral oxygen requirement ($CMRO_2$). Thiopentone is given by infusion while monitoring the EEG to produce burst suppression. Increased temperature results in increased metabolic requirements and increased cerebral blood flow. Hypothermia to temperatures of around 33°C has been used and there is some evidence that suggests an improved outcome following severe head injury. Temperatures of less than 34°C are associated with coagulopathy which may have a negative effect on outcome, particularly in those patients with multi-trauma.

Investigations

- Blood glucose, urea, creatinine, electrolytes and osmolality.
- Blood alcohol level.
- Arterial blood gases.

Computerized tomography

CT scanning is the most informative radiological investigation in the evaluation of head injury. CT scanning is needed to exclude lesions that require surgical intervention; the scans obtained have therapeutic and prognostic significance. The opportunity should also be used to scan the first and second cervical vertebrae and other areas of the cervical spine that are abnormal or inadequately seen on plain films. Adequate access to the patient, monitoring, and sedation must be ensured during CT scanning.

Monitoring

1. **ICP** monitoring should be commenced in all patients with severe head injury who are being managed actively. The gold standard remains a surgically placed intraventricular catheter which also allows the removal of CSF to reduce ICP. Prolonged periods with ICP > 25 mmHg are associated with a poor outcome. Monitoring ICP allows cerebral perfusion pressure (CPP) to be measured (CPP $=$ MAP$-$ICP). A CPP < 70 mmHg is associated with a poor outcome. Therefore, CPP is maintained at > 70 mmHg and it is usual for a vasopressor (e.g., noradrenaline) to be required to maintain this level.

2. **SjO_2** is measured by a fibreoptic catheter placed retrogradely in the internal jugular vein at the level of the C_1 vertebral body. Saturation measurements allow some assessment of global cerebral ischaemia or hyperaemia. Monitoring allows targeted hyperventilation, CPP management and osmotherapy. Saturations $< 55\%$ are associated with a poor outcome.

3. **Transcranial Doppler** allows assessment of CBF velocity. A pulsatility index can be derived which with SjO_2 can be used to define the optimum CPP.

4. **Evoked potentials and the electroencephalogram** (EEG) are used in selected patients to assess activity and gauge level of sedation in thiopentone coma. Regular assessment of GCS is mandatory. Deterioration in the GCS and/or the onset of lateralizing signs necessitates urgent investigation.

Adjunctive therapy

- Fluid balance should be carefully adjusted. Dramatic osmolar shifts, hyponatraemia and fluid overload should be avoided.
- Electrolyte disturbances are common in severe head injury patients as a result of fluid therapy, the stress response, osmotic and loop diuretics, and diabetes insipidus.
- Physiotherapy is important in preventing chest infection and limb contractures, but adequate sedation is required to prevent increases in ICP.
- Prophylactic antibiotics are required only for invasive procedures.
- Prophylactic anticonvulsants are often commenced in severe head injury. However, there is little evidence that anticonvulsant therapy has an impact on the development of late seizures. The relationship of early seizures to outcome is unclear.
- Early enteral nutrition reduces the incidence of gastric erosions, nosocomial chest infection and reduces the negative nitrogen balance that accompanies severe head injury.

- DVT prophylaxis should be initiated early. Compression stockings and calf compression devices may be used shortly after admission. Heparin therapy is often delayed because of the presence of intracerebral blood and the risk of further bleeding.

Outcome

Outcome is determined largely by the initial mechanism of injury. The post injury GCS provides a prognostic guide. Roughly a third of patients that survive a head injury with an initial GCS of less than 9 will never regain independent activity. The remainder of survivors can be expected to be independent or requiring some assistance.

Further reading

Chesnut RM. Guidelines for the management of severe head injury. In: Vincent JL (Ed). *Yearbook of Intensive Care and Emergency Medicine*. 1997. Berlin, Springer, pp. 749–765.

Bullock R *et al*. Guidelines for the management of severe head injury. Brain Trauma Foundation. *European Journal of Emergency Medicine* 1996 **3**: 109–127.

Related topics of interest

Brain stem death and organ donation, p. 48; Coma, p. 96; Convulsions, p. 100; Trauma – anaesthesia and critical care, p. 263; Scoring systems, p. 219; Trauma – primary survey and resuscitation, p. 257; Trauma – secondary survey, p. 260

HYPERTHERMIA

Richard Protheroe

Hyperthermia is a core temperature $> 37.5°C$. Severe hyperthermia is defined as a core temperature $> 40°C$ or an increase in body temperature at a rate greater than 2°C per hour. Hyperthermia leads to an increased metabolic rate and oxygen consumption which in turn requires an increase in cardiac output and minute ventilation to meet demand. With increased carbon dioxide production the patient starts to develop an acidosis, initially compensated for by tachypnoea. As the oxygen debt worsens a metabolic acidosis develops secondary to lactic acid production. Subsequent sweating and vasodilatation result in a relative hypovolaemic state and worsening of the metabolic derangement if left untreated. Neurological damage, seizures, rhabdomyolysis, acute renal failure, myocardial ischaemia and damage may all follow.

The aetiology of hyperthermia falls into two categories: increased heat production or decreased heat loss.

Increased heat production

1. Pyrogens/toxins. For example in sepsis, following burns, or blood transfusion reactions.

2. Drug reactions. As a consequence of excessive dosage of the drug or as an abnormal reaction to normal doses. Potential triggers include methylenedioxy-methamphetamine (MDMA, 'ecstasy'), thyroxine, monoamine oxidase inhibitors, tricyclic antidepressants, amphetamines, and cocaine. Hyperthermia following a drug reaction may manifest as the neuroleptic malignant syndrome (NMS) or serotonin syndrome.

3. Endocrine. Associated with hyperthyroidism or phaeochromocytoma.

4. Hypothalamic injury following cerebral hypoxia, oedema, or head injury/ trauma.

5. Malignant hyperthermia (MH).

Decreased heat loss

1. Excessive conservation especially in neonates and children.

2. Heat stroke.

3. Drug effects. As a predicted effect of anticholinergic administration, for example.

Management

1. General cooling measures. Decrease ambient temperature, exposure of the patient, skin wetting in combination with cold air fans provides efficient cooling. Application of ice packs to extremities may be used but is less efficient. Other measures include cold fluid given intravenously or intraperitoneally, cardiac bypass and cooling of blood volume.

2. Definitive treatment of underlying condition using dantrolene (e.g., in MH, NMS, MDMA poisoning) and mannitol (rhabdomyolysis, acute renal failure).

3. **General critical care.** Invasive monitoring to optimize fluid balance, sedation and ventilation if required.

MDMA; 'ecstasy'

An amphetamine derivative, first used as an appetite suppressant, and now a recreational substance of abuse. There is a range of adverse effects unrelated to dose or frequency of use. Psychosis, sudden cardiac death, seizures, tachycardia, hepatitis, subarachnoid haemorrhage, and acute renal failure may all occur. An acute syndrome comprising hyperthermia, DIC, rhabdomyolysis, acute renal failure and death may present in patients with a pre-existing metabolic myopathy or a genetic predisposition. Hyperpyrexia and myoglobinuria are triggered by a combination of sympathetic overactivity and vigorous muscular activity, as well as disturbance of central control. The aetiology appears to be an augmentation of central serotonin function by stimulation of neuronal serotonin release.

The peak temperature and duration of hyperthermia are important prognostic factors and any temperature > 40°C must be treated aggressively. Due to the similarity between this condition and MH, intravenous dantrolene has been accepted as part of the treatment. Serotonin antagonists or inhibitors of serotonin synthesis have been suggested as alternative therapies.

Serotonin syndrome

A potentially severe adverse drug reaction characterized by a triad of altered mental state, autonomic dysfunction (including hyperthermia) and neuromuscular abnormalities. The syndrome may follow the administration of selective serotonin re-uptake inhibitors such as sertaline, fluoxetine, peroxetine and fl006uroxamine. It occurs either in overdosage, in interaction with excess serotonin precursors or agonists (tryptophan, LSD, lithium, L-dopa), in interaction with agents enhancing serotonin (MDMA) or in drug interactions with non-selective serotonin re-uptake inhibitors such as clomipramine or impramine, or with monoamine oxidase inhibitors.

The cause of the syndrome appears to be excessive stimulation of serotonin receptors and as such the syndrome shows a similarity to both MDMA poisoning and the neuroleptic malignant syndrome. Treatment involves withdrawal of the precipitating agents and general supportive measures, although in severe cases serotonin antagonists such as chlorpromazine, cyproheptadine and methysergide as well as dantrolene may be used.

Neuroleptic malignant syndrome

This is an idiosyncratic complication of treatment with neuroleptic drugs such as the butyrophenones and phenothiazines. Patients are usually catatonic with extrapyramidal and autonomic effects including hyperthermia. The aetiology is unknown but appears to be related to antidopaminergic activity of the precipitating drug on dopamine receptors in the striatum and the hypothalamus suggesting a possible imbalance between noradrenaline and dopamine. There is no evidence of an association with malignant hyperthermia.

Clinical features include hyperthermia, muscle rigidity and sympathetic over-activity. Treatment involves withdrawal of the agent and general supportive and cooling measures.

Malignant hyperthermia

This is a rare pharmacogenetic syndrome with an incidence of between 1:10 000 and 1:200 000. It shows autosomal dominant inheritance with variable penetrance. The associated gene is on the long arm of chromosome 19. Other gene sites have been proposed and there may be considerable genetic heterogenicity. MH presents either during or immediately following general anaesthesia, (although it may occasionally be induced by severe exercise). The cardinal signs are hyperthermia, and a combined respiratory and metabolic acidosis often with associated muscle rigidity. Dysfunction of the sarcoplasmic reticulum increases intracellular ionic calcium, and results in depletion of high energy muscle phosphate stores, increased metabolic rate, hypercapnia and heat production, increased oxygen consumption and a metabolic acidosis. It results from exposure to the trigger agents, namely suxamethonium and the volatile anaesthetic agents.

On suspicion of MH, all trigger agents must be stopped immediately. The temperature, ECG, BP and end-tidal CO_2 levels should all be monitored and arterial blood gas analysis performed. Venous blood should be sampled intermittently for potassium, creatinine kinase and myoglobin, as well as FBC and a clotting screen. The urine output should be monitored and urine tested for myoglobin.

Dantrolene should be given in bolus doses of 1 mg kg^{-1} at 10 min intervals until the patient responds, up to a maximum dose of 10 mg kg^{-1}. Dantrolene is a muscle relaxant which acts by uncoupling the excitation-contraction mechanism. It is a yellow/orange powder stored in a vial of 20 mg with 3 g of mannitol and sodium hydroxide. It is stored below 30°C and protected from light. Reconstitution is with 60 ml of sterile water (it takes some time to dissolve) and forms an alkaline solution of pH 9.5.

General cooling measures should be undertaken and any hyperkalaemia treated with insulin and dextrose, calcium chloride and hyperventilation. Rehydration with intravenous fluids and promotion of a diuresis with frusemide or mannitol will help to prevent myoglobin-induced renal damage. DIC may develop.

Further reading

Halsall P, Ellis F. Malignant hyperthermia. *Current Anaesthesia and Critical Care* 1996; 7: 158–166.
Martin T. Serotonin syndrome. *Annals of Emergency Medicine*. Nov 1996; 28: 520–526.

Related topics of interest

Drug overdose, p. 109; Hypothermia, p. 136

HYPOTHERMIA

David Lockey

Normal body temperature is maintained between 36 and 37.5°C. Hypothermia is defined as a core temperature of less than 35°C and can be divided into mild (35–32°C), moderate (31–29°C) or severe (28°C or less). It may be induced or accidental. Induced hypothermia has been used for cerebral protection in neurosurgery, cardiac surgery and critical care to reduce the cerebral metabolic oxygen requirement. In the UK 0.7% of all hospital admissions and 3% of elderly patients admitted suffer from hypothermia. Internationally, death rates attributable to hypothermia vary widely and do not seem to depend only on the ambient temperature.

Aetiology

Accidental hypothermia can occur in individuals with normal thermoregulation exposed to severe cold. When thermoregulation is impaired it may occur following only a mild cold insult. Common causes include environmental exposure and water immersion. Patients with trauma, burns and neurological impairment (strokes, head injuries, diabetic coma and spinal cord injury) are at high risk. Patients with impaired thermoregulation include the elderly, babies, those with debilitation from any cause, and those taking depressant drugs especially alcohol.

Clinical signs

Most organ systems exhibit a progressive depression of function with increasing hypothermia.

1. Cardiovascular effects. Mild hypothermia causes sympathetic stimulation leading to vasoconstriction, tachycardia and increased cardiac output. As the temperature drops further there is progressive cardiovascular depression. ECG changes are common. Progressive bradycardia and prolonged PR and QT intervals occur. Widening of the QRS complex is a late finding. The 'J' wave at the junction of the QRS and T wave is a relatively constant finding below a core temperature of 33°C. It is not, however, specific to hypothermia. Atrial fibrillation is common in hypothermia. Below 28°C, VF may occur spontaneously and asystole usually occurs below 20°C. Arrhythmias are more likely at low temperatures because conducting tissues lose their conduction advantage over surrounding tissues.

2. Respiratory effects. Mild hypothermia causes respiratory stimulation then progressive depression occurs. Both respiratory rate and tidal volume decrease. Respiratory drive ceases at 24°C. There is also early depression of the cough reflex which makes aspiration more likely.

3. Central nervous system effects. Mild hypothermia causes confusion. Loss of consciousness usually occurs at around 30°C. Cerebral blood flow decreases by 7% per °C but there is a corresponding decrease in cerebral metabolic rate. In severe hypothermia electoencephalographic activity ceases (below 20°C) and muscle rigidity occurs.

4. Metabolic effects. Shivering occurs between core temperatures of 35°C and 30°C. This involves intense energy production and large increases in oxygen consumption and basal metabolic rate. Shivering can be limited by fatigue and glycogen depletion. Below 30°C, shivering ceases and thermoregulatory failure occurs. Basal metabolic rate decreases by approximately 6% per °C drop in temperature. Oxygen consumption drops accordingly. Blood gases are usually measured at 37°C. This will result in errors when judging the physiological state of a hypothermic patient. Gases are more soluble in blood at lower temperatures. Correcting values measured at 37°C to the actual patient temperature may reveal significant hypoxaemia. A mixed respiratory (decreased ventilation) and metabolic (decreased tissue perfusion) acidosis is usual. The oxyhaemoglobin dissociation curve is shifted to the left by decreased temperature with a consequent decrease in oxygen delivery. This effect may be offset by the right shift secondary to acidosis.

5. Renal effects. Initially renal blood flow increases. This leads to a diuresis and causes haemoconcentration. This relative hypovolaemia can be unmasked by rewarming. Electrolyte changes are variable and often reflect underlying comorbidity.

6. Haematological effects. At 35°C, clotting factor and platelet function is compromised. Clotting is increasingly impaired at lower temperatures and in severe cases there may be disseminated intravascular coagulation. Neutropenia and thrombocytopenia may result from splenic sequestration.

7. Endocrine effects. Pancreatic function is suppressed and there is reduced insulin secretion. There is also peripheral insulin resistance. Early hyperglycaemia may proceed to hypoglycaemia in prolonged hypothermia. Plasma cortisol levels are usually high. Hypopituitarism, hypoadrenalism and hypothyroidism predispose to hypothermia.

8. Infection. Hypothermia impairs the immune responses and chest infections are particularly common.

Drowning

Hypothermia caused by immersion in cold water has some specific features. When immersed in cold water in outdoor clothing core temperature falls slowly (1 hour to fall 2°C in water temperature of 5°C in laboratory conditions). When core temperature falls to 33–35°C muscles are usually considerably colder. This means that neuromuscular performance is poor and there is significant risk of aspiration and hypoxia long before any temperature related cerebral protection, which only occurs at much lower temperatures. Head immersion speeds cooling and children cool more quickly because of their large surface area to mass ratio and lack of subcutaneous fat. Even so, the cerebral protection sometimes seen in immersed children cannot be explained by cerebral hypothermia alone. The primitive mammalian diving reflex where sudden cooling of the face causes intense vasoconstriction, bradycardia and decreased metabolic rate may play a part in these rare cases. Hypothermia is said to be a good prognostic sign in unconscious drowning victims.

Diagnosis

A high index of suspicion and a low reading thermometer aids diagnosis. Investigations to detect the cause of unexplained hypothermia should include blood glucose, amylase, drug and toxin screen and thyroid function tests. The difference between death and hypothermia can be hard to distinguish. Many units operate a 'not dead until warm and dead' policy where patients are resuscitated until a core temperature of 34°C is achieved. Without extracorporeal rewarming this may be impossible. Patients should not be resuscitated if obviously lethal injuries are present or chest wall depression impossible.

Management

The underlying cause must be treated. General measures include removal from the cold environment and prevention of further heat loss. Rough handling may precipitate cardiac arrhythmias and tracheal intubation may rarely result in VF. Compromised patients should be carefully intubated and ventilated with high concentrations of warmed oxygen. Cardiac massage, though less effective in hypothermia, should be carried out in the normal way. Defibrillation is often ineffective below 30°C. Three shocks should be delivered and further shocks delayed until core temperature is increased. Drugs often have decreased effects in hypothermia and may have delayed and occasionally toxic effects on rewarming.

Rewarming

The aim of rewarming is to restore body temperature without fatal side effects. Rewarming may be passive external, active external or active internal (core rewarming). Passive external rewarming consists of placing the patient in a warm environment under insulating covers. This will not rewarm an arrested patient and is only recommended for mild hypothermia. The most effective active external is forced air warming. Internal or core rewarming is used to rewarm patients with severe hypothermia and those in cardiac arrest. Many techniques have been described including the use of warmed humidified gases, and irrigation of the stomach, colon, bladder or pleural cavity with warmed fluid. Peritoneal dialysis or haemodialysis are effective and may also be used to dialyse drugs or toxins if present. Cardiopulmonary bypass is the most rapid rewarming technique. It is the method of choice in arrested patients since it supports the circulation while rewarming. In trauma patients systemic anticoagulation should be avoided. A significant coagulopathy is usually present and heparin bonded systems are available to allow cardiac bypass in these circumstances. There have been no clinical trials of outcome to determine the best technique of rewarming.

Outcome

Widely different mortality rates are published for severe hypothermia. Patient populations are diverse. Low core temperature and the presence of significant co-morbidity are predictors of poor outcome.

Further reading

Larach MG. Accidental hypothermia. *Lancet* 1995; **345**: 493–498.
Lloyd EL. Accidental hypothermia. *Resuscitation* 1996; **32**: 111–124.

Related topics of interest

Coma, p. 96; Hyperthermia, p. 133

INFECTION CONTROL

S. Kim Jacobson

Infection control is an essential and an integral part of the running of any health care service whether or not it is in a hospital setting. For infection control to be effective it must be inter-disciplinary and interdepartmental. There is mounting evidence that controlling nosocomial infection not only improves morbidity and mortality, but also helps in the cost containment of medical procedures. Organisms multiply resistant to antibiotics such as MRSA, vancomycin resistant enterococci (VRE), multi-resistant *Mycobacterium tuberculosis* (MRTB) and extended spectrum beta-lactamase (ESBL) producing enterobacteriaceae are an increasing problem.

Alert organsims

These organisms are those that alert the infection control team to potential hazards in the ward. Other organisms, if a particular problem in an individual unit, can be added to the list as appropriate.

- MRSA.
- Group A beta-haemolytic streptococci (*Streptococcus pyogenes*).
- VRE.
- Muti-resistant Gram-negative organisms (e.g., ESBLs).
- *Clostridium difficile.*
- *Salmonella* spp., *Shigella* spp., *E. coli* 0157.
- *Mycobacterium tuberculosis.*
- Influenza A.
- Varicella zoster (chicken pox).
- Creutzfeldt–Jakob disease, and other prion diseases.

Risk factors for acquiring an infection

- Critical care unit admission for more than 48 hours.
- Trauma.
- Mechanical ventilation.
- Urinary catheterization.
- Vascular cannulae.
- Stress ulcer prophylaxis (where gastric pH is raised).
- Poor general condition of patient e.g., malnutrition, organ failure.
- Contaminated surgical procedure.

The antibiotics administered to the patient will drive the selection of organisms to those resistant to the drugs used, but the likelihood of the patient becoming infected is dependant on the above risk factors and the infection control practices adhered to in the unit.

Policies and procedures

Effective infection control in the critical care unit requires the following policies and procedures to be in place and adhered to:

- Antibiotic policies tailored to individual units.
- Asepsis and antisepsis policies tailored to individual procedures.

- Isolation procedures and indications.
- Disinfection and sterilization policies.
- Disposal of waste policies.
- Major outbreak procedures.

Hygiene

*1. **Environmental.*** The patient and the medical staff are the most likely source of surgical site infection. However, the quality of the environment has some part to play. The air quality of a critical care unit must be of a high standard and the air in most units is filtered. Some critical care units utilize high-efficiency particulate air filtration (HEPA) which filters out matter down to 0.5 mm and have a higher number of air exchanges per hour.

In addition to the quality of the air, the cleanliness of the environment is also important. Obvious dirt and dust are highly contaminated and are strongly linked with outbreaks of MRSA and *Clostridium difficile*.

*2. **Hand washing.*** The choice of hand preparation (hand wash, antiseptic hand preparation, or surgical scrub) is dependant on the degree of hand contamination and whether or not it is important to merely remove dirt and transient flora, or whether it is also important to reduce residual flora to minimum counts. This decision is ultimately dependant on the procedure about to be undertaken. Fundamentally, however, all clinical staff should perform hand washing before and after contact with a patient. Hand washing is defined as the removal of soil and transient organisms from the hands. For simple hand washing, plain soap and water should be used. There is no evidence that antibacterial soaps are of superior benefit. Soap does not kill the resident flora but does reduce transient flora, hence the importance of hand washing to reduce the transfer of pathogenic transient flora. The duration of hand washing is also important as the anti-microbial agents must be allowed enough time to be effective. All soap must then be rinsed off and the hands dried thoroughly with paper towels. Cloth towels harbour organisms. The tap should be turned off using either elbows or a paper towel which is then discarded.

When even greater reduction of transient organisms is required, hand antisepsis is necessary. This is achieved at the same time as hand washing by using soaps or detergents that contain antiseptics. It can also be achieved by using alcohol hand rub after removal of dirt, i.e., when hands are clean after initial hand washing. Large amounts of organic matter reduces the efficacy of alcohol. When dealing with more than one patient, hands can be cleansed between patients with alcohol alone provided all dirt is removed initially. The application of 70% ethanol to hands will reduce viable organism counts by 99.7%.

Preparations that contain emollients bind to the stratum corneum, prolonging the duration of action, and prevent excessive drying and damage of the skin.

Surgical hand scrub is the process used to remove or destroy transient microorganisms and reduce resident flora for the duration of the procedure. The optimal duration of surgical scrub is unclear and may be agent dependant, but approximately 5 min is usually appropriate. The agents used should be those that have demonstrated persistence. The moist and warm atmosphere inside latex surgical gloves is ideal for the proliferation of micro-organisms. This risk is reduced by agents that have a prolonged duration of action. Alcohol-based lotions are preferred in Europe and chlorhexidine or iodophors are more popular in the United States.

Poor compliance with these basic procedures is the most serious obstacle to adequate hand hygiene. Many studies have shown that health care workers do not wash their hands as thoroughly or as frequently as they should and audits indicate that doctors and nurses over estimate the efficacy of their hand washing.

3. Gloves. Gloves are not a substitute for careful hand hygiene and inappropriate use of gloves is a hazard. The appropriate use of gloves is during invasive procedures when they provide a barrier against microbial transmission to and from the patient. Gloves may not be necessary when examining patients as they are often not changed frequently enough. Transmission of organisms has been reported even when gloves are used. Thus, hands should be washed after removal of gloves, particularly after examining patients at risk of carrying hazardous organisms.

Further reading

Abrutyn F, Goldmann DA, Sheckler WE. *Saunders Infection Control Reference Service*. Saunders, 1998.
Mandell GL, Bennett JE, Dolin R. *Principles and Practice of Infectious Diseases*. 4th edn, Churchill Livingstone, 1995.

Related topic of interest

Infection in critical care, p. 143

INFECTION IN CRITICAL CARE

Susan Murray

Infection is a major cause of morbidity and mortality in the critically ill. Patients may have an infection at the time of admission to the critical care unit (acquired either from the community or hospital) or the infection may be acquired while on the unit. Community or early hospital acquired infections are more likely to be caused by relatively antibiotic sensitive organisms. However, late infections may be due to antibiotic resistant nosocomial (hospital acquired) bacteria or the patient's endogenous resistant flora selected by previous antibiotic therapy.

Patients in critical care units are at particularly high risk of nosocomial infection because of:

- Susceptibility to infection due an to underlying condition e.g., burns, trauma, surgery.
- Invasive procedures e.g., mechanical ventilation, intravascular and urinary catheterization.
- Underlying disease or drugs which depress natural barriers to bacterial colonization.
- Damage to the gut mucosa allowing bacteria and their products (e.g., endotoxins) to enter the blood stream.

Results from the European Prevalence of Infection in Intensive Care (EPIC) study show that 21% of patients had at least one infection acquired in a critical care unit. The major types of infection were pneumonia (47%), other lower respiratory tract infections [LRTI (18%)], urinary tract infection [UTI (18%)] and bacteraemia (12%) reflecting the difference from infection acquired on the ward where UTI predominates. This study also showed the increasing importance of Gram-positive bacteria in these infections (e.g., *Staphylococcus aureus*, coagulase-negative staphylococci and enterococci), which are often multi-resistant. The classic nosocomial pathogens such as *Pseudomonas* and *Acinetobacter* species still remain major problems on critical care units. They have a propensity to survive and transfer in this environment and have an innate resistance to antibiotics. There has been an emergence of Gram-negative bacteria which produce extended spectrum beta-lactamase (ESBL) (e.g., klebsiellae and *E. coli*) This is of concern as ESBL confers resistance to most beta-lactams including the newer cephalosporins. The use of broad-spectrum antibiotics accounts also for the increasing number of fungal infections on critical care units.

Most critically ill patients will need antibiotic therapy before the microbiological diagnosis is confirmed. The choice of antibiotics will be influenced by:

- The most likely site of infection and therefore the infecting organism.
- The patient's condition including age, allergies, previous antibiotics, and renal or hepatic dysfunction.
- Local and national resistance patterns of bacteria and fungi.
- The pharmacokinetic properties of each antibiotic

Close co-operation between microbiologists and critical care physicians to formulate and operate an antibiotic policy will help to prevent the overuse of broad-spectrum antibiotics. However, antibiotic guidelines are not a substitute for frequent discussions between these teams about individual patients. Suitable microbiological specimens (e.g., blood cultures, sputum and relevant swabs) must be taken before starting or changing antibiotics.

Respiratory tract infections

Epiglottitis (see p. 118)

Severe facial or chest trauma may lead to infection with respiratory tract flora such as *Staph. aureus, Strep. pneumoniae,* and *Haemophilus influenzae.* Environmental Gram-negatives and anaerobes may also be involved in the case of penetrating trauma. Initial therapy with a 2nd or 3rd generation cephalosporin with or without metronidazole is appropriate. This can be rationalised when culture results are known.

Late onset nosocomial pneumonia (see p. xx) needs careful consideration for appropriate treatment, and local resistance patterns must be taken into account. In many critical care units methicillin resistant *Staph. aureus* (MRSA) is a problem and is implicated in nosocomial pneumonia. A glycopeptide (i.e., vancomycin or teicoplanin), often with additional anti-staphylococcal treatment, such as rifampicin or fusidic acid, is used for treatment. The choice depends on renal and hepatic function and the ability to monitor serum levels, which are essential for vancomycin.

Gram-negatives (e.g., *Pseudomonas* spp. or enterobacteriaceae) are frequently involved and should be covered with empirical therapy (e.g., quinolones, extended spectrum cephalosporins, carbapenems or beta-lactams + inhibitors). Amino-glycosides do not penetrate well into respiratory secretions and should only be used if optimal levels can be achieved. More intrinsically resistant flora such as *Acineto-bacter* spp. and *Stenotrophomonas maltophilia* (inherently resistant to carba-penems) are now also implicated. ESBL producing strains of enterobacteriaceae, resistant to all beta-lactams except the carbapenems are increasingly being found and may also be resistant to quinolones or aminoglycosides. Long courses of antibiotics and invasive therapies such as parenteral nutrition will help to select for fungal (particularly candida) infections. Species other than *Candida albicans* tend to be more resistant to the imidazole group of antifungals e.g., fluconazole.

Viral pneumonias e.g., chickenpox, influenza and respiratory synctial virus may need admission to a critical care unit and specific antiviral treatment (e.g., acyclovir, amantidine, ribavirin).

Immunocompromised patients with pneumonia should be considered on an individual patient basis as cytomegalovirus or pneumocystis may be involved.

Urinary tract infection

Most patients in critical care units will have a urinary catheter *in situ.* The likelihood of the catheter becoming colonized with nosocomial bacteria increases with the duration of catheterization. Asymptomatic bacteriuria should not be treated, but if the patient becomes septic UTI should be considered along with other possible sources. Empirical broad-spectrum antibiotic therapy should cover likely urinary tract pathogens (e.g., an aminoglycoside or quinolone plus ampicillin). An extended spectrum cephalosporin, carbapenem or other beta-lactam + inhibitor combination may also be used.

Nosocomial bacteraemia

Nosocomial bacteraemia may occur in association with pneumonia, UTI, or localized sepsis, or it may be device related. Intravascular catheters are a significant source of bacteraemia in critically ill patients and lead to high rates of Gram-positive infections. The most frequently isolated bacteria are coagulase-negative staphylococci which are normally skin flora but produce an extra-cellular slime substance which allows them to adhere to foreign materials. It also inhibits access by antibiotics. These staphylococci are often multiply resistant and treatment is usually with a glycopeptide. Blood cultures should be taken both through the line and peripherally. Successful treatment may not be achieved with antibiotics and often line removal is necessary. *Staph. aureus*, Gram-negatives or *Candida* spp. may be the cause of line associated sepsis, and should be treated according to sensitivity along with early removal of the line.

Central nervous system infection

In general, patients with CSF leak are not treated prophylactically but in the presence of a pyrexia upper respiratory tract flora, especially *Strep. pneumoniae*, should be covered.

Meningitis (see p. 151)

Abdominal sepsis

In the surgical patient, treatment guidelines to cover bowel flora will depend on any antibiotics used as prophylaxis and the interval after surgery. Appropriate broad spectrum cover is provided by gentamicin (e.g., in a once daily dosage of 4 mg kg^{-1}), combined with ampicillin and metronidazole. Ciprofloxacin may be substituted for gentamicin. Alternatively agents with anaerobic activity (i.e., a carbapenum or piperacillin/tazobactam) or an extended spectrum cephalosporin combined with metronidazole may be used. However, local resistance patterns must always be taken into account.

Orthopaedic infection

Likely infecting organisms post-orthopaedic surgery are *Staph. aureus* and β haemolytic streptococci (groups A, C, G). If the patient has been admitted to hospital recently, the staphylococci are likely to be sensitive and would be covered by flucloxacillin. If the patient is allergic to penicillin or at risk of MRSA infection, a glycopeptide is most appropriate. If there is a likelihood of heavy environmental contamination, especially in compound fractures with exposed bone, cover should be extended to include Gram-negatives and anaerobes (e.g., with a once daily aminoglycoside, a quinolone or broad spectrum beta lactam agent, and metronidazole). Appropriate specimens, including blood cultures, tissue or bone at operation or wound swabs, should be taken.

The epidemiology of infection on critical care units must be monitored closely for increasing antibiotic resistance. Infection control measures are extremely important to help prevent the spread of multi-resistant bacteria. Antibiotic guidelines may be useful to help prevent the overuse of very broad-spectrum agents, but often therapy needs to be individualized and changed to narrow spectrum antibiotics on the basis of culture results.

Further reading

Bergmans DCJJ, *et al.* Indications for antibiotic use in ICU patients: a one year prospective surveillance. *Journal of Antimicrobial Chemotherapy* 1997; **39**: 527–535.

Brown EM. Empirical antimicrobial therapy of mechanically ventilated patients with nosocomial pneumonia. *Journal of Antimicrobial Chemotherapy* 1997; **40**: 463–468.

Flanagan PG. Diagnosis of ventilator associated pneumonia. *Journal of Hospital Infection* 1999; **41**: 87–99.

Infection in Neurosurgery Working Party of the British Society for Antimicrobial Chemotherapy. Antimicrobial prophylaxis in neurosurgery and after head injury. *Lancet* 1994; **344**: 1547–1551.

Vincent J-L, Bihari DJ, *et al*. The prevalence of nosocomial infection in intensive care units in Europe. Results of the European Prevalence of Infection in Intensive Care (EPIC) Study. *JAMA* 1995; **274**: 639–644.

Williamson ECM, Spencer RC. Infection in the intensive care unit. *British Journal of Intensive Care* 1997; 187–197.

Related topics of interest

Epiglottitis, p. 118; Infection control, p. 140; Meningitis, p. 151; Pneumonia – community acquired, p. 173; Pneumonia – hospital acquired, p. 177

LIVER DYSFUNCTION

James Low

Although liver dysfunction associated with critical illness is common, liver failure is rarely the primary reason for admission to a critical care unit. The principles behind the management of acute liver failure (ALF) and acute on chronic liver failure are broadly similar. Liver enzymes and plasma bilirubin are markers of liver disease. Characteristic responses of these markers in specific conditions are shown in *Table 1*.

Table 1. Patterns of liver function tests associated with liver disease

	AST/ALT	GGT	ALP	Bilirubin
Cholestasis				
Intrahepatic	++	++	++	+++
Extrahepatic	+	++++	++++	++++
Cirrhosis				
Alcoholic	N/+	++++	N/+	N/+
Primary biliary cirrhosis	+	+++	++	++
Hepatitis				
Chronic active hepatitis	++	++	+	+
Acute viral hepatitis	++++	++	N/+	++
Drug induced hepatitis	++	++	N/+	++
ICU Jaundice	N/+	N/+	N/+	++

AST, Aspartate aminotransferase; ALT, Alanine aminotransferase; GGT, Gamma-glutamyltransferase; ALP, Alkaline phosphatase.

Acute liver failure

1. Definition. ALF is the onset of hepatic encephalopathy within 8 weeks of presentation and in the absence of pre-existing liver disease. More recently the terms 'hyperacute' (encephalopathy within 8 days from the onset of jaundice), 'acute' (jaundice to encephalopathy 8–28 days), and 'subacute' (jaundice to encephalopathy 4–26 weeks) have been proposed. Hepatic encephalopathy is classified clinically into 4 grades:

1. Altered mood; impaired intellect, concentration, and psychomotor function, but rousable and coherent.
2. Inappropriate behaviour; increased drowsiness and confusion, but rousable and conversant.
3. Stuporous but rousable, often agitated and aggressive.
4. Coma; unresponsive to painful stimuli

2. Aetiology. In the UK, paracetamol overdose is the most common cause of ALF, followed by viral hepatitis and drug induced hepatotoxicity.

Prognosis of ALF

Mortality is as high as 80%. The main causes of death are cerebral oedema and multiple organ failure. Bad prognostic features are:

- Age < 10 or > 40 years
- Aetiology   Cryptogenic
- Degree of encephalopathy   Grade 3 or 4
- PT > 50 sec
- Plasma factor V $< 20\%$
- Serum bilirubin $> 300\ \mu mol\ l^{-1}$
- Serum creatinine $> 350\ \mu mol\ l^{-1}$
- Alpha fetoprotein   low
- Arterial pH < 7.3
- Arterial ketone body ratio < 0.6

Chronic liver failure

The commonest cause of chronic liver disease is alcohol abuse. Other causes include infections (hepatitis B and C), drugs (methotrexate), autoimmune (primary biliary cirrhosis), and hereditary conditions such as Wilson's disease. Common causes of acute decompensation of a patient with chronic liver disease include occult or overt GI bleeding, infection (commonly spontaneous bacterial peritonitis), hypokalaemia, constipation, systemic alkalosis, excess dietary protein, use of psychoactive drugs or benzodiazepines, porto-systemic shunts, progressive hepatic parenchymal damage.

Common to all these causes is increased production of ammonia or increased diffusion of ammonia across the blood–brain barrier (BBB). Many of these events are reversible with good recovery of liver function.

Clinical presentation and investigations. Most patients with severe chronic liver disease have subclinical hepatic encephalopathy and commonly present with mental deterioration. They are also immune suppressed and will not demonstrate the usual signs and symptoms of sepsis. Features of encephalopathy include asterexis and confusion. Other variable findings are those of underlying chronic liver disease, worsening ascites, hypoalbuminaemia, and signs of thrombocytopenia or coagulopathy (prolonged PT). Investigations are aimed at excluding common causes of acute decompensation (listed above), establishing the cause of the chronic liver disease, and excluding other non-hepatic causes of acute deterioration (e.g., stroke, meningitis, alcohol intoxication, hypoglycaemia).

Management of acute and chronic liver failure

1. General considerations. Patients with liver failure are critically ill and have a predictably high mortality. They should be managed in a specialist unit with access to appropriate facilities for managing the complications and to provide transplantation if required. They will usually require intubation and ventilation to protect the airway and optimize oxygenation. Invasive cardiovascular monitoring with fluid resuscitation and inotropic support should be instituted. Hypokalaemia and alkalosis are common in both conditions, often secondary to diuretics or vomiting. All electrolyte and acid–base abnormalities must be corrected aggressively. Diagnostic procedures such as CT scans, endoscopy and paracentesis should be carried out urgently to establish the aetiology and any possible complications.

Acute liver failure	Chronic liver failure

Cardiovascular

Hypovolaemia secondary to vomiting is common.

Stability may improve with n-acetyl cysteine infusions.

Hypovolaemia is very common.

Occult GIT bleeding should be excluded.

CVP pressures may be very high secondary to high portal and intra-abdominal pressures.

Renal

Acute renal failure secondary to fluid depletion is common.

The combination of ALF and ARF carries a very poor prognosis and early renal support should be considered.

ARF secondary to sepsis and MOF may occur but generally occurs later.

Hepatorenal syndrome is common. It is a functional renal failure characterized by oliguria, high urinary osmolality and low urinary sodium. The hepatorenal syndrome must be distinguished from dehydration and invasive monitoring is essential. The prognosis is related to the severity of the liver disease.

Bleeding

A severe coagulopathy usually occurs due to decreased synthesis and increased consumption of clotting factors. Coagulopathy is an important prognostic factor. Transfuse clotting factors only after consultation with the local transplant centre.

Patients often have a long-standing coagulopathy due to the pre-existing liver disease and poor synthetic function. This may be exacerbated by hypersplenism due to portal hypertension and the consumption of clotting factors due to sepsis. Give clotting factors as required.

Encephalopathy

Cerebral oedema is a significant factor in the pathogenesis. Avoid hyperventilation, which will aggravate cerebral ischaemia. Give mannitol as required. Raised intracranial pressure may develop suddenly and without clinical signs; ICP monitoring may improve the outcome.

Cerebral oedema is not a common feature. There is increased production of ammonia and/or increased diffusion across BBB. Oral lactulose, neomycin or metronidazole may decrease ammonia production while correction of electrolyte and acid–base abnormalities will reduce diffusion across the BBB. Eradication of *H. pylori* will reduce ammonia production and may help.

Infection

Sepsis commonly complicates ALF but is rarely the initiating event.

Systemic infection is a common cause of acute deterioration in CLF. In patients with ascites, spontaneous bacterial peritonitis is a common source. A diagnostic tap should be performed, as clinical signs of peritonitis may be absent.

Nutrition

Enteral feeding can be used. The use of feeds with branched-chain amino acids is controversial and has not been shown to improve outcome.

High calorie, low protein enteral nutrition is indicated. Restrict dietary protein to 20 g a day and slowly increased until tolerance is established.

2. **Indications for liver transplantation in ALF.** The 5 year survival rates for liver transplantation are now 50–85%. Criteria defining those patients with a poor prognosis who are most likely to benefit from transplantation are:

(a) PT > 100 sec.

or

(b) Any three of the following:

- Age less than 10 or greater than 40 years.
- PT > 50 sec.
- Serum bilirubin > 300 μmol l^{-1}.
- Non-A, non-B hepatitis, halothane, or other drug aetiology.
- Duration of jaundice before onset of encephalopathy > 2 days.

If ALF is induced by paracetamol

- pH < 7.30.

or

- Grade 3 or 4 hepatic encephalopathy and creatinine >300 μmol l^{-1} with PT > 100 sec.

Hepatic dysfunction in acute illness

Hepatic dysfunction and jaundice are common in critically ill patients. This 'ICU jaundice' is precipitated typically by sepsis, trauma, or major surgery and develops 1–2 weeks later. Plasma bilirubin rises to 150–300 μmol l^{-1} and is 70–80% conjugated. Plasma ALP may be normal or moderately elevated. Concurrent hepatic ischaemia may elevate plasma aminotransferase concentrations. Other causes of jaundice, such as extrahepatic biliary obstruction, must be excluded. The use of TPN may contribute to liver dysfunction in critically ill patients; typically plasma concentrations of ALT and ALP are doubled and the plasma bilirubin is variable. Histologically, there is fatty infiltration of the liver.

Drug induced liver dysfunction can present with a variety of patterns: acute hepatitis (paracetamol, halothane), acute cholestatic hepatitis (flucloxacillin, erythromycin), and cholestasis without hepatitis (oral contraceptives).

The management of hepatic dysfunction in acute illness is largely supportive and aimed at treating the initiating event. Hepatic failure in association with multiple organ failure carries a very poor prognosis.

Further reading

Fontana JF. Acute liver failure. *Current Opinion in Gastroenterology* 1997; **13**: 271–279.
Riordan SM, Williams R. Treatment of hepatic encephalopathy. *New England Journal of Medicine* 1997; **337**: 473–479.

Related topics of interest

Drug overdose, p. 109; SIRS, sepsis and multiple organ failure, p. 228

MENINGITIS

Jeff Handel

Bacterial infection is the usual cause of meningitis in patients admitted to critical care units. A variety of viruses (particularly herpes simplex) may cause meningo-encephalitis and opportunistic organisms, including protozoa and fung, may cause meningitis in immunocompromised patients. Non-infective processes, such as connective tissue disorders and malignant infiltration, may also cause meningitis.

Epidemiology

Bacterial meningitis is more common in childhood. The peak incidence of about 1:1000 occurs in children under 1 year of age. The likely causative organism depends upon the age group. Group B streptococci (*Streptococcus agalactiae*), K1 capsulate *Escherichia coli* and *Listeria monocytogenes* are the commonest organisms in neonates. In older children bacterial meningitis is usually caused by *Neisseria meningitidis* (meningococcus) and *Streptococcus pneumoniae* (pneumococcus). The incidence of *Haemophilus influenzae* meningitis has declined dramatically since the introduction in Britain in 1992 of an effective conjugated vaccine against this organism.

In adults the most common infecting organisms are meningococci and pneumococci, the latter being more common in elderly patients. Small numbers of cases are caused by Gram-negative bacilli and *Listeria monocytogenes* following ingestion of contaminated food such as unpasteurized soft cheeses. Infection with *listeria* is more common at the extremes of age, in pregnant women, and in immunocompromised patients. Post-traumatic meningitis is usually caused by pneumococcus whilst device (CSF drains and shunts) associated meningitis is usually caused by coagulase negative staphylococci or *Staphylococcus aureus*. Tuberculous meningitis is more common in children, the elderly, the immunocompromised, and the immigrant population.

Pathology

An intense inflammatory process in the meninges, extending into the brain, results from the presence of bacteria and their fragments in the CSF. The inflammatory reaction causes cell damage and death as a result of oedema, the generation of cytotoxic free radicals and the release of excitatory neurotransmitters in the presence of tissue hypoxia. These effects are compounded by intracranial hypertension which impairs cerebral perfusion and, ultimately, may cause brain stem herniation.

Clinical features

The classical features of meningism; headache, neck stiffness, fever, reduced conscious level, Kernig's and Brodzinski's signs, are common in adults but not reliably present in children. Infants with meningitis and raised intracranial pressure (ICP) may have a bulging anterior fontanelle. In tuberculous meningitis symptoms and signs may develop insidiously over several weeks. A characteristic petechial rash usually accompanies meningococcal meningitis if there is concomitant septicaemia.

Investigation

The diagnosis of meningitis is made by examination of CSF obtained by lumbar puncture. If ICP is raised this procedure carries a risk (1–8%) of causing brain stem herniation, particularly in the presence of a focal space occupying lesion. If there are signs of raised ICP (e.g. reduced conscious level or papilloedema) or focal neurological signs, a CT scan may be useful to identify cerebral oedema, mass lesions, or other differential diagnoses such as subarachnoid haemorrhage. It should be remembered, however, that a CT scan might appear normal in the presence of raised ICP. When there is clinical and/or CT scan evidence of raised ICP the diagnostic benefits of lumbar puncture should be weighed against the risks. If the risk of brain stem herniation is high it may be safer to treat the patient empirically. In a few centres, rapid antigen testing and DNA PCR testing of blood may be available.

The CSF in bacterial meningitis characteristically has a high neutrophil count, low glucose and high protein concentrations. A raised lymphocyte count is seen in early bacterial meningitis, *Listeria monocytogenes*, tuberculous, and viral meningitis, and, importantly, may be seen in partially treated bacterial meningitis.

If organisms are not seen on microscopy culture may take days or, in the case of tuberculosis, even weeks.

Treatment

Antibiotic therapy is usually started empirically, before the diagnosis and organism are confirmed. The choice of antibiotic is determined by the likely pathogen considering the patient's age. Microscopy, culture and sensitivity will later confirm the appropriateness of the antibiotic given. Expert microbiological advice should always be sought. In practice, a third generation cephalosporin such as cefotaxime is appropriate for adults and children older than neonates.

Complications

*1. **Seizures**.* Treatment with benzodiazepines, phenytoin, or phenobarbitone alone or in combination is usually effective. Resistant seizures and status epilepticus may require thiopentone which usually necessitates intubation and ventilation.

*2. **Raised ICP**.* This may result from cerebral oedema and/or hydrocephalus, brain abscess, sterile subclinical effusion, or empyema for which specific neurosurgical treatment may be indicated. Strategies for the management of raised ICP include intubation and control of ventilation to prevent hypercapnia and hypoxia, and resuscitation with fluids and vasoactive drugs to maintain blood pressure and cerebral perfusion pressure. Nursing the patient in a slightly head up posture will reduce venous pressure and enhance cerebral perfusion. Pyrexia should be controlled and active cooling may reduce the cerebral metabolic demand. Hyperglycaemia may worsen ischaemic brain damage and should be treated. Osmotic diuretics can reduce cerebral oedema, but repeated administration in conditions such as meningitis, where the blood brain barrier is impaired, may worsen cerebral oedema.

Various nerve palsies and learning difficulties may persist in patients recovering from meningitis. Nerve deafness is particularly common. The role of steroid therapy is not fully understood but administration in the acute illness may reduce the incidence of permanent hearing loss in children with *Haemophilus influenzae* or pneumococcal meningitis.

Prophylaxis

Prophylaxis is not usually considered necessary for contacts of patients with pneumococcal meningitis. For meningococcal meningitis see page xx.

Prognosis

With current antibiotic regimens and treatment strategies the mortality of bacterial meningitis in the UK is 10% or less, with 10% of survivors suffering permanent neurological damage.

Further reading

Quagliarello VJ, Scheld WM. Treatment of bacterial meningitis. *New England Journal of Medicine* 1997; 336: 708–716.
Tauber MG. Management of bacterial meningitis in adults. *Current Opinion in Critical Care* 1998; 4: 276–281.

Related topics of interest

Infection control, p. 140; Infection in critical care, p. 143; Meningococcal sepsis, p. 154; SIRS, sepsis and multiple organ failure, p. 228

MENINGOCOCCAL SEPSIS

Jeff Handel

Meningococcal sepsis is caused by the Gram-negative coccus *Neisseria meningitidis*. The group B subtype causes two thirds of cases and group C about one third. Although 10% of the population have chronic asymptomatic nasopharyngeal carriage of pathogenic meningococci, invasive disease probably results from recent acquisition of the organism.

Meningococcal sepsis may occur at any age but it most commonly affects children and younger adults. It presents as a septicaemic illness which ranges in severity from a mild condition to fulminant septic shock with severe systemic inflammatory response and MOF. Death may occur in a matter of hours from intractable cardiovascular failure. Meningococcal meningitis and septicaemia can occur separately or as part of the same illness. The prognosis of meningococcal sepsis may be worse when meningitis is not present. Occasionally, meningococcal sepsis can present as a subacute condition with mild symptoms lasting several weeks. There may be a focus of infection such as septic arthritis.

If meningitis is present typical signs of meningism may occur.

Clinical features

Meningococcal sepsis begins usually as a non-specific illness with fever, influenza-like symptoms and sometimes diarrhoea. This may evolve rapidly into profound shock and MOF.

The skin rash consists typically of spreading petichiae and ecchymoses. It is caused by capillary thrombosis and extravasation of red cells. It may cause large areas of skin infarction with loss of digits or limbs. Meningococci can often be detected in the skin lesions.

Management

Suspected meningococcal sepsis must be treated promptly and aggressively. Antibiotic therapy should be started immediately. The organism is almost always sensitive to penicillin G and cefuroxime. If there is a clear history of sensitivity to penicillin, chloramphenicol is an alternative. It has been suggested that antibiotics may increase endotoxin levels by lysing bacteria but treatment should not be delayed.

Aggressive cardiovascular resuscitation with fluids and inotropes is invariably necessary. Haemodynamic monitoring with a pulmonary artery flotation catheter may help to guide therapy. Patients frequently require intubation and ventilation for cardiorespiratory and neurological failure.

Adrenocortical infarction has been well described in meningococcal sepsis, and dysfunction with reduced glucocorticoid and mineralocorticoid production may occur as part of the SIRS. The role of steroid replacement therapy is controversial.

New therapies

Plasma exchange and haemofiltration to remove the mediators of septic shock, and ECMO to treat intractable cardiovascular failure, have both been recommended as adjunctive therapies. However, no benefit to outcome has been shown from either of these treatments.

A multicentre trial of recombinant bactericidal/permeability increasin protein, an endotoxin binding agent to block the inflammatory cascade, is currently being undertaken. Similarly, the effects of protein C, which may inhibit intravascular thrombosis and reduce organ damage, are also being assessed in meningococcal sepsis.

Mortality

The mortality from meningococcal sepsis is approximately 19% overall and 40–50% in patients who are shocked. Scoring systems have been developed to predict mortality for groups of patients. The most common is the Glasgow Meningococcal Score which uses seven weighted factors:

- Blood pressure.
- Skin/rectal temperature difference.
- Coma score.
- Absence of meningism.
- Rash.
- Base deficit.
- Deterioration in the last hour.

The maximum score is 15. A score of 8 predicts a 73% probability of death.

Vaccination

Effective vaccines have been developed against groups A and C meningococci. Unfortunately group B meningococcus is not sufficiently immunogenic to produce an effective vaccine yet.

Meningococcal sepsis is a notifiable disease. Antibiotics (rifampicin or cipro-floxacin) to eradicate carriage are offered to household contacts of individual cases. In the case of a cluster (two cases in a community within a 4 week period), antibiotics are offered to all members of the community. Vaccine is offered to contacts of patients with disease due to group A or C meningococcus.

Further reading

Weir PM. Meningococcal septicaemia. *Current Anaesthesia and Critical Care* 1997; **8**: 2–7.

Related topics of interest

Infection control, p. 140; Infection in critical care, p. 143; Meningitis, p. 151; SIRS, sepsis and multiple organ failure, p. 228

MYASTHENIA GRAVIS

Myasthenia gravis (MG) is an autoimmune disease. The majority of patients (~90%) have antibodies to the nicotinic acetylcholine receptors in the post-synaptic membrane of the neuromuscular junction, although the correlation between absolute antibody levels and disease severity is weak. Muscarinic acetylcholine receptors, and thus the autonomic nervous system, are spared. Thymus disease is associated with MG; 75% of patients have histological evidence of an abnormality (e.g., germinal centre hyperplasia) whilst 10% have a benign thymoma. Other autoimmune disorders are associated with MG (e.g., thyroid disease, pernicious anaemia) as are certain HLA subgroups. The prevalence of MG is around 5 per 100 000 population with young women being affected most commonly (peak onset 20–30 years of age). Men over the age of 50 are the next most commonly affected, though most patients with a thymoma associated with MG fall into this group. Critical care may be required for patients with MG under the following circumstances;

- In crisis (myasthenic or cholinergic).
- With resultant respiratory failure.
- Following pulmonary aspiration.
- With a complication of immunosuppressive therapy.
- For post-operative care following a thymectomy.

Clinical features

The muscle weakness of MG is typically made worse by exertion and improved by rest. The characteristic distribution of affected muscles, in descending order, is extra-ocular, bulbar, cervical, proximal limb, distal limb and trunk. Thus patients frequently complain of ptosis and diplopia, and dysphagia. Severe bulbar weakness leaves them at risk from frequent pulmonary aspiration.

The Eaton–Lambert syndrome, by contrast, is characterized by muscle weakness which improves on exertion and spares the ocular and bulbar muscles. It is a condition associated with small-cell carcinoma of the bronchus and sufferers, like myasthenics, are exquisitely sensitive to non-depolarizing muscle relaxants.

Investigations

1. Edrophonium test. The diagnosis of MG is established by administering an intravenous dose of the short-acting anticholinesterase edrophonium. Anticholinesterases increase the amount of acetylcholine available at the neuromuscular junction. An improvement in muscle function following edrophonium thus supports the diagnosis. Prior to administering the drug, intravenous access, continuous ECG monitoring, and full resuscitation facilities should be established. Patients weak due to cholinergic crisis may become apnoeic after edrophonium. A muscle group appropriate for the patient (i.e., where they are weak) is chosen for assessment. For those with respiratory weakness, forced vital capacity is measured. A test dose of 2 mg of edrophonium is administered intravenously, followed, in the absence of adverse effects, by 8 mg 1 min later. Muscle function is assessed prior to, and 1 and 10 min following the administration of edrophonium.

2. Electromyography. A decremental response in the size of the compound motor action potential after repeated electrical stimulation of a motor nerve can confirm the diagnosis. This is true even in the majority of those with only ocular symptoms.

Treatment

1. Anticholinesterases. Pyridostigmine bromide 60 mg is given four times a day and increased until an optimal response is achieved. It may not be possible to abolish all weakness and increasing the dose in an attempt to do so may precipitate a cholinergic crisis.

2. Anticholinergics. May be required to control side effects of anticholinesterase administration such as salivation, colic, and diarrhoea. They are not used as a matter of routine in all patients.

3. Immunosuppression. Corticosteroids may benefit those patients with pure ocular symptoms and those whose response to anticholinesterases is suboptimal. Their administration may be associated with an initial deterioration and improvement may take several weeks. Plasma potassium levels should be monitored to ensure that steroid induced hypokalaemia (enhanced renal potassium loss) is not adding to muscle weakness. Azathioprine has been used in those with severe myasthenia unresponsive to other measures.

4. Plasma exchange. Some patients show a short lived but dramatic improvement in weakness following plasma exchange. Maximum response is usually seen about a week after a series of five or so daily exchanges. Improvement lasts for around a month. It may be a useful technique for those in severe myasthenic crisis or to allow weaning from ventilation.

5. Thymectomy. Thymectomy results in clinical improvement in around 80% of all myasthenics. It produces a more rapid onset of remission and is associated with a lower mortality than medical therapy alone. Patients due to undergo thymectomy should have their respiratory function optimized pre-operatively. Plasma exchange and steroids may help with this. The dose of pyridostigmine should be reduced as much as possible without compromising respiratory function. This is because thymectomy often leaves patients more sensitive to the effects of anticholinesterases and cholinergic crisis may ensue after surgery. Also, the intraoperative management of neuromuscular blockade is easier in the presence of a mildly myasthenic patient.

Myasthenic crisis

This is a severe life threatening worsening of MG. It can progress rapidly to respiratory failure necessitating urgent tracheal intubation and respiratory support. Myasthenic crisises can be precipitated by infection, pyrexia, surgical or emotional stress, and certain drugs. These drugs include aminoglycoside (e.g., gentamicin) and polymixin (e.g., neomycin) antibiotics, membrane stabilizing anti-arrhythmics (e.g., quinidine, procainamide lignocaine), anticonvulsants (e.g. phenytoin), and antidepressants (e.g., lithium). If the patient's FVC falls below $10-15$ ml kg^{-1}, or they are unable to adequately expectorate secretions, they require intubation and respiratory support. Many then withdraw all anticholinesterase therapy and rest the patient, believing that the sensitivity of the motor end plate to acetylcholine will increase under such circumstances.

Subcutaneous heparin should be given for prophylaxis against thrombo-embolism. Plasma exchange or immunosuppressive therapy may be required to wean the patient from mechanical ventilation.

The differential diagnosis of an acutely weak patient with MG includes cholinergic crisis.

Cholinergic crisis

A cholinergic crisis is caused by an excess of acetylcholine available at the neuro-muscular junction and usually follows excessive administration of anticholinergics. It too may present with respiratory failure, bulbar palsy and virtually complete paralysis. It may be difficult to distinguish from a myasthenic crisis but often includes an excess of secretions, which may worsen the respiratory failure. Other symptoms more likely during a cholinergic crisis include abdominal pain, diar-rhoea, and blurred vision. The differential may be made by administering a small dose of intravenous edrophonium. Patients in myasthenic crisis should improve, where as those with a cholinergic crisis will get worse.

Further reading

Drachman DB. Myasthenia gravis. *New England Journal of Medicine* 1994; **330**: 1797–1810.

Related topic of interest

Respiratory support – weaning from ventilation, p. 210

NUTRITION

Martin Schuster-Bruce

Nutritional support is a routine part of critical care. Malnutrition is a common problem in critically ill patients and is associated with increased morbidity and mortality. It may be present on admission or can develop during the course of critical illness. In starvation, fat and protein are lost, but the protein loss is minimized and fat oxidation becomes the principle source of energy. However, in critical illness, with hypermetabolism, accelerated protein catabolism occurs. The rationale for providing nutritional support for critically ill patients is to prevent the breakdown of muscle and visceral protein.

Nutritional requirements

1. Energy. Existing body mass is the major determinant of total energy requirement. This can be measured directly using a metabolic chart or estimated using either a nutritional index (e.g., Harris Benedict) or on a simple weight basis. Twenty-five to 30 kcal kg^{-1} body weight day^{-1} is adequate in most patients. Thirty to 70% of the total energy can be given as carbohydrate, 15–30% as fat and 15–20% as protein sources.

2. Nitrogen. Nitrogen intake should be 0.1–0.3 g kg^{-1} day^{-1} and can be given as protein (1.2–1.5 g kg^{-1}) or amino acids.

3. Micronutrients. The precise requirements for vitamins, minerals and trace elements have yet to be determined.

Route of administration

Enteral. There is good evidence that enteral nutrition (EN) has additional affects, beyond the supply of energy and protein. These include modulation of the host's immune response, improved splanchnic perfusion, maintenance of gut integrity and possibly prevention of bacterial translocation and multiple organ dysfunction (MODS). Therefore, current data support the initiation of EN as soon as possible after surgery or resuscitation.

Standard 500 ml proprietary feeds are iso-osmotic solutions containing 1–1.5 kcal ml^{-1} of energy, 45% of which is as carbohydrate, 20–35% as lipid and 15–20% as protein. Feeds are gluten and lactose free and contain substrates similar to those found in a normal diet (i.e., polymeric). They provide the normal requirements of electrolytes, vitamins and trace elements. Elemental feeds are available, but polymeric feeds are preferred since they are less likely to induce diarrhoea. Feeds are administered continuously with a daily 4-hour rest period to allow restoration of gastric pH, which may prevent bacterial overgrowth in the stomach.

The nasogastric route is used most commonly, but impaired gastric emptying can limit infusion rates. Prokinetics may improve gastroparesis or, alternatively, the small bowel can be fed directly via nasojejunal or surgical jejunostomy tubes.

There are few absolute contraindications (intestinal obstruction, anatomic disruption and severe intestinal ischaemia). Enteral nutrition can be successful in virtually all critically ill patients even after major surgery and in acute pancreatitis. The main complications of EN are failure to achieve nutritional targets, abdominal pain, distension and diarrhoea. Nutritional targets are more likely to be met if EN is administered by strict protocol.

Enteral nutrition is no longer a therapy simply to prevent malnutrition.

Prokinetic agents

Metoclopromide promotes normal gastric emptying by dopamine antagonism. Erythromycin has a direct contractile effect via the motilin receptor and normalises gastric emptying in diabetic induced gastroparesis. Cisapride increases physiological release of acetylcholine in the myenteric plexus without dopamine antagonism, to improve gastric emptying. It may cause prolongation of the QT interval. Imidazole antifungals and macrolide antibiotics inhibit its metabolism and co-administration should be avoided.

Parenteral. Failure of EN alone is not an indication for parenteral nutrition. Parenteral nutrition does not share the additional benefits of EN and there is good evidence that it may increase morbidity and mortality in critically ill patients. Parenteral nutrition is indicated only in the small group of patients who are unable to be enterally fed for up to 7 days. Patients who are malnourished before their critical illness and are unable to tolerate early EN may require parenteral nutrition immediately.

Intravenous fat emulsions have replaced glucose as the main energy source since they cause less metabolic derangement. Nitrogen is delivered as amino acids. Most hospitals use parenteral nutrition solutions, which have been prepared aseptically in the hospital pharmacy and contain all the requirements for a 24-hour period in a single bag. The feeds are non-physiological, hyperosmolar and irritant and are therefore administered into a central vein.

Complications include all those of central venous access. The risk of venous thrombosis and catheter related sepsis is substantially increased. Catheter related sepsis is reduced by the use of a dedicated lumen, minimizing handling of the line and the use of anti-microbial coatings. Subcutaneous tunnelling does not seem to be of benefit. Other complications of parenteral nutrition include gut mucosal atrophy, hyperglycaemia and hepatobiliary problems, particularly fatty infiltration and intrahepatic cholestasis. Compared to EN, parenteral nutrition is nutritionally incomplete and dietary deficiencies can occur.

Immunonutrition

During severe illness, there is an alteration in the immune response, metabolic homeostasis and the inflammatory response. Specific dietary substrates have been evaluated for their individual effects on metabolic and immune functions.

Glutamine is an amino acid that facilitates nitrogen transport and reduces skeletal and intestinal protein catabolism. It is the major fuel for the enterocyte and preserves intestinal permeability and function. Arginine is an amino acid that improves macrophage and natural killer cell cytotoxicity, stimulates T-cell function and modulates nitrogen balance. Omega-3-polyunsaturated fatty acids are derived from fish oil and are potent anti-inflammatory agents and immune modulators. Nucleotides have immunostimulant properties on natural killer cells and T-lymphocytes.

An enteral feed supplemented with arginine, nucleotides and omega-3-polyunsaturated fatty acids is commercially available. Randomized clinical trials suggest that immune-enhanced feeds may improve outcome.

Further reading

Applied Nutrition in ICU patients. A Consensus Statement of the American College of Chest Physicans. *Chest* 1997; **111**: 769–778.

Jolliet P, Pichard C, Biolo G, *et al.* Enteral nutrition in intensive care patients: a practical approach. *Intensive Care Medicine* 1998; **24**: 848–859.

Zaloga GP. Immune-enhancing enteral diets: Where's the beef? *Critical Care Medicine* 1998; **26**: 1143–1146.

Related topics of interest

Infection in critical care, p. 143; SIRS, sepsis and multiple organ failure, p. 228

OBSTETRIC EMERGENCIES – MAJOR HAEMORRHAGE

Jenny Tuckey

In the UK between 1994 and 1996, 12 deaths were due to obstetric haemorrhage (5.5 per million maternities). This comprised three cases of placenta praevia, four of abruptio placenta and five patients with post-partum haemorrhage. Haemorrhage becomes life threatening when blood loss exceeds 40% of the blood volume.

Obstetric haemorrhage may occur antepartum (APH) or post-partum (PPH). Consideration of the fetus will be necessary in the case of an APH. The principles of resuscitation are similar for APH or PPH. The obstetric intervention required will depend upon the cause of the blood loss.

Antepartum haemorrhage

Defined as bleeding from the birth canal after 20th week of pregnancy and before the birth of the baby. An ultrasound scan will help differentiate the cause.

The main causes are:

- Placental abruption.
- Placenta praevia/accreta.
- Uterine rupture.
- Placental conditions e.g., circumvallate formation, vasa praevia.

Placental abruption

1. **Definition.** Separation of a normally implanted placenta (usually by haemorrhage into decidua basalis) from the 20th week of pregnancy.

2. **Incidence.** Occurs in 1–1.5% pregnancies and accounts for 20–25% APH. Recurs in 10–15% pregnancies. Associations include smoking, cocaine abuse, low socioeconomic status, poor nutritional status, advancing age, advancing parity.

3. **Aetiology.** The cause is identified in only the minority of cases. Causes include severe hypertensive disorders, trauma (e.g., RTA, external cephalic version), and sudden reduction in size of uterus which may cause premature separation of the placenta e.g., second twin.

4. **Clinical features.** Bleeding may be revealed, concealed or a mixture of the two. The fetus suffers as a direct reduction in the functioning intervillous space as well as indirect effects of maternal vasoconstriction and uterine spasm. If retroplacental haemorrhage > 500 ml occurs, fetal death is likely; if > 1000 ml, serious maternal sequelae are likely, including shock and disseminated intravascular coagulation (DIC).

With increasing placental separation there is increasing abdominal tenderness, pain, rigidity and increased likelihood of fetal death. The uterine fundus may be higher than expected for gestational age.

Placental praevia

1.   **Definition.** The placenta is situated partly or wholly in the lower uterine segment of the uterus.

2.   **Incidence.** 0.5–1% of pregnancies and is responsible for 15–20% APH.

3.   **Types of placenta praevia**
- First degree: part of the placenta is in the lower segment but does not reach the internal os.
- Second degree: the lower margin of the placenta reaches the internal os but does not cover it.
- Third degree: the placenta covers the os when closed but not completely when dilated.
- Fourth degree: the placenta lies centrally over the os.

The significance of these gradings is that morbidity and mortality for mother and fetus increase the more the placenta encroaches upon the os. Because the endometrium is less well developed in the lower uterine segment, the placenta is more likely to become attached to the underlying muscle (placenta praevia accreta). This may cause problems during the third stage of delivery when placental separation should occur.

4.   **Aetiology.** Implantation low in the uterine cavity increases with age, parity, multiple pregnancy, previous LSCS or termination and smoking.

5.   **Clinical features.** Painless vaginal bleeding in the latter stages of pregnancy. The onset may be spontaneous or precipitated by coitus, coughing or straining. Any painless bleeding in the second half of pregnancy is placenta praevia until proved otherwise. Definitive diagnosis is by means of ultrasound scan. If there is a major degree of placenta praevia, Caesarean section (LSCS) will be required for safe delivery. There is often difficulty in delivering the placenta. This is because there is poorer contraction of the lower segment muscle, high vascularity and risk of placenta accreta. There is a higher than normal risk of PPH.

6.   **Management.** After significant APH, hospitalize women with placenta praevia in 3rd trimester. Pursue conservative management until the fetus is mature. Deliver by LSCS by senior obstetric and anaesthetic personnel. Anterior placenta praevia may be under the incision site. Cross match six units of blood, site two large intravenous cannulae and use a fluid warming device. If the placenta is anterior and especially if there has been a previous LSCS, general anaesthesia is the technique of choice. The placenta may be morbidly adherent. Anticipate PPH.

Post-partum haemorrhage

PPH may be primary or secondary.

Primary PPH

1.   **Definition.** Bleeding of 500 ml or more from the birth canal in the first 24 hours after delivery. Major PPH is blood loss > 1000 ml in the 24 hours after delivery.

2. Incidence. There is an increased incidence if very short or prolonged labour, macrosomia or multiple gestation, magnesium used in severe pre-eclampsia, operative delivery, LSCS, previous PPH, chorioamnionitis and in obesity.

3. Aetiology. Retained products of conception, uterine atony, trauma (e.g., uterine rupture or lacerations of the birth canal), bleeding diathesis.

Retained products of conception

Occurs in 2–5% pregnancies. It is obvious if the entire placenta is retained. It is less obvious if the placenta is ragged and a small cotyledon retained. Treatment includes evacuation of the uterus under anaesthesia, regional or general. If there is placenta accreta, either wholly or in part, there will be no plane of cleavage and the risk of uterine rupture will be high. Haemorrhage may require embolization or ligation of the uterine or iliac arteries. Hysterectomy may be required.

Uterine atony

Less common now with routine use of oxytocic drugs. Exacerbated by volatile anaesthetics, β-blockers, and magnesium sulphate. Normal uterine contraction is inhibited by a full bladder, uterine sepsis, exhaustion from a long labour and high parity.

Management. Obstetric manoeuvres such as uterine massage, bimanual compression, administration of oxytocin, ergometrine. If these fail, intramyometrial injection of 1–2 mg of prostaglandin F2 is appropriate. Compression of bleeding points is also possible using uterine packing or Sengstaken-Blakemore balloon inflated with 300 ml saline, in the short term.

Trauma

1. Uterine rupture. Occurs in multiparous women with large fetus or malpresentation e.g., brow, injuditious use of oxytocics, operative and other trauma e.g., external version with uterine scar, breech extraction, mid forceps delivery.

- Clinical. Pain, tenderness on abdominal palpation and shock. Contractions decrease. Fetal distress. Symptoms more extreme if upper segment rupture. Treatment includes uterine repair and, if necessary, hysterectomy.

2. Local trauma to the lower birth canal. Rarely causes life-threatening haemorrhage.

Coagulation defect

In obstetric practice, DIC is the commonest cause of failure of blood clotting. Predisposing factors include severe abruption, intrauterine death, severe pre-eclampsia, amniotic fluid embolism, sepsis, and shock.

Management should involve discussion with senior haematologist.

Secondary PPH

Defined as excessive bleeding after first 24 hours post-partum until end of puerperium. Generally caused by retained products of conception which act as a nidus for infection.

Treatment. Antibiotics.

Unusual sequelae of obstetric haemorrhage

Sheehan (pathologist England 1937) reported infarction of anterior and occasionally posterior lobe of pituitary gland. The first clinical manifestation is failure of lactation, then amenorrhoea. Later there will be failure of thyroid and adrenal axes.

Principles of management of obstetric haemorrhage

The principle goal is successful maternal resuscitation. All fetal issues are secondary to this. The aim is to maintain or restore adequate oxygen delivery to all organs including the uteroplacental unit.

Further reading

Jouppila P. Postpartum haemorrhage. *Current Opinion in Obstetrics and Gynecology* 1995; 7: 446–450.

William Stones R, Paterson CM, Saunders NJ. Risk factors for major obstetric haemorrhage. *European Journal of Obstetrics and Gynecology and Reproductive Biology* 1993; **48**: 15–18.

Related topics of interest

Blood coagulation, p. 34; Obstetric emergencies – medical, p. 166

OBSTETRIC EMERGENCIES – MEDICAL

Jenny Tuckey

Pulmonary thromboembolism (PE)

There were 48 deaths due to thromboembolism reported to the Confidential Enquiry into Maternal Deaths (CEMD) during 1994–1996 (rate 21.8 per million pregnancies). Of the 48 deaths, 46 were due to PE and two to cerebral embolism secondary to DVT. Thromboembolism is the single greatest cause of direct maternal deaths in the UK and occurs in approximately 1 in 2000 pregnancies. (see page 189)

Pregnancy-induced hypertension

There were 20 direct deaths due to pregnancy-induced hypertension reported to the CEMD during 1994–1996 (rate 9.1 per million pregnancies). Pre-eclampsia may be defined as 'gestational proteinuric hypertension developing during pregnancy or for the first time in labour'. It occurs in approximately 10% of pregnancies, most commonly between 33 and 37 weeks gestation. The only cure is delivery of the placenta. Pre-eclampsia generally resolves within 48–72 hours of delivery. The commonest causes of death due to hypertensive diseases of pregnancy (CEMD 1994–1996) are: ARDS, cerebral oedema, intracranial haemorrhage, pulmonary oedema and ruptured liver.

The American College of Obstetricians and Gynecologists use any one of the following to define severe pre-eclampsia: systolic blood pressure (BP) > 160 mmHg, diastolic BP > 110 mmHg, mean arterial pressure > 120 mmHg, proteinuria (5 g in 24 hours or +3/+4 on 'dipstick' testing), oliguria (< 500 ml in 24 hours), headache or cerebral disturbance, visual disturbance, epigastric pain or raised liver enzymes (transaminases), pulmonary oedema or cyanosis, HELLP (haemolysis, elevated liver enzymes, low platelets).

The prognosis in mild pre-eclampsia is good. Severe pre-eclampsia is associated with morbidity and mortality.

Eclampsia

Eclampsia is diagnosed if one or more grand mal convulsions (not related to other conditions) occurs in pre-eclampsia. The incidence, (according to the British Eclampsia Survey Team, 1994), is 4.9 per 10000 maternities. Two per cent of eclamptics die, whilst 35% suffer major complications. Eclampsia is commoner in teenagers and in cases of multiple pregnancy.

HELLP syndrome

The HELLP syndrome is one form of severe pre-eclampsia and is associated with a maternal mortality of up to 24%. HELLP syndrome presents with malaise in 90%, epigastric pain (90%) and nausea and vomiting (50%). Physical signs include right upper quadrant tenderness (80%), weight gain and oedema. Blood pressure may be normal and proteinuria may be absent. Resolution of symptoms following delivery may be slow. These patients may require dialysis. Corticosteroids may normalize platelets and liver enzymes and hasten recovery.

1. *Management of pre-eclampsia.* The general aims are to minimize vasospasm, improve perfusion of uterus, placenta and maternal vital organs, and assess fetal maturity.

-   Antihypertensive agents are given if the diastolic blood pressure persistently exceeds 100 mmHg (e.g., labetolol, nifedipine or hydralazine).
-   Regular assessment of proteinuria, urate, platelet count, and the fetus is required.
-   If the pregnancy is < 34 weeks two doses of dexamethasone (12 mg) are given to aid maturation of the fetal lungs. Delivery is ideally delayed for 48 hours for maximal benefit.
-   Magnesium sulphate may be given as prophylaxis against convulsions. It is a central nervous system depressant, cerebral vasodilator and mild antihypertensive. It increases prostacyclin release by endothelial cells, increases uterine and renal perfusion, and decreases platelet aggregation. Conversely, its tocolytic effect may prolong labour and increase blood loss. A bolus dose of 4 g is given followed by an infusion of 1–3 g h^{-1}. Tendon reflexes, respiratory rate, SpO_2 and mental state should all be monitored. Therapeautic blood levels are 2.0–3.5 mmol l^{-1}. Heart block and respiratory paralysis occur at 7.5mmol l^{-1}. The antidote is calcium gluconate.

2. *Fluids in severe pre-eclampsia.* In severe pre-eclampsia, CVP correlates poorly with left ventricular end diastolic pressure. If the CVP is zero, there is scope for a fluid challenge. Measurement of pulmonary artery occlusion pressure may be useful if there is evidence of pulmonary oedema, if blood products are required because of haemorrhage, or if there is prolonged oliguria.

Amniotic fluid embolism (AFE)

Between 1994 and 1996, there were 17 maternal deaths due to AFE (7.7 per million maternities). The incidence is 1 in 8000 to 1 in 80000 live births. Mortality is as high as 86%, with 50% dying within the first hour. Amniotic fluid embolus can occur in early pregnancy, at the time of termination of pregnancy or amniocentesis, or following closed abdominal trauma. It can also occur during Caesarean section or artificial rupture of the membranes, as well as during the more widely described oxytocic driven vigorous labour of an elderly multip with a large baby.

Pathophysiology

Amniotic fluid or fetal matter enters the maternal circulation. This can occur asymptomatically. The presence of meconium worsens prognosis. For amniotic fluid to enter the maternal circulation there must be rupture of membranes and breach of uterine veins.

Clinical features

Typically, there is a sudden onset of dyspnoea, cyanosis and hypotension out of proportion to blood loss, followed quickly by cardiorespiratory arrest. Up to 20%

will have seizures and up to 40% will have DIC with bleeding from the vagina, surgical incisions, and intravenous cannula sites. Non-cardiogenic pulmonary oedema will follow in up to 70% of initial survivors.

Management of AFE is symptomatic and supportive.

Intracranial bleed

Between 1994 and 1996 there were 24 maternal deaths reported due to intracranial haemorrhage (14 subarachnoid haemorrhage and nine primary intracerebral).

Cardiac arrest in pregnancy

This is almost always an unexpected event and attendant personnel usually have little experience of resuscitation of cardiac arrest. Hypoxia develops rapidly due to the reduced FRC and increased oxygen consumption of pregnancy. Early intubation is essential to prevent aspiration and because of the reduced pulmonary compliance. Caval compression should be avoided and chest compressions performed with a wedge beneath the victim's right hip, or the gravid uterus displaced manually. If spontaneous circulation is not restored rapidly the fetus should be delivered by immediate Ceasarean section. Resuscitation should not be abandoned until after delivery of the fetus.

Local anaesthesia toxicity

Circumoral numbness, tinnitus, light-headedness, confusion and a sense of impending doom are typical complaints. Muscle twitching and grand mal convulsions may occur. All these symptoms and signs are exacerbated by acidosis and hypoxia. Central nervous system symptoms usually occur before cardiovascular collapse.

Further reading

Department of Health, Welsh Office, Scottish Office Department of Health and Social Services, Northern Ireland. *Report on Confidential Enquiries into Maternal Deaths in the United Kingdom 1994–1996.* Norwich; Her Majesty's Stationery Office, 1998, pp. 48–55.

Related topics of interest

Convulsions, p. 100; Obstetric emergencies – major haemorrhage, p. 162; Pulmonary embolism, p. 189; Resuscitation – cardiopulmonary, p. 213; Subarachnoid haemorrhage p. 245

PANCREATITIS

Inflammation associated with acute pancreatitis may also involve tissues around the pancreas and/or remote organs. Approximately 80% of cases of acute pancreatitis are mild and resolve with simple fluid and electrolyte replacement and analgesia. However, the remaining 20%, representing those with severe acute pancreatitis, are subject to organ failure and/or local complications (e.g., necrosis, pseudocysts, fistulae). Severe disease carries a mortality of 10–20%.

Causes

Alcohol abuse and gallstones account for 80% of cases of acute pancreatitis. Acute idiopathic pancreatitis occurs in about 10% of cases. However, biliary sludge can be found in two thirds of these and they often respond to endoscopic sphincterotomy. Many other conditions make up the remaining 10% of causes (e.g., drugs, trauma, infections, and tumours).

Pathogenesis

For reasons that remain incompletely understood (possibly related to duodeno-pancreatic reflux), pancreatic enzymes are activated prematurely. This results in autodigestion of pancreatic tissue. In severe cases, circulating enzymes cause a systemic inflammatory response syndrome (SIRS).

Clinical features

Continuous, epigastric pain that radiates through to the back is a typical presentation of acute pancreatitis. It is often accompanied by nausea and vomiting and a low grade fever. Abdominal distension, due to an associated ileus, is common. Evidence of retroperitoneal bleeding in the form of periumbilical (Cullen's sign) or flank (Grey–Turner's sign) bruising is rare but should be sought as a prognostic indicator. There may be evidence of basal pleural effusions and atelectasis.

There are two phases in the clinical course of severe acute pancreatitis. The early toxaemic phase (0–15 days) is characterized by SIRS associated with marked fluid shifts. In the later, necrotic phase, intra-abdominal necrosis with or without subsequent infection causes local and systemic complications.

Investigations

1. Amylase. The appropriate clinical features in combination with a serum amylase of > 1000 U will confirm the diagnosis of acute pancreatitis. If the upper limit of the normal range for serum amylase is used as the cut-off value, the specificity is reduced to 70%. Amylase is a small molecule and is cleared rapidly by the kidneys. Serum lipase takes longer to clear and may be a better 'historical' indicator of pancreatitis. The combination of both serum amylase and lipase will provide sensitivity and specificity of 90–95% for detecting acute pancreatitis.

2. Ultrasound. Abdominal ultrasound will identify gallstones, although bowel gas associated with an accompanying ileus may make the examination technically difficult.

3. *Computerized tomography.* Contrast enhanced computerized tomography (CT) of the abdomen is the best method of imaging the pancreas. It may show pancreatic necrosis, and/or pseudocysts. CT is indicated:

- Where the initial diagnosis is in doubt.
- In the presence of severe pancreatitis, fever and leucocytosis, CT-guided fine needle aspiration will help with the diagnosis of infected pancreatic necrosis.

Prognostic indicators

A number of scoring systems have been used to help to assess the severity of pancreatitis. The APACHE II system allows rapid determination of prognosis but is relatively complex. Ranson's criteria form the most popular system. They are divided into five criteria that are assessed on admission and a further six that are evaluated at 48 hours:

1. *On admission*
- Age > 55 years.
- White blood count $> 16\,000$ mm^{-3}.
- Glucose > 11 mmol l^{-1}.
- Lactate dehydrogenase > 350 IU l^{-1}.
- Aspartate aminotransferase > 250 U l^{-1}.

2. *During initial 48 hours*
- Haematocrit decrease $> 10\%$.
- Blood urea increase > 1.8 mmol l^{-1}.
- Serum calcium < 2 mmol l^{-1}.
- $PaO_2 < 8$ kPa.
- Base deficit > 4 mmol l^{-1}.
- Fluid sequestration > 6 l.

The presence of fewer than 3 Ranson's criteria indicates a mild pancreatitis and a mortality of $< 1\%$. The mortality increases to 16% in the presence of 3–4 criteria and $> 40\%$ with 5 or more criteria. The presence of 3 or more of Ranson's criteria indicates a likely need for admission to a critical care unit. The Imrie score reduces the number of Ranson's criteria by 3 (LDH, base deficit, and fluid deficit) without losing predictive power.

Management

The general principles of management are metabolic and nutritional support, control of symptoms, and prevention and treatment of vital organ dysfunction.

1. *Resuscitation.* Patients with acute pancreatitis will require aggressive fluid resuscitation with CVP guidance, and correction of hyperglycaemia and electrolyte disorders. Patients with SIRS associated with severe pancreatitis will often require inotropic support. Abdominal distension, basal pleural effusions, and atelectasis all contribute to significant respiratory embarrassment even in the absence of ARDS. The level of respiratory support required will range from simple oxygen therapy to intubation and mechanical ventilation.

2. **Calcium.** The rationale for correcting hypocalcaemia associated with pancreatitis is not entirely clear. Total serum calcium does not correlate well with ionized calcium and any replacement should be titrated against the latter. Correction of hypocalcaemia will improve arterial pressure but may not enhance cardiac index and oxygen delivery.

3. **Nutrition.** Oral feeding is withheld and nasogastric drainage is usually instituted, although there is little hard data to support either of these therapies. Most patients with mild uncomplicated pancreatitis do not benefit from nutritional support. However, patients who have moderate to severe pancreatitis should receive early nutritional support. State of the art consensus indicates that a trial of nasojejunal feeding should be initiated and parenteral nutrition given only if this is not tolerated. It is likely that deeply entrenched dogma will prevent this approach from becoming accepted for some time.

4. **Analgesia.** The severe pain associated with acute pancreatitis will require systemic opioids or thoracic epidural analgesia. The latter is more effective and in the absence of contraindications is the method of choice. Theoretical concern that morphine causes spasm of the sphincter of Oddi has led to the recommendation of pethidine for systemic analgesia. In reality, morphine is probably a better choice.

5. **Antibiotics.** Prophylactic antibiotics are indicated for those patients who are predicted to develop severe pancreatitis. Bacterial infection of necrotic pancreatic tissue occurs in 40–70% of patients with acute necrotizing pancreatitis. Prophylactic high dose cefuroxime, a quinolone or a carbapenem have been shown to reduce morbidity, though not mortality.

6. **Gallstone extraction.** Endoscopic retrograde cholangiopancreatography (ERCP) and extraction of gallstones is indicated in the acute setting only when increasing jaundice or cholangitis complicates severe pancreatitis.

7. **Surgery.** The precise role of surgery in acute pancreatitis remains controversial. It usually reserved for one or more of the complications discussed below.

Complications

The systemic complications of MODS or failure are well-recognized sequelae of SIRS. Local complications include pancreatic necrosis, pseudocysts, and fistulas.

1. **Pancreatic necrosis.** Pancreatic necrosis is detected by lack of enhancement of the pancreatic tissue on contrast-enhanced CT scan. Once necrosis develops the presence of bacterial contamination and the general condition of the patient will determine the outcome. The role of surgical intervention in sterile necrotizing pancreatitis is undecided. However, if the patient is improving medical treatment is probably sufficient. If necrosis is detected in the deteriorating patient, CT-guided aspiration of pancreatic tissue is indicated. If Gram stain and culture confirm infection the patient should undergo some form of surgical debridement.

2. **Pseudocyst.** A pseudocyst is a collection of pancreatic secretions that lacks an epithelial lining. Drainage should be considered in the following circumstances:

- Larger than 5–6 cm in diameter.
- Pain.
- Gastric outlet obstruction.
- Infection or haemorrhage into the cyst.

Drainage may be undertaken percutaneously or at laparotomy. Ultrasound- or CT-guided percutaneous drainage is an effective method for decompression although there is a significant risk of recurrence.

3. Fistulas. Disruption of the pancreatic duct may cause pancreatic fistulas. A pancreaticopleural fistula will result in an extensive pleural effusion. A pancreaticoperitoneal fistula should be suspected in patients with massive ascites. Persistent pancreatic fistulas will require surgery.

Further reading

Baron TH, Morgan DE. Acute necrotizing pancreatitis. *New England Journal of Medicine* 1999; **340:** 1412–1417.
Mergener K, Baillie J. Acute pancreatitis. *BMJ* 1998; **316:** 44–48
Wyncoll DL. The management of severe acute necrotising pancreatitis: an evidence based review of the literature. *Intensive Care Medicine* 1999; **25:** 146–156.

Related topic of interest

SIRS, sepsis and multiple organ failure, p. 228

PNEUMONIA – COMMUNITY ACQUIRED

Pneumonia is an acute septic episode with respiratory symptoms and radiological shadowing, which was neither pre-existing nor of other known cause. The criteria for precise clinical definition are:

1. The presence of a new radiographic pulmonary infiltrate.
2. Acute onset of at least one 'major' and two 'minor' clinical findings suggestive of pneumonia.

The 'major' criteria are cough, sputum production and fever. The 'minor' criteria are dyspnoea, pleuritic chest pain, altered mental status, lung consolidation (on physical examination), and a total leukocyte count of over $12\,000\ mm^{-3}$.

Community-acquired infection is defined as an infection that occurs in a patient who has not been hospitalized in the preceding 2 weeks or one that occurred within 48 hours of admission to hospital. Approximately 80–95% of adults with pneumonia are treated at home by general practitioners. One per thousand of the population are admitted to hospital with pneumonia annually. Of those patients requiring admission to a critical care unit, the mortality is 30–50%. Community-acquired pneumonia (CAP) occurs more commonly in those over 65, smokers, and those with other non-respiratory illnesses. The pathogenesis of CAP differs from pneumonia acquired while the patient is in hospital (nosocomial pneumonia). Although antibiotic strategies differ, the general approach to critical care management of pneumonia is the same regardless of the aetiology.

Epidemiology

Streptococcus pneumoniae is the commonest cause of CAP. It is isolated in about 30% of cases and probably accounts also for the third of cases in which no causative organism is found. Other organisms commonly found are listed below. Although *Legionella* is relatively rare as a cause of CAP in the UK, it is the second commonest cause after *Strep. pneumoniae* in the United States and Spain.

Pathogens in CAP in the UK:

Streptococcus pneumoniae	30%
Mycoplasma pneumoniae	15%
Haemophilus influenzae	8%
Influenza viruses	8%
Legionella species	5%
Chlamydia species	2–3%
Staphylococcus aureus	3%
Moraxella catarrhalis	1–2%
Other organisms	5–8%
No pathogen found	30%

H. influenzae is the commonest cause of bacterial exacerbation of COPD. The possibility of *Staph. aureus* should be considered during an influenza epidemic, particularly if there is radiological evidence of cavitation. *Mycoplasma* is commonly associated with cough, sore throat, nausea, diarrhoea, headache, and myalgia. On the whole, clinical features are not sensitive or specific enough to predict the microbial aetiology. As legionellosis has become increasingly recognized, and less severely ill patients are seen earlier in the course of the disease, clinical features of unusual severity once considered distinctive of legionnaire's disease are now known to be non-specific. However, hyponatraemia does occur more frequently in legionnaire's disease than in other types of pneumonia.

Assessment of severity

There is a 20-fold increase in the risk of death or need for critical care when two or more of the following factors are present:

- Respiratory rate $\geqslant 30$ min^{-1}.
- Diastolic blood pressure $\leqslant 60$ mmHg.
- Serum urea > 7 mmol l^{-1}.

A more comprehensive list of features associated with an increased risk of death is given below:

1. *Clinical features*
- Respiratory rate $\geqslant 30$ min^{-1}.
- Diastolic blood pressure $\leqslant 60$ mmHg.
- Age $\geqslant 60$ years.
- Underlying disease.
- Confusion.
- Atrial fibrillation.
- Multilobar involvement.

2. *Laboratory features*
- Serum urea > 7 mmol l^{-1}.
- Serum albumin < 35 g l^{-1}.
- Hypoxaemia: PaO$_2$ $\leqslant 8$ kPa.
- Leucopenia: WBC $\leqslant 4000 \times 10^9$ l^{-1}.
- Leucocytosis: WBC $\geqslant 20\,000 \times 10^9$ l^{-1}.
- Bacteraemia.

Investigations

Investigations should be undertaken to assess severity and identify aetiology:

- CXR.
- Arterial blood gas analysis.
- Full blood count: a white cell count $> 15\,000 \times 10^9$ l^{-1} makes a bacterial pathogen likely. A normal count is often seen in atypical or viral infection, but this is not specific enough to be of diagnostic value.
- Urea, electrolytes and liver function tests
- Sputum Gram stain, culture and sensitivity. The presence of Gram-positive diplococci implies pneumococci. Results of sputum culture must be interpreted cautiously; many of the organisms responsible for pneumonia are normal upper respiratory tract commensals.

- Urine antigen test. *Legionella* antigen can be detected in urine. The test has a sensitivity of 70% and a specificity of almost 100%.
- Blood culture.
- Serology is available for influenza A and B viruses, respiratory syncytial virus, adenovirus, *C. burnetti*, *C. psittaci*, *M. pneumoniae* and *L. pneumophila*, but does not often provide diagnostic changes early enough to be clinically useful. However, the majority of patients with *Mycoplasma* pneumonia will have a positive *Mycoplasma*-specific immunoglobulin M titre on admission to hospital.
- Bronchoscopy is normally reserved for those with very severe pneumonia. This will allow sampling by protected specimen brush (PSB) or by bronchoalveolar lavage (see nosocomial pneumonia). Bronchoscopy will also allow the diagnosis of any underlying lung disease such as a bronchial tumour.

Management

All patients with severe CAP should be given oxygen to maintain arterial $PaO_2 > 8$ kPa, and antibiotics as indicated below. On the ward, the minimum monitoring should include regular pulse, blood pressure and respiratory rate, pulse oximetry and repeat blood gas sampling. Physiotherapy is helpful for those patients with copious secretions. These patients will often be dehydrated and may require intravenous fluid replacement. According to the British Thoracic Society, the indications for transfer to the ICU include:

- Severe pneumonia (as defined above).
- Arterial $PaO_2 < 8$ kPa with $FiO_2 > 0.6$.
- Arterial $PaCO_2 > 6.4$ kPa.
- Exhausted, drowsy or unconscious patient.
- Respiratory or cardiac arrest.
- Shock.

These criteria are relatively extreme; a patient with severe CAP should be admitted to a HDU (when available) before they have deteriorated to this level. Mask CPAP and/or NIPPV will improve oxygenation and may prevent the need for tracheal intubation. However, if the patient's admission to the critical care unit has been delayed until they are exhausted, non-invasive techniques are unlikely to be successful.

Antibiotic therapy

The infecting organism is usually unknown when treatment is initiated. Empirical therapy should always cover *Strep. pneumoniae*. Penicillin-resistant pneumococci are relatively rare in the UK but are increasing in other parts of the world. A second- or third-generation cephalosporin (e.g., cefuroxime or cefotaxime) combined with clarithromycin is appropriate empirical therapy. Antibiotic treatment should be continued for 5–7 days and then reviewed. If *Legionella* is suspected clarithromycin should be combined with rifampicin or ciprofloxacin. Staphylococcal pneumonia is treated with flucloxacillin.

Further reading

Brown PD, Lerner SA. Community-acquired pneumonia. *Lancet* 1998; **352**: 1295–1302.

Hosker HSR, Jones GM, Hawkey P. Management of community acquired lower respiratory tract infection. *British Medical Journal* 1994; **308**: 701–705.

The British Thoracic Society. Guidelines for the management of community-acquired pneumonia in adults admitted to hospital. *British Journal of Hospital Medicine* 1993; **49**: 346–350.

Related topics of interest

Arterial blood gases – analysis, p. 28; Chronic obstructive pulmonary disease, p. 91; Infection control, p. 140; Infection in critical care, p. 143; Pneumonia – hospital acquired, p. 177; Respiratory support – non-invasive, p. 200; Respiratory support – invasive, p. 205

PNEUMONIA – HOSPITAL ACQUIRED

Introduction

Nosocomial infection is defined as an infection occurring more than 48 hours after hospital admission, or within 48 hours of discharge. Nosocomial pneumonia accounts for 15% of all hospital acquired infections and 40% of infections acquired in the ITU. It is a cause of considerable morbidity and mortality.

Pathogenesis

The aetiology of nosocomial pneumonia is influenced significantly by the patient's length of stay in hospital. The early onset (< 5 days) hospital acquired pneumonias are likely to be caused by potentially pathogenic micro-organisms (PPM) that were carried by the patient at the time of hospital admission. Patients admitted to hospital with a reduced conscious level and impaired airway reflexes (e.g., trauma) represent those most likely to succumb to this primary endogenous infection. The organisms concerned are likely to be upper respiratory tract commensals such as *Streptococcus pneumoniae, Haemophilus influenzae* and *Staphylococcus aureus*.

In health, an intact mucosal lining, mucus, normal gastrointestinal motility, secretory IgA, and resident anaerobes inhibit colonization of the gastrointestinal tract by aerobic bacteria. In the critically ill, impairment of these protective mechanisms leads to colonization of the gastrointestinal tract by aerobic Gram-negative bacteria (e.g., *E. coli, Psuedomonas aeruginosa, Klebsiella* spp., *Proteus* spp.), *S. aureus* and yeasts (e.g., *Candida* spp.). Secondary endogenous infection is caused by PPMs acquired in the critical care unit. These have variable patterns of resistance and are a significant cause of pneumonia developing after 5 days in hospital (late onset). There are a number of risk factors for colonization and infection by abnormal flora:

- Prolonged intubation bypasses the natural mechanical host defences, causes mucosal damage and facilitates entry of bacteria into the lung. Nasotracheal intubation increases the risk of sinusitis. Approximately two thirds of ITU patients with sinusitis will develop pneumonia.
- Nasogastric tubes encourage gastro-oesophageal reflux, bacterial migration and sinusitis.
- Opiates, high FIO_2, inadequate humidification, and tracheal suctioning impair mucociliary transport.
- A gastric pH > 4.0 encourages colonization by Gram-negative organisms. Thus, H_2blockers are more likely than sucralfate to contribute to nosocomial pneumonia.
- The supine position encourages microaspiration.
- Patients over the age of 60 years and those with chronic lung disease are more likely to develop nosocomial pneumonia.

Diagnosis

A variety of clinical criteria have been used for diagnosis of nosocomial pneumonia but the most popular are:

- New or progressive consolidation on the chest X-ray.
- Fever.
- Leukocytosis.
- Purulent tracheobronchial secretions.

There are significant limitations in using these criteria alone to diagnose noso-comial pneumonia:

- Purulent tracheal aspirates are commonly produced by colonization of the upper airway alone.
- The radiological appearances of pneumonia are non-specific.
- There are many causes of fever in the critically ill.

The use of clinical signs alone will lead to overdiagnosis of nosocomial pneumonia. Excessive use of antibiotics will encourage the selection of multi-resistant organisms.

Diagnostic techniques. Simple aspiration of the tracheal tube or tracheostomy has good sensitivity but poor specificity for diagnosing pneumonia. Although these specimens are less likely to be contaminated than expectorated sputum, there will still be frequent false positive cultures from organisms colonizing the upper airway and tracheal tube. Quantitative cultures of tracheal aspirates using 10^5 to 10^6 colony forming units per ml (cfu ml^{-1}) as the cut off may have an acceptable diagnostic accuracy.

There are a number of techniques that bypass the upper respiratory tract and allow a relatively uncontaminated sample to be obtained from the lower airways. This may improve diagnostic accuracy. The PSB is passed through a fibreoptic bronchoscope and allows collection of uncontaminated specimens from suspected areas of infection. Bacteria cultured in concentrations higher than 10^3 cfu are considered pathogenic. Alternatively, with the bronchoscope wedged in a distal airway, bronchoalveolar lavage (BAL) with 20 ml aliquots of saline will sample a larger area of lung. This method is more sensitive than the PSB, but contamination of the bronchoscope with organisms from the upper airway, reduces its specificity. Thus, following BAL only cultures of $> 10^4$ cfu are considered significant. The protected mini-BAL technique has been described recently. This combines attributes from the PSB and BAL techniques and offers excellent sensitivity (97%) and specificity (92%) in diagnosing pneumonia. The ultimate invasive diagnostic technique, open lung biopsy, is rarely indicated in the diagnosis of nosocomial pneumonia, except for immunosuppressed patients.

Prevention

Every effort must be made to minimize colonization by PPM and reduce spread of infection. Use of early enteral nutrition and controlled use of H_2-blockers will reduce colonization of the gastrointestinal tract. Close suction systems may reduce contamination of the patient's airway. Avoid long-term nasotracheal intubation. Selective decontamination of the digestive tract (SDD) is a controversial strategy that was developed to reduce the incidence of Gram-negative pneumonia in the critically ill. A variety of non-absorbable antibiotics are given enterally in an effort to preserve the normal aerobic flora of the gastrointestinal tract and reduce colonization and secondary infection by aerobic organisms. A few doses of a broad-spectrum, parenterally administered antibiotic (e.g., cefuroxime) are given to prevent infection by primary endogenous organisms. The many clinical studies of SDD have produced conflicting conclusions. Most have shown a reduction in the incidence of nosocomial pneumonia but with no significant reduction in mortality. The use of SDD is expensive and there is a theoretical risk of selecting resistant organisms. Few critical care units are using SDD.

Treatment

Seriously ill patients with nosocomial pneumonia will require treatment with empirical therapy after samples have been taken. An immediate Gram-stain of sample may be helpful. Some critical care units run a programme of micro-biological surveillance. Regular samples are taken from all patients in the unit and sent for culture. This helps to define the local flora and will direct appropriate empirical therapy for severe nosocomial pneumonia. Early onset pneumonia can be treated with a 2nd or 3rd generation cephalosporin (e.g., cefuroxime or cefo-taxime). Metronidazole is added if aspiration is a possibility. If the patient has received a cephalosporin previously or the nosocomial pneumonia is late in onset (> 5 days), therapy may be changed to use ciprofloxacin in combination with amoxycillin. This will cover Gram-negatives and *S. aureus* as well as many community-acquired organisms. Other possibilities are a carbapenem (imipenem or meropenem) or piperacillin/tazobactam.

Prognosis

The European Prevalence of Infection in Intensive Care (EPIC) study showed that ITU-acquired pneumonia almost doubled the risk of ITU death. It is likely that most of this contribution to increased mortality comes from late-onset nosocomial pneumonia.

Further reading

Estes RJ, Meduri GU. The pathogenesis of ventilator-associated pneumonia: 1. Mechanisms of bacterial transcolonisation and airway inoculation. *Intensive Care Medicine* 1995; 21: 365–383.
Parke TJ, Burden P. Noscomial pneumonia. *Care of the Critically Ill* 1998; 14: 163–167.

Related topics of interest

Infection control, p. 140; Infection in critical care, p. 143; Pneumonia – community acquired, p. 173; Pulmonary aspiration, p. 185; Stress ulceration, p. 240

POTASSIUM

Angela White

Potassium is the major intracellular cation. A 70 kg adult has 3500 mmol potassium of which about 60 mmol (2%) is extracellular. The normal extracellular concentration ranges from 3.5 to 5.0 mmol l^{-1}. The intracellular concentration is 150 mmol l^{-1}. Large changes can occur in total body potassium without significant effect on plasma potassium concentration.

Potassium therapy should take account of both maintenance and replacement requirements. The daily requirement for potassium is approximately 1 mmol kg^{-1}.

Hypokalaemia – <3.5 mmol l^{-1}

Hypokalaemia is a finding in more than 20% of in-hospital patients. Severe hypokalaemia (<3.0 mmol l^{-1}) is seen in around 5% of in patients. Mild hypokalaemia is usually well tolerated in healthy patients but may be associated with increased morbidity and mortality in those with severe cardiovascular disease.

Causes

1. Gastrointestinal. Prolonged severe diarrhoea, prolonged vomiting/nasogastric suction, laxative abuse, malabsorption/malnutrition, ureterosigmoidostomy, fistulae, colonic mucus secreting neoplasms.

2. Renal. Drugs (thiazide/loop diuretics, steroids, carbenoloxone), hyperaldosteronism, Cushing's syndrome, renal tubular acidosis (type I), diuretic phase of ARF, nephrotic syndrome, metabolic alkalosis, hypomagnesaemia.

3. Other. Intravenous fluids with inadequate supplements, β_2 agonists (e.g., salbutamol), xanthines (e.g., aminophylline, caffeine), glucose/insulin infusions (overdose or treatment of DKA), metabolic alkalosis, congestive cardiac failure, cirrhosis, liver failure, hyperthyroidism, familial hypokalaemic periodic paralysis.

Clinical features

Mild hypokalaemia is usually asymptomatic, the diagnosis is made on blood analysis. Tachycardias e.g., SVT (especially with digoxin therapy) ventricular arrhythmias and cardiac arrest may occur. There may be increased blood pressure secondary to sodium retention. Muscle weakness may cause cramps, an ileus and constipation. There may be loss of tendon reflexes and the patient may be easily fatigued, complaining of apathy and sleepiness. Polyuria may be present.

Early ECG changes include large U waves whilst later there may be flattened or inverted T waves. The ST segments may be depressed. A metabolic alkalosis secondary to loss of hydrogen ion in exchange for potassium may occur.

Management

Eliminate artefact as a cause e.g., contamination by intravenous infusion fluid. Minimize unnecessary potassium wasting drugs and consider the use of potassium sparing diuretics (amiloride, spironolactone).

Potassium chloride may be given by intravenous infusion at a rate of 20–30 mmol h^{-1}, repeated according to measured levels. In profound hypokalaemia (< 2 mmol l^{-1}) more rapid rates under continuous ECG monitoring will be required. Potassium phosphate is used to provide both potassium and phosphate replacement.

If the patient is asymptomatic and the potassium is low normal (3.6 – 4.0 mmol l^{-1}), it may be sufficient to provide oral supplements or additional potassium to maintenance fluids or parenteral nutrition. Oral potassium is safer as it is slower to enter the circulation.

On average, a reduction in serum potassium of 0.3 mmol l^{-1} requires a reduction in total body potassium of 100 mmol. Magnesium will need to be supplemented at the same time.

Hyperkalaemia – > 5.5 mmol l^{-1}

Causes

1. Impaired renal excretion. For example in ARF, advanced chronic renal failure, due to potassium sparing diuretics or in steroid deficiency (Addison's disease or hypoaldosteronism)

2. Potassium shift from cells as seen in acidosis, haemolysis, massive blood transfusion, tumour lysis following chemotherapy, rhabdomyolysis, suxamethonium administration (especially in patients with neurological disease or denervation), malignant hyperthermia, and following cardiac arrest.

3. Other causes including excessive potassium administration, and familial hyperkalaemic periodic paralysis.

Clinical features

Most patients will be asymptomatic until the potassium is > 6.0 mmol l^{-1}.

Arrhythmias are related more closely to the rate of rise than the absolute values but may progress to cardiac arrest. There may be muscle weakness and loss of tendon reflexes. The patient may be confused. ECG changes include peaked T waves, flattened P waves, and wide QRS complexes.

Management

Ensure that the finding of hyperkalaemia is not an artefact. Stop the administration of all potassium containing fluids. Depending on the level of potassium, or urgency of the situation, the options are to:

- Give calcium intravenously to antagonize the cardiotoxic effects of hyperkalaemia. Calcium chloride 10% contains 0.68 mmol ml^{-1}, initial dose of 10 ml can be repeated if the effect is inadequate. It has an immediate onset and lasts up to 60 min (calcium gluconate 10% contains 0.225 mol ml^{-1}).
- Give bicarbonate 50–100 mmol over 10–20 min. Onset of action is around 5 min with a duration of effect of up to 2 hours.
- Give 50 ml of 50% glucose with 20 units soluble insulin which will increase cellular uptake of potassium.

- Infusion of a β_2 agonist may also be used to drive potassium into the cells but there is a risk of arrhythmias.
- Ion exchange resins e.g., calcium resonium can be used orally (15 g 6 hourly) or rectally (30 g 12 hourly).

Renal losses of potassium may be increased with the use of a loop diuretic and dialysis can be used to both decrease plasma potassium and correct acidosis.

Further reading

Halperin Mh, Kamel KS. Potassium. *Lancet* 1998; **352**: 135–140.

Gennari FJ. Hypokalemia. *New England Journal of Medicine* 1998; **339**: 451–458.

Related topics of interest

Adrenal disease, p. 8; Calcium, magnesium and phosphate, p. 56; Resuscitation – cardio-pulmonary, p. 213; Fluid-therapy, p. 122; Renal replacement therapy, p. 197; Sodium, p. 231

PSYCHOLOGICAL ASPECTS OF CRITICAL CARE

Jas Soar

The critical care environment can be psychologically stressful for patients, relatives and staff. Inevitably, care focuses the physical needs of the patient. The psychological, social and spiritual aspects of care are often overlooked. The needs of the family and staff must also be acknowledged and addressed.

Patient problems can be considered in the following categories.

1. Problems associated with the disease resulting in admission.
2. Specific aspects unique to the critical care environment.
3. Long term effects manifesting after discharge.

Problems associated with the disease resulting in admission

Pain and distress associated with difficulty in breathing are common. Careful use of sedation and analgesia is needed to minimize this. Patients may present to the critical care unit with the whole range of organic and functional psychiatric disorders. Anxiety and mild to moderate depression are common. Syndromes associated with delirium have been described in patients after cardiopulmonary bypass and major surgery. Features include clouding of consciousness, disorientation, and intellectual dysfunction. This can extend to hallucinations (usually visual) and paranoid delusions. Drugs, hypoxia and metabolic abnormalities contribute. This psychological impairment usually resolves but can contribute to morbidity and mortality especially in the elderly patient.

Specific aspects unique to the critical care environment

The high technology environment of the critical care unit has a profound impact on the patient which may result in fear, anxiety, vulnerability and dependency. Depression may hinder improvement in the patient's condition. Some patients develop ICU psychosis. Symptoms include disorientation, hallucinations, paranoia, restlessness and combativeness. Contributing factors include:

1. Physical factors. Exposure to multiple procedures which are often painful. Noise is a common problem. Noise levels of less than 45 decibels (dB) are required to facilitate restful sleep. This rarely occurs in the critical care environment where noise levels range from 55 to 65 dB with peaks reaching 90 dB. Alarms, pagers, and staff conversation have been rated as highly annoying. Lighting around the clock disrupts normal circadian rhythms. Odours are also troublesome.

2. Psychological factors include loss of privacy and invasion of personal space. Sensory disturbance occurs due to lack of familiar sights and sounds together with an increase in abnormal stimuli. Isolation from friends and family if visiting is limited can cause worry.

3. Sleep disturbance and sleep fragmentation results in disorientation and fatigue. Alterations in the amount of REM and non-REM sleep may be detrimental to the patients medical condition.

Preventative measures including privacy, noise control and disturbance-free rest periods may help. Keeping the patient orientated in time and space as well as adequately informed of what is happening is beneficial. Patients may benefit from treatment with antidepressants. Selective serotonin re-uptake inhibitors (e.g., fluoxetine) are well tolerated in the critically ill.

Long term effects manifesting after discharge

Many patients have little recall of events whilst on the critical care unit. Lack of sleep, pain, anxiety and noise are common complaints. Physical disability will have an ongoing psychological impact.

A small but significant proportion of patients has recurrent and frightening memories of the critical care unit. These patients may go on to develop a post-traumatic stress disorder (PTSD). Traumatic events are persistently re-experienced. This may result in terror, guilt, hostility, anxiety and depression. Symptoms may result in significant impairment of daily function. In motor vehicle accident victims, chronic PTSD was related to the severity of trauma, on going medical problems, perceived threat, dissociation during the accident, female gender, previous emotional problems and litigation. Education, social support, cognitive therapy and antidepressant drugs may benefit these patients.

Further reading

Hofhuis J, Bakker J. Experiences of critical ill patients in the ICU: what do they think of us? *International Journal of Intensive Care* 1998; 5: 114–117.

Related topics of interest

Analgesia – basic, p. 14; Analgesia – advanced, p. 18; Sedation, p. 223

PULMONARY ASPIRATION

Andrew Padkin

Pulmonary aspiration is the passage of foreign liquids or solids into the lower respiratory tract. Aspiration of gastric contents causes up to 20% of all anaesthetic related deaths. Mortality associated with aspiration varies widely between 7.5 and 85% depending on the aspirate (type and volume), the number of pulmonary lobes involved, and the patient's underlying clinical condition and treatment.

Predisposing factors

1. Impaired cough and gag reflexes
(a) Decreased conscious level e.g., overdose, anaesthesia, head injury, meningitis, seizures, metabolic coma, cerebrovascular accident, severe illness
(b) IX and X cranial nerve disease:
- Brain stem e.g., motor neurone disease, syringobulbia, polio.
- Pressure effects/invasion near the jugular foramen e.g., glomus tumour, nasopharyngeal carcinoma.
- Demyelination e.g., Guillain–Barré syndrome, diphtheria.
- Neuromuscular junction disease e.g., myasthenia gravis.

2. Increased risk of vomiting/regurgitation
(a) Increased intra-abdominal pressure (pregnancy, bowel obstruction, obesity).
(b) Slow gastric emptying (labour, trauma, opiates, alcohol, intra-abdominal sepsis, pyloric stenosis).
(c) Abnormal lower oesophageal sphincter (reflux disease, pregnancy, hiatus hernia, presence of nasogastric tube).
(d) Abnormal oesophageal anatomy (oesophagectomy, oesophageal stricture, tracheo-oesophageal fistula).
(e) Abnormal oesophageal motility (achalasia, scleroderma).

Substances aspirated

1. Solids
(a) Large solids (e.g., meat in adults, peanuts in children) may cause large airway obstruction that is immediately life threatening. These must be removed immediately (e.g., by back blows).
(b) Smaller solids (e.g., teeth, peanuts in adults) can cause lower airway obstruction. If partial obstruction occurs a monophonic wheeze may be heard. Atelectasis distal to the obstruction may be followed by persistent infection, abscess formation and bronchiectasis. Vegetable matter causes particular problems by producing a localized inflammatory reaction.

2. Liquids
(a) Non-infected fluids:
- Sterile acid. Gastric acid causes direct lung damage within minutes. Injury severity increases with increasing acidity and volume, though critical values for these are difficult to determine. Many authors suggest that a pH < 2.5 and

volume greater than 25 ml (or 0.4 ml kg^{-1}) are associated with severe injury, though the evidence for these values is weak.

Four effects may occur early:

1. Laryngospasm.
2. Vagally-mediated bronchospasm.
3. Surfactant dysfunction leading to patchy atelectasis.
4. Alveolar-capillary breakdown leading to interstitial oedema and haemorrhagic pulmonary oedema. Enough fluid may be lost from the circulation to cause hypotension.

Following aspiration lung volume is decreased, pulmonary compliance is decreased, there is an increase in pulmonary vascular resistance and a large intra-pulmonary shunt develops. The initial acute inflammatory process usually starts to resolve by 72 hours and is followed by a fibroproliferative phase.

A prolonged clinical course with the development of ARDS occurs in 15%. Aspiration of acid particulate matter causes the most severe damage.

- Non-acidic fluids (e.g., blood, saliva). Although alveolar damage and acute inflammatory changes are usually less severe, severe hypoxia due to laryngospasm, bronchospasm and surfactant dysfunction may be life threatening.

(b) Infected fluids. Immediate effects are similar to those caused by non-infected fluids. In previously healthy patients gastric contents are sterile and infection is unusual in the early stages following aspiration. If it develops later it is often due to anaerobic oral flora. In contrast, the upper GI tract often becomes colonized by Gram-negative aerobes and anaerobes in those who are hospitalized, use antacids or use H$_2$ antagonists. This is thought to be due to a lack of the normal protective acidic gastric environment. If pulmonary infection develops in these patients following aspiration it is likely to be due to the above organisms.

Clinical presentation

In acute aspiration there may be soiling of the pharynx or trachea. Dyspnoea, coughing, wheeze and severe hypoxaemia all occur. If large volumes of acid have been aspirated signs of hypovolaemia may be present. Fever and leucocytosis may occur in the absence of infection.

Diagnosis

Usually clinical, though tracheal suction can be used to detect acid pH. Testing tracheal samples for glucose is unreliable.

CXR may reveal a small solid if it is radio-opaque, or simply show distal collapse or consolidation.

Acid aspiration usually leads to diffuse bilateral pulmonary infiltrates. Isolated right upper lobe changes may be seen after supine aspiration, and right middle/lower lobe changes after semi-recumbent aspiration.

Management

Prevention of aspiration of gastric contents:

1. *Posture.* All spontanously breathing unconscious patients should be placed in the recovery position unless contraindicated until airway protection is achieved.

2. *Airway protection.* Tracheal intubation or tracheostomy provides the best airway protection for patients at risk of aspiration.

3. *Reduction of volume of gastric contents.* Nasogastric tubes are used for aspiration of gastric contents in those patients with gastric stasis though they impair oesophageal sphincter function and should be removed immediately prior to anaesthesia.

4. *Anaesthesia.* Anaesthesia in those at risk of aspiration should be planned carefully. Pre-operatively, gastric contents should be minimized and neutralized e.g., by nasogastric suction as above, or by using a prokinetic agent, an H_2 antagonist or proton pump inhibitor and sodium citrate. Regional anaesthesia may be possible, allowing surgery without compromising the airway. If general anaesthesia is necessary, tracheal intubation should be performed either awake or after a rapid sequence induction with cricoid pressure.

Treatment

1. *Position.* If the airway is not protected and there are no contraindications, the patient should be placed laterally, head down.

2. *Airway clearance.* Any pharyngeal soiling should be cleared. If the patient is intubated the trachea can be suctioned to clear semi-solid material (liquid disperses quickly). Physiotherapy will aid clearance of the lower airways.

3. *Oxygen.* High concentration oxygen should be given to maintain oxygen saturation.

4. *Tracheal intubation.* If the patient is at risk of further aspiration, the airway should be protected by intubation.

5. *Mechanical ventilation.* There should be a low threshold for mechanical ventilation as delay may worsen outcome. PEEP is necessary to maintain alveolar recruitment and diminish shunt. It also decreases pulmonary vascular resistance (unless excessive PEEP is used causing overdistension).

6. *Cardiovascular support.* Fluid balance should be carefully monitored as intravascular volume can be significantly decreased. Inotropes are often necessary.

7. *Bronchodilators.* Bronchospasm may be severe, and bronchodilators should be given though may not be particularly effective.

8. *Bronchoscopy.* Small particles may be removed by flexible FOB. Lavage is not useful unless the aspirated matter is particulate. Even then only small amounts of saline should be used. Rigid bronchoscopy allows wide-bore suctioning and the passage of large grasping forceps, and is the procedure of choice for the removal of most inhaled objects.

9. *Antibiotics.* Early treatment with antibiotics should be considered only when infected fluid has been aspirated (e.g., faecal aspiration in bowel obstruction).

Secondary bacterial infection occurs in 20–30% and antibiotics should be directed at the responsible organism.

10. Steroids. Steroids have no proven benefit after aspiration, and may slow pulmonary healing.

Microaspiration

Microaspiration is thought to be a major cause of ventilator-associated pneumonia (VAP). It occurs in intensive care patients when colonized secretions pool in the subglottic above the tracheal cuff space then leak around the cuff along longitudinal folds in the wall.

Prevention

1. Decreasing the bacterial colonization of upper GI secretions. Sucralfate or H_2 blockers are often used as prophylaxis against upper GI bleeding in critically ill patients. Sucralfate is protective to gastric cells without altering gastric pH, so would be expected to be associated with less upper GI and tracheobronchial colonization with pathogenic bacteria, and hence fewer episodes of VAP. This has been confirmed in some observational studies. However, a recent large multi-centre randomized controlled trial has shown no significant difference in the incidence of VAP in patients treated with ranitidine compared to those treated with sucralfate, with ranitidine providing greater protection against GI bleeding.

2. Decreasing reflux of gastric contents. Providing enteral nutrition by gastrostomy or jejunostomy rather than via a nasogastric tube may decrease the incidence of VAP, though it does not completely prevent it.

3. Decreasing the amount of fluid that leaks past the cuff. Nursing intensive care patients semi-recumbent rather than supine may decrease microaspiration.

Further reading

Leroy O, Vandenbussche C, Collinier C, *et al*. Community-acquired aspiration pneumonia in intensive care units. Epidemiological and prognosis data. *American Journal of Respiratory Critical Care Medicine* 1997; **156**: 1922–1929.

Lomotan JR, George SS, Brandselter RD. Aspiration pneumonia. Strategies for early recognition and prevention. *Postgraduate Medicine* 1997; **102**: 225–231.

Related topics of interest

Acute respiratory distress syndrome, p. 5; Coma, p. 96; Nutrition, p. 159; Stress ulceration, p. 240; Pneumonia – community acquired, p. 173; Pneumonia – hospital acquired, p. 177; Tracheostomy, p. 250

PULMONARY EMBOLISM

Pulmonary embolism (PE) is a complication of DVT. Almost all pulmonary emboli result from thromboses of the lower limbs, deep pelvic veins, or inferior vena cava. Most of these episodes of thrombosis are asymptomatic. The mortality of patients with PE is lower in those who are treated than in those who are not or in whom the diagnosis was not suspected.

Aetiology

The aetiology of PE is that of DVT. Virchow's triad describes the predisposing factors for the development of a DVT. They are (i) stasis of blood flow, (ii) damage to blood vessels and (iii) abnormal coagulation. Patients at high risk include:

1. Inherited. Antithrombin III deficiency, protein C deficiency, protein S deficiency, dysfibrinogenaemias.

2. Acquired. Lupus disease, nephrotic syndrome, malignancy, low cardiac output states, polycythaemia, obesity, advancing age, oestrogen therapy, sepsis, stroke (75% incidence of DVT in paralysed leg), peripheral vascular disease.

3. Surgical. Orthopaedic patients represent the highest risk group with those undergoing hip or knee reconstructive surgery being at particular risk. Other operative risks are gynaecological surgery, surgery for malignancy and prolonged surgery. Duration of operation has been positively correlated to the incidence of DVT in neurosurgical patients.

Clinical presentation

PE may present with one of three clinical syndromes:

1. Pulmonary infarction/haemorrhage (60% of diagnosed cases of PE).
2. Isolated shortness of breath (25% of diagnosed cases of PE).
3. Sudden circulatory collapse (10% of diagnosed cases of PE). One third of these patients die within a few hours of presentation.

The three most common symptoms are dyspnoea, tachypnoea, and pleuritic chest pain.

There may be little in the way of positive clinical signs. Those that are present are usually non-specific and at best support the diagnosis. They include signs of right heart strain, pulmonary hypertension, and DVT. The ECG may show non-specific ST segment changes, axis changes, or rarely, and only in the case of a large PE, an S wave in lead I, a Q wave and T wave inversion in lead III ('S_1, Q_3, T_3'). The CXR often shows a parenchymal abnormality (e.g., atelectasis). There may also be an elevated hemidiaphragm. The patient may have a mild pyrexia and elevated white cell count. The finding of a low PaO_2 also supports the diagnosis.

Specific investigation

The most useful investigation is probably a combination of a pulmonary ventilation/perfusion (V/Q) scan and measurement of the plasma D-dimer levels.

D-dimer is formed when plasmin digests cross-linked fibrin. A low D-dimer level is strong evidence against the diagnosis of a PE.

V/Q scan

Pulmonary perfusion scans are usually performed using intravenous albumin labelled with technetium-99m. A ventilation scan is performed following the inhalation of xenon-133. A pulmonary perfusion scan which is interpreted as showing a high probability of a PE is no less sensitive a predictor of PE than a combined V/Q scan. If the result of the perfusion scan is of intermediate probability a subsequent V/Q scan may change the interpretation to a more definitive probability. The Prospective Investigation of Pulmonary Embolism Diagnosis (PIOPED) study defined five categories for V/Q scans; high, intermediate, low, and very low probability, and normal.

Leg studies

A patient with a non-diagnostic V/Q scan requires further investigation. A venogram or compression ultrasound will determine the presence of a DVT. The finding of a DVT guides therapy since the treatment of PE and DVT is the same. Absence of a DVT combined with a low probability V/Q scan usually permits withholding treatment. A negative leg-study in a patient with an intermediate probability scan will normally necessitate pulmonary angiography.

Pulmonary angiography

This remains the diagnostic standard for PE. The finding of an intraluminal filling defect is specific. Fewer than 2% of patients suffer serious adverse effects during pulmonary angiography.

Contrast-enhanced spiral CT

Early evidence suggests that this imaging technique may be of high specificity and selectivity if the PE is in the central pulmonary vessels. Its value in diagnosing PE in more peripheral vessels is less clear and the true role of contrast-enhanced spiral CT in the investigation of possible PE has yet to be fully defined.

Management

1. Anticoagulation. Patients with an uncomplicated PE should be treated with heparin to maintain the APTT (activated partial thromboplastin time) at 1.5–2 times the control. Oral anticoagulation may be commenced at the same time or shortly after starting heparin. There should be a 5 day overlap with both therapies and the INR maintained at approximately 2–3 times normal before the heparin is stopped. LMWH has advantages over unfractionated heparin. These include greater bioavailabilty when given by subcutaneous injection, more predictable anticoagulant effects (permitting the administration of a fixed dose and removing the need for laboratory monitoring), and an increased duration of action. The use of LMWH results in less heparin-induced thrombocytopenia, osteoporosis, and bleeding. Some centres now manage uncomplicated DVT and PE with administration of LMWH and commencement of oral anticoagulation at home, thus avoiding hospital admission altogether. Early follow up of patients managed in this way has shown comparable rates of fatal and non-fatal PE compared with patients treated with unfractionated heparin.

2. *Inferior vena cava (IVC) filters.* IVC filters should be inserted in patients with a proximal DVT or PE in whom anticoagulation is contraindicated or if PE has recurred despite adequate anticoagulation. A caval filter may also be inserted if the PE is severe (hypotension or right ventricular failure) or if recurrent PE is likely to be fatal. IVC filters are inserted percutaneously.

3. *Thrombolytic therapy.* Lysis of PE occurs more rapidly when thrombolytics are given than with anticoagulation alone. In patients who have not had a massive PE, long term survival is the same for both groups, however. Thrombolysis has been shown to alter outcome in patients with a massive PE. They had a lower in hospital mortality and rate of PE recurrence but higher incidence of major haemorrhage than similar patients treated with anticoagulation alone.

4. *Pulmonary embolectomy.* Patients who have suffered a massive PE, and are shocked despite resuscitative measures and thrombolysis, may benefit from open embolectomy. Mortality remains high even in patients offered surgery.

Further reading

Simonneau G, Sors H, *et al.* A comparison of low molecular weight heparin with unfractionated heparin for acute pulmonary embolism. *New England Journal of Medicine* 1997; **337**: 663–669.
Stein PD, Hull RD. Acute pulmonary embolism. *Current Opinion in Critical Care* 1998; **4**: 322–330.
The PIOPED Investigators. Value of ventilation/perfusion scan in acute pulmonary embolism. Results of the Prospective Investigation of Pulmonary Embolism Diagnosis (PIOPED). *JAMA* 1990; **263**: 2753–2759.

Related topics of interest

Blood coagulation, p. 34; Resuscitation – cardiopulmonary, p. 213

RENAL FAILURE – RESCUE THERAPY

Appropriate and aggressive management of pre-renal failure may avoid the onset of established renal failure and the requirement for renal replacement therapy (RRT). Every factor contributing to pre-renal failure must be addressed:

Nephrotoxic drugs

NSAIDs inhibit the synthesis of renal prostaglandins that would normally dilate the afferent arterioles. In the presence of low renal blood flow NSAIDs may cause acute renal failure (ARF). These drugs are contraindicated in patients with impending renal failure. ACE inhibitors are also contraindicated in these patients; they reduce the production of angiotensin-2 that normally constricts the efferent arterioles.

Circulating volume

Fluid loading will tend to reverse many of the physiological mechanisms that maximize fluid retention (e.g., release of aldosterone and antidiuretic hormone). Single, independent CVP measurements are poor indicators of intravascular volume; differences in myocardial compliance and venous tone make interpretation very difficult. The dynamic process of assessing the response of the CVP to a fluid challenge (e.g., 200 ml of colloid) is more useful, but high venous tone will still tend to mask hypovolaemia. A low dose nitrate infusion (e.g., GTN 2 mg h^{-1}) will reduce venous tone and may reveal hypovolaemia. Simple clinical signs, such as rewarming of the peripheries, will also help to indicate restoration of adequate circulating volume.

Cardiac output and oxygen delivery

If oliguria persists despite an appropriate circulating volume, an inotrope such as dobutamine can be added to increase cardiac output. A haemoglobin concentration of > 10 g dl^{-1} and appropriate oxygen saturation will help to ensure adequate renal oxygen delivery.

Renal perfusion pressure

Renal blood flow and glomerular filtration rate (GFR) are normally autoregulated over a wide range of mean arterial pressure. However, in the presence of ischaemic ATN and/or sepsis, autoregulation may be impaired significantly. Thus, in the critically ill, adequate renal blood flow may depend on achieving the patient's normal premorbid systolic blood pressure. In the presence of an adequate circulating volume and cardiac output, a noradrenaline infusion can be titrated to achieve this 'normal' blood pressure. The increase in urine output often seen with this approach may be accounted for by: (a) the increase in renal perfusion pressure, and (b) the relatively greater increase in arteriolar resistance on the efferent side of the glomerulus in comparison with the afferent side (increasing filtration fraction).

Frusemide

Oxygen tension is particularly low in the outer medulla. At this point blood flow is slow to maintain the medullary osmotic gradient. The ion pumps in the medullary thick ascending limb of the loop of Henle (mTAL) are high oxygen consumers. Frusemide reduces the activity of the $Na^+ K^+ 2Cl^-$ co-transporter in the tubular cell, thus reducing oxygen consumption. Animal studies have shown that frusemide increases renal medullary oxygen tension. Frusemide also stimulates production of vasodilator prostaglandins, thereby increasing afferent arteriolar flow. A bolus of 10 mg of frusemide, followed by an infusion of $1-10$ mg h^{-1} may produce an adequate urine output. Although the use of frusemide in this way undoubtedly enhances urine output and is theoretically sound, there is little evidence that it prevents renal failure. However, the prevention of fluid overload alone may be enough to postpone or prevent the need for RRT in some critically ill patients.

Dopamine

Until recently, a low dose dopamine infusion ($1-3$ μg kg^{-1} min^{-1}) was the most popular treatment for oliguria in the presence of an adequate circulating volume. The increase in renal blood flow was thought to be a specific effect mediated through dopamine receptors. In reality, this dose of dopamine has significant inotropic and chronotropic effects and the increase in renal blood flow is probably secondary to a general increase in cardiac output. Furthermore, dopamine may induce gut mucosal ischaemia. Like frusemide, dopamine will often induce a diuresis but has not been shown to be 'protective' against the onset of ARF. As dopamine has potentially harmful effects, in the presence of an adequate circulating volume and appropriate blood pressure, a low dose frusemide infusion is a more logical choice for the treatment of oliguria.

Abdominal compartment syndrome

Intra-abdominal hypertension ($> 20-25$ mmHg) may occur in a variety settings, including:

- Severe acute pancreatitis.
- Faecal peritonitis.
- Retroperitoneal haematoma (aortic aneurysm, pelvic fracture).
- Intestinal obstruction.

High intra-abdominal pressure (IAP) may cause oliguria by reducing total renal blood flow (increased venous resistance) or by direct compression of renal parenchyma. If other causes of oliguria have been eliminated and the IAP (measured from the bladder) exceeds 20 mmHg, surgical decompression of the abdomen should be considered.

Further reading

Cordingley J, Palazzo M. Renal rescue: management of impending renal failure. In: Vincent JL (ed). *Yearbook of Intensive Care and Emergency Medicine*. Berlin: Springer, 1996, pp. 675–689.

Related topics of interest

Fluid therapy, p. 122; Renal failure – acute, p. 194; Renal replacement therapy, p. 197

RENAL FAILURE – ACUTE

A variety of definitions have been applied to acute renal failure (ARF); 'a recent, reversible or potentially reversible deterioration in renal function' is one of the most practical.

Incidence

Approximately 1% of patients at the time of admission to hospital. Increasing to 2–5% during hospitalization.

Causes

In most cases ARF is multifactorial but the classification of potential causes encourages a systematic approach to investigation and treatment.

1. **Pre-renal.** Inadequate perfusion of otherwise normal kidneys:

- Hypovolaemia (haemorrhage, sepsis, gastrointestinal losses, burns, inadequate intake);
- Hypotension (hypovolaemia, cardiac failure, vasodilatation);
- Functional acute renal failure (NSAIDS, hepatorenal syndrome);
- Abdominal compartment syndrome.

2. **Renal.** Intrinsic parenchymal renal disease can be classified according to the primary site of injury:

- Acute tubular necrosis (ATN) accounts for 85% of the intrinsic causes (50% due to ischaemia and 35% due to toxins) of renal failure. Toxins causing ATN include inflammatory mediators, aminoglycosides, paracetamol, heavy metals, and myoglobin. The thick ascending limb (TAL) of the Henle's loop is particularly predisposed to ischaemia for two reasons: (a) Although total blood flow to the kidneys is very high (25% of cardiac output), the majority is directed to the renal cortex. Medullary blood flow is limited so that the concentration gradient of osmolality is preserved. (b) Active ion pumps in the TAL are high oxygen consumers. The combination of poor blood supply and high oxygen demand leaves this section of the tubule very vulnerable to ischaemia. Thus, the onset of ATN is commonly related to an episode of reduced renal blood flow. Renal ischaemia and toxic insults act synergistically to invoke ATN. Non-steroidal anti-inflammatory drugs will compound the problem by blocking the production of prostaglandin, a substance that offers renal protection during low flow states.
- Interstitial nephritis accounts for fewer than 10% of the causes of intrinsic ARF. It may be caused by an allergic reaction to a drug or by autoimmune disease, infiltrative diseases (e.g., sarcoidosis), or infection.
- Glomerulonephritis is an infrequent cause of ARF (5%) and may be related to systemic illness such as SLE or Goodpasture's syndrome.
- Small or large vessel renal vascular disease is another cause of ARF. The vascular disorder may be embolic or thrombotic.

3. Post-renal. Obstruction to both urinary outflow tracts will result in ARF. The obstruction, which can be at any level within the urinary tract, must be detected and resolved quickly. This optimizes the likelihood of complete recovery.

- Intrarenal obstruction may be caused by proteins (e.g., haemoglobin, myoglobin), or drugs (e.g., methotrexate).
- Renal pelvis – calculi, tumours or blood clot.
- Ureter – stones, accidental ligation.
- Bladder – prostatic enlargement, bladder tumour.
- Urethra – stricture.

Diagnosis and investigations

1. History. The patient's history and examination will indicate the likely cause of ARF. The patient's notes may reveal a period of hypovolaemia and/or hypotension. In critical care patients, oliguria (< 0.5 ml kg^{-1} min^{-1}) is usually the first indication of acutely impaired renal function.

2. Plasma biochemistry. Rising blood urea and creatinine levels, a metabolic acidosis, with or without hyperkalaemia, confirm the diagnosis. Pre-renal factors are excluded by ensuring normovolaemia and a mean arterial pressure within the patient's normal range (see Renal failure – rescue therapy).

3. Exclude urinary outflow obstruction. Urinary outflow obstruction must also be excluded, particularly if the patient is anuric. Correct location of a urinary catheter must be confirmed. Ultrasound may reveal a dilated urinary system. Small kidneys indicate a degree of chronic renal disease. If the patient is anuric following any recent surgery that could conceivably involve the renal arteries, renography is indicated.

4. Urinalysis. Plasma and urine osmolality, urine sodium and protein content, and urine microscopy are valuable investigations for ARF. Typical urine findings in pre-renal ARF and ATN are listed in the *Table 1*. In pre-renal ARF the tubules attempt to 'restore intravascular volume' by reabsorption of salt and water. Loss of tubular concentrating ability in intrinsic ARF results in urine and plasma that are iso-osmolar. Urinary sodium concentration is high. Pigmented granular casts are associated with ATN, and red cell casts with glomerulo-nephritis.

Table 1 Typical urine findings in pre-renal ARF and ATN

Parameter	Pre-renal ARF	ATN
Urine osmolarity (mosm l^{-1})	> 500	< 350
Urine sodium (mmol l^{-1})	10–20	> 20
Urine urea (mmol l^{-1})	> 250	< 150
Urine : plasma ratio osmolarity	> 1.5	< 1.1
Urine : plasma ratio urea	> 20	< 10
Fractional excretion of sodium	$< 1\%$	$> 1\%$

5. *Renal biopsy.* Renal biopsy is rarely necessary in the evaluation of ARF. It may be indicated if the history, clinical features, and laboratory and radiological investigations have excluded pre- and post-renal causes and an intrinsic cause, other than ATN, is likely.

Further reading

Thadhani R, Pascual M, Bonventre JV. Acute renal failure. *New England Journal of Medicine* 1996; 334: 1448–1460.

Tovison CRV, Plant WD. ATN and selected syndromes. *Key Topics in Renal Medicine.* Oxford, BIOS Scientific Publishers, 1997, pp. 7–10.

Related topics of interest

Renal failure – rescue therapy, p. 192; Renal replacement therapy, p. 197

RENAL REPLACEMENT THERAPY

Indications

In critically ill patients, renal replacement therapy (RRT) is generally started early after the onset of ARF. It simplifies fluid and nutritional management and early use of RRT may improve outcome. Indications for RRT include:

- Fluid overload.
- Hyperkalaemia (> 6.0 mmol l^{-1}).
- To create space for drugs and nutrition.
- Creatinine rising > 100 μmol l^{-1}day^{-1}.
- Creatinine > 300–600 μmol l^{-1}.
- Urea rising > 16–20 mmol l^{-1} day^{-1}.
- Metabolic acidosis (pH < 7.2) caused by renal failure.
- Clearance of dialysable nephrotoxins and other drugs.

Principles of dialysis and filtration

Dialysis describes the *diffusion* of solute across a semi-permeable membrane and down a concentration gradient. Filtration is the movement of solute by *convection* across a semi-permeable membrane. Dialysis is particularly efficient for small molecules such as K^+, Na^+, and urea. Dialysis can be undertaken by using an artificial membrane or the peritoneum. It can be performed continuously or intermittently. The size of the molecules removed by filtration will depend on the cut off point (size of the holes) of the artificial membrane. Membranes designed for dialysis or filtration are most commonly made of polyacrylynitrile. This is a biocompatible material and is unlikely to cause significant complement activation.

Renal replacement therapy techniques

Methods of renal replacement include:

- Peritoneal dialysis.
- Intermittent haemodialysis.
- Continuous haemodialysis and/or haemofiltration.

Peritoneal dialysis

In critical care units peritoneal dialysis (PD) has been largely replaced by more advanced techniques of RRT. It may be used where haemodialysis is contraindicated or where the appropriate equipment is unavailable.

Intermittent haemodialysis

Intermittent haemodialysis (IHD) is rarely undertaken in critical care units within the United Kingdom. Continuous techniques (described below) are more widely available and, in the critically ill patient with multiple organ failure, are more haemodynamically stable. Critically ill patients do not tolerate the rapid changes in plasma osmolality and intravascular volume which can occur with IHD. Renal units treating patients with 'single-organ' ARF or chronic renal failure typically use

IHD. Many American intensivists also prefer to use IHD for managing renal failure in the critical care unit.

Continuous renal replacement therapies

The following techniques are used for continuous RRT:

- Continuous arteriovenous haemofiltration (CAVH).
- Continuous venovenous haemofiltration (CVVH).
- Continuous arteriovenous haemodialysis (CAVHD) or haemodiafiltration (CAVDF).
- Continuous venovenous haemodialysis (CVVHD) or haemodiafiltration (CVVDF).

Arteriovenous techniques rely on the patient's own cardiac output to generate adequate flow through the filter.

Venovenous techniques employ a pump to deliver blood to the filter.

1. CAVH. Vascular access is achieved with femoral arterial and venous cannulae or with a surgically fashioned distal limb Scribner arteriovenous shunt. The rate of filtrate removal depends on the characteristics of the filter membrane and its vertical position in relation to the patient. The patient's fluid balance is maintained by giving replacement fluid with an appropriate electrolytic composition.

2. CAVHD. The relatively poor clearances achieved with CAVH can be improved by running dialysis fluid in a direction counter current to the blood flow on the opposite side of the membrane.

3. CVVHD and CVVHDF. Venous access is obtained with a single, wide-bore, double-lumen cannula placed in the subclavian, internal jugular or femoral vein. The excellent urea clearance achieved with CVVHDF is sufficient for even the most catabolic patients. Modern machines allow control of blood, dialysate, filtrate, and replacement fluid flows, thus providing total control of the patient's fluid balance. The rate of fluid replacement is determined by the desired fluid balance.

Replacement fluid

Bicarbonate is unstable in solution thus most replacement fluids contain either lactate or acetate instead of bicarbonate. In the presence of significant liver dysfunction, lactate or acetate may not be metabolized to bicarbonate and the use of standard replacement fluids may result in an increasing metabolic acidosis. Bicarbonate replacement solutions are now available. If prepared immediately before use, the bicarbonate will remain in solution for about 12 hours.

Anticoagulation

Unless the patient has a significant coagulopathy anticoagulant therapy is necessary to prevent clotting of the filter and extracorporeal circuit. Following a bolus of 3000 units, a heparin infusion is started at 10 U kg^{-1} and adjusted to maintain an APTT at 1.5–2 times the control value. In those few patients who develop heparin-induced thrombocytopaenia and in other high-risk cases, prostacyclin (2.5–5 ng $kg^{-1} min^{-1}$) is an alternative.

Nutrition

Modern techniques of RRT enable critically ill patients to receive protein and calories in quantities required by their catabolic state. Wherever possible, this should be given by the enteral route. A significant quantity of non-urea nitrogen is lost across the filter thus it may be appropriate to increase the nitrogen content of feeds given to patients receiving RRT.

Diuretic phase

The oliguric or anuric phase of ATN lasts typically for 2–4 weeks, although there is considerable spread either side of this average. The return of renal function presents with a diuresis. Although at this stage, urine output is high, renal function may still be poor. A rising urea and creatinine may indicate the need for a few more days of RRT.

Further reading

Forni LG, Hilton PJ. Continuous hemofiltration in the treatment of acute renal failure. *New England Journal of Medicine* 1997; **336**: 1303–1309.

Ronco C, Bellomo R. The evolving technology for continuous renal replacement therapy from current standards to high-volume hemofiltration. *Current Opinion in Critical Care* 1997; **3**: 426–433.

Related topics of interest

Renal failure – rescue therapy, p. 192; Renal failure – acute, p. 194

RESPIRATORY SUPPORT – NON-INVASIVE

Stephen Fletcher

Respiratory failure is impairment of pulmonary gas exchange sufficient to cause hypoxaemia with or without hypercarbia. Non-invasive respiratory support encompasses a variety of techniques that aim to produce adequate oxygenation and acceptable carbon dioxide excretion.

Hypoxaemic (Type I) respiratory failure

Hypoxaemia is due to ventilation/perfusion (V/Q) mismatch, true shunt (areas of zero V/Q) or, most often, a combination of the two. True shunt occurs when alveoli are completely collapsed, totally consolidated or filled with oedema fluid.

V/Q mismatch is caused by regional variations in compliance, and perfusion abnormalities. With inspired oxygen concentrations in excess of 35%, perfusion of alveoli with low (but not zero) V/Q ratios has relatively little effect on arterial oxygen tension (PaO_2). If the effective shunt (venous admixture) is greater than 30–50% of CO then it may be impossible to increase the PaO_2 by increasing the inspired oxygen concentration (FIO_2).

Ventilatory (Type II) respiratory failure

Inadequate alveolar ventilation (ventilatory failure) with resultant hypercarbia may be due to:

- Reduced ventilatory effort.
- Inability to overcome an increased resistance to ventilation.
- Failure to compensate for increased carbon dioxide production.
- Failure to compensate for an increase in dead space.
- A combination of these factors.

In the patient breathing air only hypoventilation will inevitably cause hypoxaemia (alveolar gas equation). However, this is easily corrected by increasing FIO_2. Thus, in the patient breathing air, pulse oximetry is a fair monitor of alveolar ventilation; when oxygen is given, pulse oximetry will not reflect hypoventilation. An increase in dead space, either physiological dead space or dead space due to inappropriate breathing system design will result in hypercarbia if the patient is unable to increase minute ventilation to compensate. It is important to consider excessive equipment dead space when hypercarbia occurs in a patient receiving any form of respiratory support.

Simple measures to improve respiratory function

Prevention of respiratory complications should be seen as a high priority. Particular groups of patients at high risk include those with known respiratory disease, depressed level of consciousness, impaired cough, chest trauma, and post-operative upper-abdominal and thoracic surgery. Attention should be directed to:

1. Treat the underlying condition. In practice there may be difficulties in identifying underlying pathology e.g., differentiating infection from heart failure. Empirical treatment in these situations may be justifiable.

2. *Airway manoeuvres.* Airway obstruction may sometimes be subtle and must be excluded.

3. *Posture.* Sitting the patient up reduces the weight of the abdominal contents on the diaphragm, increases FRC, reduces the central blood volume, improves ventilation and reduces left ventricular diastolic pressure.

4. *Analgesia.* Pain, particularly that following thoracic or abdominal surgery or trauma, inhibits diaphragmatic movement, deep breathing and sighing, and results in a reduced FRC and lung collapse. Inhibition of coughing leads to sputum retention. Pain should therefore be managed aggressively with a multimodal approach, involving simple analgesics, opioids, NSAIDs and neural blockade, as appropriate.

5. *Physiotherapy.* Physiotherapy is an important part of respiratory support. Deep breathing exercises, particularly in conjunction with incentive spirometry, improve lung expansion and FRC. Chest percussion and coughing improve sputum clearance.

6. *Humidification.* Adequate humidity should always be provided in conjunction with oxygen therapy. Humidification will result in preservation of mucociliary clearance, reduces the viscosity of secretions and reduces collapse and infection.

7. *Infection control.* Infection control should be scrupulous to reduce the chances of cross-infection and nosocomial pneumonia.

Oxygen therapy

Oxygen is indicated in any patient with hypoxia; there are no absolute contra-indications. In some patients with severe COPD oxygen-induced release of hypoxic vasoconstriction increases V/Q mismatch. The subsequent increase in dead space may then cause hypercarbia. This mechanism, and not the removal of 'hypoxic drive', explains why some COPD patients become progressively hypercarbic with high concentration oxygen. Oxygen should be given when it is needed and the concentration should be titrated against an appropriate end point (usually the SaO_2).

Variable performance devices

These devices comprise the facemask (e.g., 'MC' mask, 'Hudson' mask) and nasal prongs, and are so called because they do not deliver a constant FIO_2. Most oxygen delivery systems allow a maximum flow of 15 l min^{-1}. The patient's peak inspiratory flow may reach 30 l min^{-1}, even during quiet breathing. Thus, a variable amount of air is inspired along with the delivered oxygen.

In the acutely dyspnoeic patient, peak inspiratory flow may be many times that of the normal subject and the actual FIO_2 will be lower and less predictable. Despite this, these devices are safe as long as oxygenation is being monitored. They have the advantage of being simple and inexpensive.

When using a facemask the oxygen flow should be greater than 6 l min^{-1} as a low flow will not wash the expired alveolar gas out of the mask dead space and rebreathing may occur, with resultant hypercarbia. This is of particular concern in children. The FIO_2 probably varies from about 0.35 to 0.55 with oxygen flows of 6–10 l min^{-1}.

Nasal prongs have the advantage of being comfortable and not interfering with eating and drinking. They are not as effective in mouth breathing patients. A flow of more than 2–4 l min^{-1} is uncomfortable.

Fixed performance devices.

A constant FIO_2 can be achieved by delivering the air/oxygen mixture at flows that exceed the patient's peak inspiratory flow, or by providing a reservoir bag of gas mixture from which the patient breathes. Despite their classification as fixed performance, these devices may not perform as expected in the presence of high peak inspiratory flows or abnormal breathing patterns.

The Venturi mask uses the Bernoulli principle; a moving gas has a lower pressure than stationary gas. Oxygen is forced through a small orifice producing a high velocity jet which 'sucks' ambient air into the entrainment chamber. The volume of air entrained and thus FIO_2 is a fixed function of the oxygen flow and the characteristics of the Venturi.

The Ventimask has separate Venturis for each FIO_2 and the correct oxygen flow must be given. Other systems employ a fixed Venturi but with a variable aperture to regulate air intake. Typically, to achieve an FIO_2 of 0.6, the oxygen flow is set at 15 l min^{-1} and the total gas mixture flow is 30 l min^{-1}, which exceeds peak inspiratory flow for the normal patient.

The 'non-rebreather' mask uses a collapsible bag into which high flow fresh oxygen is delivered and from which the patient inspires. Valves prevent inspiration of ambient air and prevent expiration into the reservoir bag. The system is designed to provide as high a FIO_2 as possible. In practice there is inspiratory leakage of ambient air and thus a FIO_2 of 1.0 cannot be achieved.

Continuous positive airway pressure

CPAP is indicated in any patient with hypoxia unresponsive to simple methods of oxygen delivery. Failure of alveolar ventilation may also be an indication for CPAP if improvement in compliance and reduction in the work of breathing significantly improve alveolar ventilation. Patients with profound hypoventilation should receive mechanical ventilation. CPAP does not benefit the apnoeic patient. Patients with disturbances of consciousness may not be appropriate candidates.
CPAP has a number of effects:

1. Increase in FRC. A low FRC results in atelectasis and lung collapse, leading to V/Q mismatch and reduced pulmonary compliance with increased airway resistance, which increases the work of breathing. Restoration of a normal FRC will improve oxygenation and reduce the work of breathing.

2. Reopening closed alveoli (recruitment). This occurs as part of the general improvement in FRC.

3. Reduction in left ventricular transmural pressure. This is of value in left ventricular failure and may be the main way in which CPAP improves oxygenation in acute cardiogenic oedema. CPAP does not necessarily drive pulmonary oedema fluid back into the circulation and total lung water may not change despite clinical improvement.

4. Reducing threshold work. In patients with auto-PEEP or dynamic hyper-inflation, the inspiratory muscles have to work to drop the alveolar pressure from its positive, end-expiratory value to less than the upper airway pressure (normally zero) before gas flow occurs. This is termed threshold work and may be significant. By increasing the airway pressure CPAP reduces the work required to initiate inspiratory flow.

5. Airway splinting. CPAP is a specific treatment for obstructive sleep apnoea and is often of value in patients with temporary airway problems.

6. Delivery of high FiO_2. Because CPAP systems are closed, with no rebreathing, the chosen inspired oxygen concentration can be reliably delivered, up to and including 100% oxygen.

Adverse effects:

1. Hypotension. An increase in intrathoracic pressure reduces right ventricular end diastolic volume and can precipitate hypotension in the presence of hypo-volaemia.

2. Barotrauma. As with any form of pressure therapy, over-inflation and gas trapping are possible, although frank barotrauma is rare.

3. Discomfort. Patients frequently find the CPAP mask uncomfortable and claustrophobic; patient refusal of mask CPAP is common.

4. Gastric distension. When CPAP is delivered by facemask, gastric inflation can occur. Although this is an indication for gastric decompression, prophylactic placement of a nasogastric tube is not required in every patient.

5. Pulmonary aspiration. Vomiting or regurgitation into a tight-fitting CPAP mask may result in massive aspiration.

6. Pressure necrosis. This may be helped by the use of a hydrocolloid or similar dressing placed over vulnerable areas such as the bridge of the nose.

When used in the treatment of obstructive sleep apnoea, a nasal mask is often effective and is better tolerated by the patient. In patients with manifest respiratory failure, a full facemask is usually necessary.

Airway pressure is kept at a specified level (typically 5–15 cm H_2O) throughout the respiratory cycle of spontaneously breathing patients. This is achieved by supplying the inspiratory gas at flow rates well in excess of the patient's maximal inspiratory flow capacity and placing a threshold resistor in the expiratory limb of the breathing system. In such a system the continuity of the positive pressure can be checked by examining the expiratory valve; it should stay open throughout the respiratory cycle. An alternative, but less efficient, method for providing CPAP utilizes a pressurized reservoir of fresh gas such as a spring-loaded concertina-style reservoir bag.

Non-invasive ventilation

Non-invasive positive pressure ventilation (NIPPV) via a facemask or nasal mask can be used instead of conventional ventilation via a tracheal tube. NIPPV may permit patients with chronic conditions such as muscular dystrophy to stay at home. In acute respiratory failure, for example, an exacerbation of chronic bronchitis and emphysema, use of NIPPV may avoid conventional ventilation. In some patient categories (e.g., COPD) NIPPV may improve outcome by avoiding the complications of tracheal intubation and reducing the incidence of nosocomial infections. Although full mandatory ventilation can be provided non-invasively, candidates for NIPPV should be awake and breathing spontaneously.

NIPPV can be provided by conventional ventilators and by simpler, specifically designed ventilators. The preferred mode is CPAP with pressure support. Pressure support ventilation minimizes peak inspiratory mask pressure and air leakage, and is better tolerated.

Further reading

Brochard L. Noninvasive ventilatory support. *Current Opinion in Critical Care* 1999; **5**: 28–35.
Hillberg RE, Johnson DC. Noninvasive ventilation. *New England Journal of Medicine* 1997; **337**: 1746–1752.

Related topics of interest

Arterial blood gases – analysis, p. 26; Respiratory support – invasive, p. 205; Respiratory suppport – weaning from ventilation, p. 210; Tracheostomy, p. 250

RESPIRATORY SUPPORT – INVASIVE

Stephen Fletcher

The provision of respiratory support by positive pressure ventilation is a core function of the ICU. As ventilator technology has progressed, new, and often more complex modes of ventilation, have been developed. Using the equipment available, and in the light of current knowledge, the clinician must attempt to select the safest and most appropriate mode of ventilation for any given patient.

Indications for mechanical ventilation

Despite didactic lists of indications for ventilation and trigger values of PaO_2 and $PaCO_2$, in practice the combination of respiratory failure, patient fatigue and conscious level will dictate the need for mechanical ventilation.

Complications of mechanical ventilation

Although mechanical ventilation often produces improvement in oxygenation and carbon dioxide removal, it has a number of adverse effects:

- The increase in pleural pressure reduces right ventricular diastolic volume and CO, and causes hypotension. Thus, tissue oxygen delivery may fall despite an increase in red cell oxygen content. Transmission of airway pressure to the pleural space depends on lung and chest wall compliance. In the presence of low lung compliance (e.g., ARDS) there is little transmission. There is increased pressure transmission in patients with low chest wall compliance (e.g., COPD, abdominal distension). Thus, positive pressure ventilation in these patients produces significant cardiovascular impairment.
- High airway pressures, particularly when transmitted to the distal airways can cause barotrauma. Peak pressure may be a poor indicator of risk of barotrauma. End-inspiratory plateau pressure reflects alveolar pressure and may be a better indicator of the risk of barotrauma. Pulmonary damage is related more closely to changes in alveolar volume which results in high shear forces between open and closed lung units and loss of surfactant ('volutrauma'). Alveolar hyperinflation and subsequent disruption will result in pneumomediastinum and pneumothorax. Volutrauma will also cause pulmonary interstitial oedema.

Recent changes in ventilatory techniques have emphasized the importance of reducing distal airway pressure by encouraging the patient to maintain some spontaneous respiratory effort while gaining a degree of assistance from the ventilator. Keeping the alveoli open and eliminating large swings in alveolar pressure may reduce shear forces, thus limiting parenchymal damage.

Modes of ventilation

Mechanical ventilation can be pressure-targeted ('pressure control') or flow-controlled volume-cycled ('volume control'). The addition PEEP will improve oxygenation by alveolar recruitment. Excessive PEEP will compromise venous return and may cause hypotension.

1. *Volume control ventilation.* Standard volume-controlled mechanical ventilation is the least sophisticated ventilatory mode. Breaths are delivered at a preselected rate and volume and lung compliance determines the airway pressures generated. The main limitation of this mode is that it does not allow any contribution from the patient. Volume-targeted modes provide a preset volume unless a specified pressure limit is exceeded. Depending on the precise ventilator, the clinician may select either tidal volume and flow delivery pattern or flow delivery pattern and minimum minute ventilation. Older ventilators provided only a constant flow delivery profile. A decelerating flow will improve distribution of ventilation to the lungs.

2. *Pressure-controlled ventilation.* Inspiratory pressure is limited to a level selected by the clinician, while inspiratory flow will vary with the resistance and compliance of the patient's respiratory system. Tidal volume depends on the inspiratory flow rate and inspiratory time. The decelerating flow pattern results in a reduction of peak airway pressure. However, mean airway pressure is increased. Oxygenation can be dramatically enhanced by prolonging inspiratory time. Inverse ratio ventilation is defined by an I:E ratio greater than 1:1 and can be performed in conjunction with volume-controlled or pressure-controlled modes. The longer inspiratory time will reduce peak airway pressures. The short expiratory time will not allow for complete lung deflation, and there may be a significant increase in end-expiratory alveolar pressure (so called auto-PEEP or $PEEP_I$), even when external PEEP is zero. Mean airway pressure is increased.

3. *Assisted mechanical ventilation.* During mechanical assisted ventilation each inspiration triggered by the patient is boosted by the ventilator. Assisted modes allow much better ventilator–patient synchrony and will help to reduce respiratory muscle atrophy. This enhances patient co-operation and should eliminate the need for heavy sedation. Older ventilators have pressure triggers that require the patient to generate a negative-pressure deflection below the set level of end-expiratory pressure to initiate the machine's inspiratory phase. Modern ventilators have much improved sensitive flow triggers that will allow initiation of the inspiratory phase without a negative-pressure deflection.

The patient-initiated breaths can be pressure supported (to a predetermined peak inspiratory pressure) or volume supported (to a predetermined tidal volume). During pressure support ventilation (PSV) inspiration ends when the inspiratory flow reaches a threshold value (e.g., 25% of peak flow), which theoretically coincides with the end of the inspiratory muscle effort. This method of cycling is one of the most comfortable for the patient. The level of pressure support is adjusted to allow the patient's respiratory rate to be between 25 and 30 breaths min^{-1}.

Synchronized intermittent mandatory ventilation (SIMV) forces a number of mandatory breaths (to a preset tidal volume or pressure) in addition to the patient's own efforts. The mandatory breaths are synchronized to the patient's own inspiratory effort. SIMV ensures a minimum minute volume but there may be substantial variation in tidal volume between the mandatory breaths and the patient's unassisted breaths.

Strategies for mechanical ventilation

When initiating mechanical ventilation typical settings might be:

PEEP	5 cm H_2O
Tidal volume (VC mode)	7–10 ml kg^{-1}
Inspiratory pressure (PC mode)	20 cm H_2O (15 above PEEP)
Frequency	10 – 15 min^{-1}
I:E ratio	1:2
Pressure trigger	–1 to –3 cm H_2O
Flow trigger	2 l min^{-1}
Pressure support	20 cm H_2O (15 above PEEP)

These settings should be titrated against the patient's PaO_2 and $PaCO_2$ and comfort. Carbon dioxide elimination can be improved by increasing the tidal volume (or peak pressure) or by increasing the respiratory rate. Oxygenation of arterial blood can be improved by increasing the FIO_2, increasing external PEEP, or by prolonging the inspiratory time. The latter will raise mean airway pressure and create $PEEP_i$.

Prolonged exposure to an $FIO_2 > 0.5$–0.6 may cause pulmonary oxygen toxicity and it may be better to increase PEEP and/or prolong the inspiratory time once this concentration is required. It is not necessary to achieve 'normal' arterial blood gases; in the absence of lactic acidosis or a marked base deficit a PaO_2 of 8 kPa is often adequate. Where possible, inspiratory plateau pressure should be limited to < 35 cm H_2O. This should help to reduce overdistension of relatively compliant areas of lung. Limiting inspiratory pressure in this way may necessitate using small tidal volumes of 5–7 ml kg^{-1} and will result in hypercarbia. In the presence of adequate renal function, the rising $PaCO_2$ will be adequately compensated and the pH will remain near normal. This strategy of permissive hypercapnoea may reduce barotrauma but has yet to be shown to improve outcome.

Adjuncts to mechanical ventilation

1. Prone ventilation. In ARDS, the lung often consists of discrete healthy and diseased portions. Dependant areas become consolidated and a large V/Q mismatch results. Placing the ventilated patient prone directs more ventilation to the dorsal areas and hence improves V/Q matching. In practice, around 60% of patients will show improvement in oxygenation. This improvement may be sustained by changing periodically from front to back. The main disadvantage of prone positioning is the likelihood of tube and catheter displacement, difficulty nursing and pressure effects on the face. The results of a multicentre study to determine whether prone ventilation in ARDS improves survival are awaited.

2. Nitric oxide. In ARDS, NO causes vasodilation specifically in ventilated lung areas, secondarily reducing perfusion to poorly ventilated regions. V/Q matching improves and around 60–70% of patients experience an improvement in oxygenation. It is believed that by permitting a reduction in the 'intensity' of ventilation, NO might improve outcome in ARDS. This remains unproven.

3. Prostacyclin (PGI₂). Given intravenously or by nebulization, prostacyclin is a pulmonary vasodilator. However, there is some vasodilation in non-ventilated lung regions even when given by nebulizer and this limits its efficacy in improving V/Q matching.

Specialized modes of ventilation

1. *High frequency ventilation.* There are three modes of high frequency ventilation:

- High frequency positive pressure ventilation (HFPPV). Although some conventional ventilators can achieve the frequency that defines HFPPV (60–120 breaths min^{-1}), this mode is rarely used.
- High frequency oscillation ventilation (HFOV). This mode is practicable only in small children and requires specific equipment. A diaphragm oscillating at 3–20 Hz induces CO_2 elimination and a system of CPAP provides oxygenation.
- High frequency jet ventilation (HFJV). Jet ventilation requires both a special ventilator and a specific design of tracheal tube. High pressure gas (1–2 bar) is directed into the distal trachea at frequencies of between 1 and 5 Hz. Tidal volumes are usually unmeasurable, gas exchange occurring via poorly defined mechanisms thought to include facilitated diffusion.

Although jet ventilation is of value in the setting of massive airleak from bronchopleural fistula, none of these modes have proven superiority over conventional ventilation in adults. In addition, barotrauma, difficulty in humidifying inspired gases and other technical problems limit its usefulness.

2. *Independent lung ventilation.* The lungs of patients with severe asymmetric lung disease will have marked differences in compliance resulting in unevenly distributed ventilation. By placing a double-lumen endobronchial tube and attaching two ventilators, one to each lumen, it is possible to optimize the ventilatory parameters for each lung individually. The endobronchial tube can be difficult to position initially, and later can migrate out of position. The relatively narrow lumina of the double-lumen tube can make aspiration or suction difficult.

3. *Tracheal gas insufflation (TGI).* The simple act of infusing oxygen by catheter into the airway at the level of the carina both improves oxygenation (partly by simply increasing the mean FiO_2) and improves CO_2 elimination. The main benefit stems from an effective reduction in dead space. TGI may be of value in ventilated patients with refractory hypoxaemia.

4. *Cuirass ventilation.* An airtight rigid shell applied to the anterior thorax allows ventilation by negative pressure. The Hayek oscillator allows very high frequency cuirass ventilation. Although there are theoretical advantages, including haemodynamic stability and improved sputum clearance, in practice the cuirass systems are rarely used.

5. *Partial liquid ventilation (PLV).* Perfluorocarbon solutions (Perflubron or Fluosol-DA) have a high solubility for oxygen. In PLV these solutions are instilled into the lungs until a meniscus is seen in the tracheal tube. Oxygenation improves by a combination of improved distribution of perfusion (a function of the solution's weight) and improved alveolar stability. The technique remains experimental.

6. Intravenous oxygenation (IVOX). Pure oxygen is drawn through a mass of hollow, gas permeable fibres placed surgically in the IVC via a femoral venotomy. Unfortunately, the contribution to gas exchange is limited and this technique remains experimental.

7. Extracorporeal CO$_2$ removal (ECCO$_2$R). ECCO$_2$R is a modification of full ECMO. The lower extracorporeal blood flow enables smaller vascular catheters to be used while still maintaining high gas flows across the membrane. This optimizes CO$_2$ removal but oxygenation is still partly dependant on the lungs. Low frequency ventilation allows the lungs to 'rest'. Whilst these extracorporeal techniques are undoubtedly beneficial in neonates, their contribution to the management of adult ARDS is controversial. To date the only prospective randomized trial in adults shows no benefit in comparison with conventional respiratory support.

Further reading

Bramson RD. New modes of mechanical ventilation. *Current Opinion in Critical Care* 1999; **5**: 33–42.
Kacmarek RM. Innovations in mechanical ventilation. *Current Opinion in Critical Care* 1999; **5**: 43–51.

Related topics of interest

Arterial blood gases – analysis, p.26; Respiratory support – non-invasive, p. 200; Respiratory support – weaning from ventilation, p. 210

RESPIRATORY SUPPORT – WEANING FROM VENTILATION

Jonathan Hadfield

Mechanical ventilation is associated with complications. It is thus important to discontinue ventilator support at the earliest opportunity. More than 40% of the time that a patient receives mechanical ventilation in a critical care unit is spent trying to wean the patient from the ventilator.

Once the underlying pathological process inducing the need for mechanical ventilation has resolved, the patient gradually resumes the full ventilatory workload to allow discontinuation of mechanical support. Weaning allows gradual exercise and reconditioning of the respiratory muscles and return of co-ordinated activity.

The speed with which a patient may be weaned from ventilatory support is usually dependant on the duration of ventilation. Rapid weaning and early extubation can be expected in post-operative patients, acute asthma exacerbations and drug overdoses whereas longer weaning periods are predicted for those with more extensive dysfunction such as COPD and ARDS. The use of assist modes of ventilation at the earliest opportunity will help maintain respiratory muscle function.

Problems

- Pre-requisites – is the patient ready for weaning?
- Predictors – will the patient manage to self ventilate?
- Preparation of the patient for weaning.
- Methods or techniques of weaning.

Pre-requisites

Weaning is unlikely to be successful if:

- There is persistent hypoxia (common criteria for acceptable oxygenation are $PaO_2 > 8$ kPa, $FIO_2 < 0.5$ and PEEP $\leqslant 5$ cm H_2O).
- Patient psychological status is poor (e.g., confusion, agitation, depression).
- The original disease is still active.
- There is haemodynamic instability or a continued requirement for pressor support.
- Sepsis is present (increased O_2 consumption and CO_2 production increasing respiratory demand).
- There is severe abdominal distension producing diaphragmatic tamponade.

Predictors

Successful weaning may be predicted by:

- Vital capacity > 10–15 ml kg^{-1}.
- Tidal volume > 5 ml kg^{-1}.
- Minute volume < 10 l min^{-1}.
- Respiratory rate < 35 breathes min^{-1}.
- Maximum negative inspiratory pressure > 20 cm H_2O.

More complex means of assessment include:

- Work of breathing (computed from transpulmonary pressure and volume).
- Measurement of respiratory muscle oxygen consumption.
- Assessment of respiratory muscle function (electromyograms of diaphragm, transdiaphragmatic pressures).
- Ultrasound assessment of intercostal muscle bulk.
- Assessment of ventilatory drive using airway occlusion pressure measured at the mouth or tracheal tube in the first 0.1 s of inspiratory effort against an occluded airway.

Preparation

Administration of neuromuscular blocking agents should be ceased in anticipation of any attempt at weaning.

Pain should be controlled using regional analgesic techniques (e.g., epidural infusions) to minimize the requirement for systemic opioids which cause respiratory depression. Nutrition must be optimized to fuel the respiratory muscles and anabolic processes of the body. Malnutrition will result in atrophy and weakness of the respiratory muscles. Excessive calorific intake, especially of carbohydrate, will increase CO_2 production and exert greater demands on the respiratory muscles. Electrolytes essential to muscle function (Ca^{2+}, Mg^{2+}, K^+, PO_4^{2-}) should be within the normal ranges.

The weaning process should be explained to the patient accompanied by continuous support and encouragement to maintain motivation and co-operation.

Method

Using assist modes of ventilation (e.g., pressure support) it is possible to adjust the level of support to meet the patient's demands, whilst still allowing gradual exercise of the respiratory muscles. From the outset the ventilator settings are continually matched to the requirements of each patient. Weaning thus becomes a continuous process beginning from the time the initial pathology begins to resolve.

1. Pressure support weaning. In this mode all breaths are initiated by the patient following which the ventilator generates an inspiratory pressure in the breathing circuit to assist each breath. The inspiratory phase is terminated when the inspiratory flow reaches a threshold value (e.g., 25% of peak flow). There is no backup ventilation should the patient become apnoeic. The pressure support is gradually reduced, usually to a level of 5–10 cm H_2O (a minimum necessary to eliminate work done against resistance to airflow through a tracheal tube and ventilator breathing system), at which point a trial of CPAP may be initiated or the patient extubated.

2. CPAP/T-Piece weaning. A CPAP/T-Piece circuit is used intermittently for progressively extended periods allowing the patient to take over all the work of breathing with shortening periods of rest on the ventilator. This technique is simple but requires close observation of the patient to avoid exhaustion.

3. Intermittent mandatory ventilation (IMV) weaning. The ventilator delivers a preset tidal volume at a preset rate ensuring a minimum minute volume is delivered to the patient irrespective of their own effort. Patient generated breaths are then permitted in between. These breaths can also be pressure. The number of ventilator delivered breaths is reduced gradually allowing the patient to take on the full work of breathing. Ventilator breaths are usually synchronized to the patients own efforts (SIMV). The ventilator will deliver a mandatory breath independent of respiratory effort only if a patient initiated breath does not occur within a specified time period. Recent data suggest that SIMV and IMV are not as effective at reducing respiratory work as pressure support.

It is likely that patients who are easy to wean from mechanical ventilation will progress successfully irrespective of the technique used. Prospective randomized trials of weaning modes have reached conflicting conclusions. However, there is consensus that SIMV is the least efficient method of weaning from ventilation.

4. Adjunctive treatments

- Salbutamol: evidence suggests inhaled β_2 agonists may reduce work of breathing by 25% even if there is no evidence of bronchospasm
- Aminophylline may improve diaphragmatic contractility and may be beneficial in counteracting respiratory muscle fatigue in patients whose work of breathing is normally increased (e.g., COPD).

Failure to wean

Close observation of the patient for early signs of failure to wean is essential to avoid distress, fatigue and haemodynamic compromise. Subjective symptoms of fatigue and dyspnoea will often be the first indicators followed by evident exhaustion accompanied by a falling tidal volume and rising respiratory rate. At this point the level of support must be increased to assist the respiratory muscles and avoid fatigue. Respiratory muscles once fatigued to a state of exhaustion take many hours to recover.

It is sensible to initiate weaning early on in the day so progress can be closely monitored, possibly with planned periods of rest overnight.

Further reading

Dries DJ. Weaning from mechanical ventilation. *Journal of Trauma* 1997; **43**: 372–384.
Esteban A, Alia I. Clinical management of weaning from mechanical ventilation. *Intensive Care Medicine* 1998; **24**: 999–1008.

Related topics of interest

Analgesia – advanced, p. 18; Analgesia – basic, p. 14; Respiratory support – invasive, p. 205; Respiratory support – non-invasive, p. 200; Sedation, p. 223; Tracheostomy, p. 250

RESUSCITATION – CARDIOPULMONARY

In adults the commonest primary arrhythmia at the onset of cardiac arrest is ventricular fibrillation (VF) or pulseless ventricular tachycardia. The definitive treatment of these arrhythmias – defibrillation – must be administered promptly. Survival from VF falls by 7–10% for every minute after collapse. Advanced life support (ALS) is the process that attempts to deliver the definitive treatment for the underlying rhythm. Basic life support (BLS) extends the interval between the onset of the collapse and the development of irreversible organ damage and provides the opportunity for ALS to be effective.

Basic life support

Basic life support refers to maintaining airway patency, and supporting breathing and the circulation without the use of equipment other than a protective mouth shield. It consists of the initial assessment, airway maintenance, expired air ventilation (rescue breathing) and chest compressions. Failure of the circulation to deliver oxygenated blood to the brain for 3–4 min (less if the patient was initially hypoxic) will lead to irreversible cerebral damage. The purpose of BLS is to maintain adequate ventilation and circulation until the underlying cause of the cardiac arrest can be treated.

During two-person CPR five chest compressions (rate 100 min^{-1} with 4–5 cm sternal depression) are given for each breath of 400–600 ml.

Advanced life support

A universal adult ALS treatment algorithm has been developed. After the initial assessment it divides into two pathways; arrest in VF/VT and other rhythms. Each step in the algorithm assumes that the previous step was unsuccessful. When using the algorithm it is essential to remember that early defibrillation, adequate oxygenation and ventilation through a clear airway, and chest compressions, are always more important than the administration of drugs.

Above all, **treat the patient, not the monitor.**

Defibrillation

The initial three shocks in the treatment sequence of VF/VT should be delivered at 200 J, 200 J, and 360 J. Thereafter each shock should be at 360 J. If VF/VT recurs after a period of spontaneous circulation, the first and second shocks should be delivered at 200 J. Defibrillators should always be charged with the paddles held against the patient's chest wall or whilst housed in the defibrillator. They should never be charged with the paddles held in the air. The most commonly use transthoracic defibrillators deliver energy as a damped sinusoidal waveform. Newer defibrillators using a biphasic waveform reduce the energy requirement for successful defibrillation. Automated defibrillators that deliver a current based shock appropriate to the measured transthoracic impedance (impedance compensation) are also available.

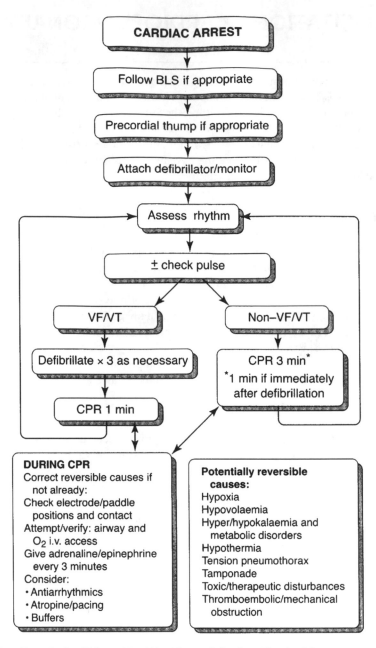

```
┌─────────────────────────┐
│     CARDIAC ARREST      │
└─────────────────────────┘
            │
            ▼
┌─────────────────────────┐
│  Follow BLS if appropriate │
└─────────────────────────┘
            │
            ▼
┌─────────────────────────────┐
│ Precordial thump if appropriate │
└─────────────────────────────┘
            │
            ▼
┌─────────────────────────┐
│ Attach defibrillator/monitor │
└─────────────────────────┘
            │
            ▼
┌─────────────────────────┐
│      Assess  rhythm      │
└─────────────────────────┘
            │
            ▼
┌─────────────────────────┐
│      ± check pulse       │
└─────────────────────────┘
```

VF/VT

Non–VF/VT

Defibrillate × 3 as necessary

CPR 3 min*
*1 min if immediately after defibrillation

CPR 1 min

DURING CPR
Correct reversible causes if
  not already:
Check electrode/paddle
  positions and contact
Attempt/verify: airway and
  O_2 i.v. access
Give adrenaline/epinephrine
  every 3 minutes
Consider:
• Antiarrhythmics
• Atropine/pacing
• Buffers

**Potentially reversible
  causes:**
Hypoxia
Hypovolaemia
Hyper/hypokalaemia and
  metabolic disorders
Hypothermia
Tension pneumothorax
Tamponade
Toxic/therapeutic disturbances
Thromboembolic/mechanical
  obstruction

Reprinted from *Resuscitation*, Volume 37, 1998 with permission from Elsevier Science.

Vasopressor agents

Adrenaline improves myocardial and cerebral blood flow and resuscitation rates in experimental animals. There is no clinical evidence that adrenaline improves neurological outcome in humans. It remains, however, the only recommended pressor agent in adult cardiac arrest.

Anti-arrhythmic drug therapy

Haemodynamically significant bradycardias should be treated with atropine. A single dose of 3 mg i.v. is sufficient to block vagal activity in fit adults with a cardiac output. There is incomplete evidence to make firm recommendations on the use of any anti-arrhythmic during VF/VT. Lidocaine (lignocaine), bretylium and amiodarone all have their proponents but defibrillation remains the treatment of choice for these rhythms.

Buffer agents

If effective BLS is performed arterial blood gas analysis does not show a rapid development of acidosis during CPR. A prospective randomized controlled trial of the use of a buffer in patients suffering out of hospital cardiac arrest failed to show an improvement in outcome. The judicious use of buffers is advocated in severe acidosis (pH < 7.1, base excess < −10) and in cardiac arrest associated with hyperkalaemia or following tricyclic anti-depressant overdose.

The denervated heart

A denervated heart (as occurs following heart transplantation) is exquisitely sensitive to the actions of adenosine. Supraventricular tachyarrythmias in a denervated heart should not be treated with adenosine. In the presence of severe bradycardia that does not respond to atropine or pacing an adenosine antagonist (e.g. aminophylline) should be considered.

Return of spontaneous circulation (ROSC)

Patients who are successfully resuscitated should be referred immediately for post resuscitation care.

Further reading

Colquhoun MC, Handley AJ, Evans TR. *ABC of Resuscitation* Third Edition. London, BMJ Publishing Group, 1995.
Parr MJA, Craft TM. *Resuscitation: Key Data – Third Edition.* Oxford: BIOS Scientific Publishers Ltd, 1998, 109 pp.

Related topics of interest

Cardiac chest pain, p. 69; Cardiac pacing, p. 80; Resuscitation – post-resuscitation care, p. 216

RESUSCITATION – POST-RESUSCITATION CARE

The objective of CPR is to produce a patient with normal cerebral function, no neurological deficit, a stable cardiac rhythm, and normal haemodynamic function, resulting in adequate organ perfusion. The return of a spontaneous circulation (ROSC) is just the first step in what may be a long process in some patients.

Aims of post-resuscitation care

- Prevent a further cardiac arrest (secondary prevention).
- Define the underlying pathology.
- Limit organ damage.
- Predict non-survivors.

Secondary prevention

To stabilize a patient who has survived initial resuscitation as many variables as possible should be corrected. Oxygenation should be optimized. Following all but the briefest cardiac arrest (e.g., ventricular fibrillation responding to immediate precordial thump or early defibrillation) this will require assisted ventilation via a tracheal tube. Even after an immediate return to full consciousness following a short cardiac arrest, patients should be given additional oxygen via a facemask.

Electrolyte disturbances, in particular of the cations K^+, Mg^{2+}, and Ca^{2+}, should be corrected. Acidaemia (high blood H^+ ion concentrations) should be corrected by addressing the underlying cause (e.g., poor peripheral perfusion) rather than by the administration of alkali such as bicarbonate. Bicarbonate may result in intracellular acidosis as it is converted to carbon dioxide with the release of H^+ ions within the cell. Exceptions, when small amounts of bicarbonate may be given following cardiac arrest, are profound acidaemia (pH $<$ 7.1, base excess $>$ −10), when the excess H^+ ions may directly depress myocardial function, cardiac arrest associated with hyperkalaemia or following tricyclic antidepressant overdose. Bicarbonate (or other alkalis) should be administered against known blood acid-base status and its effect monitored by frequent arterial blood gas analysis.

Hyperglycaemia, even in the non-diabetic, should be treated with insulin.

Define the underlying pathology

The patient's pre-arrest medical condition should be established.

Assessment of the current status requires a thorough physical examination, seeking, in particular, evidence of correct placement of tracheal tube (bilateral, equal signs of air entry), broken ribs, and pneumothorax. Listen to the heart for evidence of murmurs (valvular damage, septal rupture) and seek evidence of ventricular failure. A brief neurological assessment should be made and the GCS recorded. Investigations to support the physical findings include a CXR, 12 lead ECG, arterial blood gas analysis and baseline creatinine and electrolytes.

Limit organ damage

In those patients whose cardiac arrest is associated with a myocardial ischaemia, a supply of oxygenated blood needs to be restored to all parts of the myocardium as soon as possible. This will help prevent myocardial necrosis and limit the size of any associated acute infarct. Coronary artery reperfusion using thrombolytic agents carries its own risk of the development of arrhythmias. Protracted chest compressions are a relative contraindication to thrombolysis (see Cardiac chest pain p. 69).

A third of patients who achieve ROSC following cardiac arrest eventually die a neurological death whilst one third of long-term survivors have motor or cognitive deficit.

The extent of damage to other organs, especially the brain, after ROSC depends greatly on the ability of the heart to deliver adequate amounts of oxygenated blood to them. This in turn may influence the occurrence of a secondary hypoxic insult consequent upon microcirculatory changes. A variety of inflammatory mediators (TNF, IL-1, IL-6) may contribute to this 'post-resuscitation syndrome'. Despite extensive investigation, no specific therapy has yet been shown to improve cerebral outcome.

Predict non-survivors

Those working in critical care have a moral, ethical, and fiscal responsibility to treat only those patients who will benefit from it. Despite years of research, survival from cardiac arrest remains disappointing. Minimizing the duration of cardiac arrest and CPR correlates with more rapid ROSC and better neurological outcomes. Prognostication in those with depressed CNS after more protracted CPR remains unreliable in the first 24 hours and possibly for as long as 72 hours after ROSC. Myocardial, neurological and other organ function may all improve slowly given appropriate support over a period of time. Vigorous intensive care for at least 72 hours should thus be considered in the comatose patient with ROSC following cardiac arrest.

Long term management

All patients who have survived an acute myocardial infarction require rehabilitation and lifestyle counselling (see Cardiac Chest Pain p. 69).

Automatic implantable cardioverter defibrillators (AICDS) have been shown to reduce mortality in those patients at risk of recurrent cardiac arrest due to ventricular tachycardia or fibrillation. Such patients should be identified using electrophysiological testing and considered for implantation of an AICD.

Care of the arrest team

All attempts at resuscitation should be audited formally and the team debriefed at the earliest opportunity after cessation of the acute resuscitation, regardless of the outcome. Audit data should be recorded on a standard Utstein template so that comparable multi-centre information can be gathered. Examination of the performance of the team should take the form of positive critique and not develop a fault/blame culture. Whether the attempts at resuscitation were successful or not, the relatives of the patient will obviously require a considerable amount of support. Equally, the pastoral needs of all those associated with the arrest, no matter how hardy they may seem, should not be forgotten.

Further reading.

Nolan JP. Post resuscitation care. In: Bossaert L (ed.) *European Resuscitation Council Guidelines for Resuscitation*. Amsterdam: Elsevier, 1998, pp. 55–61.

Related topics of interest

Cardiac chest pain; p. 69; Cardiac pacing, p. 80; Resuscitation – cardiopulmonary, p. 213

SCORING SYSTEMS

Angela White

Scoring systems are designed to provide objective measurement of a patients condition at a point or particular period in time. They have a variety of uses:

- Giving an indication of current clinical state and monitoring that state over time.
- Predicting outcome given a specific disease.
- Assisting with triage of casualties.
- As a tool for comparing efficacy of ICUs.

Each scoring system depends on quantifying values for variables to produce a score that may be used independently or incorporated into some further equation.

There are a number of different scoring systems. The most frequently used in critical care include:

- GCS: Glasgow Coma Scale;
- APACHE II: Acute Physiology and Chronic Health Evaluation;
- TISS: Therapeutic Intervention Scoring System;
- ISS: Injury Severity Score.

Glasgow coma scale – GCS

Was introduced in 1974 by Teasdale and Jennett as a means of quantifying the neurological status of head injured patients. Conscious level is assessed by eye opening, verbal, and motor responses. The test is easily repeatable and can be used for continuous assessment of the patient. The GCS can also provide an indication of likely outcome.

The maximum score is 15 and is calculated in adult patients according to the following findings. In children and babies the responses are variously redefined. The minimum score is 3.

Coma is defined as GCS of 8 or less.

	Eye opening	Verbal response	Motor response
6	–	–	Obeys Commands
5	–	Orientated	Localizes to pain
4	Spontaneous	Confused	Normal flexion (withdrawal) to pain
3	To speech	Inappropriate	Abnormal flexion to pain
2	To pain	Incomprehensible	Extends to pain
1	None	None	None

Acute physiology and chronic health evaluation – APACHE II

Is a system for classifying severity of disease. It has a number of uses:

- It provides a score which can be incorporated in to an equation to calculate risk of death.
- It can be used to correct for case mix when comparing the efficacy of different therapies in specific disease states.

- It enables evaluation of hospital resources and comparisons of ICUs in different hospitals.

The score is based on 12 physiological variables (the smallest number that can convey derangement in all vital organ systems), the age of the patient and evaluation of chronic health. Severity of acute illness is quantified by recording the extent of deviation from normal.

Chronic health status and age are included as they reflect premorbid physiological reserve.

The physiological variables attract a score from 0 to 4 according to the deviation of the value from the normal range. The most abnormal values in the first 24 hours of admission to intensive care are selected. The following variables are recorded:

- Temperature.
- MAP.
- Heart rate.
- Respiratory rate.
- Oxygenation.
- Arterial pH.
- Serum sodium.
- Serum potassium.
- Serum creatinine.
- Haematocrit.
- White cell count.
- GCS (Score 15 less actual GCS).

The chronic health status is based on defined criteria for severe organ dysfunction or immunocompromise that were present before the current hospital admission.

Points are assigned according to whether the patient has received an operation or not and if so whether it was elective or emergency operative intervention. Non-operative or emergency post-operative care scores 5 points; elective post-operative scores 2 points. A surgical patient is one who is admitted direct from theatre or recovery. All others are non-operative. Sedated, ventilated patients with no anticipated neurological dysfunction score a GCS of 15 and an as yet undetected disability will not be accounted for in the assessment.

Age points are assigned as follows:

- < 44 years   0
- 45–54 years   2
- 55–64 years   3
- 65–74 years   5
- > 75 years   6

Scores from 0 to 71 are theoretically possible. The risk of hospital death increases with increasing score.

Therapeutic Intervention Scoring System – TISS

TISS is an easy method of classifying critical care patients. It has both clinical and administrative applications:

- Assessing severity of illness.
- Determining resource requirements (nursing ratios, number of critical care beds).
- Assessing use of critical care facilities and function.

As yet, TISS has not been standardized; different hospitals use different score allocations. Daily data are collected on each patient concerning about 70 possible clinical interventions. Ideally, data are collected at the same time(s) each day and by the same observer.

Each intervention is rated from 1 to 4 points and, where several related interventions have been undertaken in the assessment period points are only awarded for the highest scoring intervention.

Based on the TISS score, four classes of patients are recognized.

- Class I: < 10 points, does not require critical care.
- Class II: 10–19 points, 1:2 nurse:patient ratio.
- Class III: 20–39 points, 1:1 nurse:patient ratio.
- Class IV: > 40 points, 1:1 nurse:patient ratio (+ more nursing assistance).

A patient who is improving shows a trend of decreasing points. Conversely, an increasing number of points implies that the patient is deteriorating.

TISS can provide an estimate of the cost of an episode of care by dividing the cost of running the unit by the total number of TISS points allocated. The result, typically around £25, can then be multiplied by the number of points allocated to the intervention or episode in question.

Injury Severity Score – ISS

The ISS is designed to quantify the overall severity of injury in the multi-injured patient. Its basis is the Abbreviated Injury Scale (AIS) which details a score from 0 (no injury) to 6 (fatal injury) for over 1200 injuries.

For the purposes of the ISS the body is divided into six regions:

- Head and neck.
- Abdomen and pelvic contents.
- Bony pelvis and limbs.
- Face.
- Chest.
- Body surface area.

The score is derived by taking the AIS values for the three most severely injured body regions. The values are individually squared and then summed. The maximum value possible is $3 \times 5^2 = 75$.

An AIS of 6 is automatically allocated a score of 75.

The score correlates well with mortality. When ISS was developed, the highest score in a surviving patient was 50. Of the fatalities, the higher the score the shorter the survival time. For scores of less than 10 there were no deaths in a patient less than 50 years old and no one dead on arrival. Death rates increase with increasing number of body areas injured even though each injury in isolation may not be life threatening.

In addition to using the ISS as a predictor of patient prognosis, the score also allows evaluation of mortality in different groups of trauma patients and might be used to assist evaluation of changes in emergency management of certain patient groups.

The new ISS (NISS) has been described recently. By allowing more than one injury to be included from a single body region it may predict outcome more accurately.

Further reading

Knaus WA, *et al.* APACHE II: a severity of disease classification system. *Crit. Care Med.*, 1985; **13:** 818–829.

Steele A, Bocconi GA, Oggioni R, Tulli F. Scoring systems in intensive care. *Curr. Anaesthesia Crit. Care,* 1998, 9: 8–15.

Related topics of interest

SEDATION

Sedatives help to relieve anxiety, encourage sleep, help the patient to synchronize with the ventilator, and permit therapeutic procedures. The requirements for sedation will vary greatly depending on the patient's pathology, psychological state, and intensity of the medical and nursing procedures being undertaken. Improving the patient's environment may help to reduce the need for drugs. Effective communication and appropriate reassurance will help to relieve the patient's anxiety. Many patients receiving mechanical ventilation will require sufficient sedation to keep them comfortable yet rousable to voice. Patients with a tracheostomy who are receiving assisted modes of ventilation may not require any sedation. Where indicated, epidural analgesia will prevent the need for large doses of systemic analgesia. Those requiring unphysiological modes of ventilation (e.g., inverse ratio), prone ventilation, or control of intracranial hypertension or seizures, for example, will need heavy sedation.

The ideal sedative

The ideal sedative would possess the following properties:

- Anxiolysis.
- Analgesia.
- Hypnosis.
- Amnesia.
- Titratability.
- Predictable effect.
- Rapid elimination.
- Lack of cardiovascular and gastrointestinal side effects.
- No development of tolerance.
- Low cost.

No single agent meets all of these ideals and for this reason it is common practice to use a combination of drugs. However, even this approach rarely achieves all of the objectives.

Drug administration

Sedatives are administered usually by bolus or by continuous intravenous infusion. Inhalational sedation with isoflurane has been described but is rarely used. Continuous infusion is a convenient method of drug administration but may produce over-sedation if the patient's conscious level is not assessed frequently. Bolus dosing will reduce the incidence of over-sedation but is less convenient for nursing staff.

Drugs

1. Sedative drugs. Propofol and benzodiazepines are the commonest sedatives used in critical care. Benzodiazepines produce excellent sedation, anxiolysis, and amnesia. Midazolam is the most commonly used benzodiazepine in critical care. All benzodiazepines are extensively metabolized in the liver. Sepsis will reduce blood flow to the liver and will impair the metabolism of benzodiazepines. The active metabolite of midazolam is α-hydroxy-midazolam. This is shorter acting than the metabolites of diazepam but nevertheless will accumulate with prolonged infusion and will add to the sedative effects of midazolam.

Propofol is an intravenous anaesthetic agent. It is eliminated rapidly from the central compartment and full recovery of consciousness is achieved very quickly (minutes) even after infusions for many days. Hepatic and renal dysfunction have no clinically significant effect on the metabolism of propofol. Propofol reduces systemic vascular resistance and will tend to cause hypotension. The main disadvantage of propofol is its cost. However, the reduction in length of stay achieved by using propofol may offset its cost. Anecdotal reports of severe cardiovascular depression after prolonged propofol infusions in critically ill children have prevented its widespread use in patients under 16 years. When propofol is used in combination with an opioid, typical infusion rates to achieve adequate sedation are 1.5–3 mg kg^{-1} h^{-1}.

2. Analgesic drugs. Opioids will produce effective analgesia and anxiolysis, and will help too to reduce respiratory drive. The respiratory depression produced by opioids may help the patient to synchronize with the ventilator. However, excessive doses will cause apnoea and prevent the use of patient-triggered modes of ventilation. They will also cause gastrointestinal stasis, which will hamper the ability to feed the patient enterally. Morphine is cheap and remains a popular choice for analgesia and sedation in critical care. It is metabolized mainly in the liver to produce morphine-3-glucuronide and morphine-6-glucuronide. The latter is a potent analgesic and is excreted in the urine. Considerable accumulation of this metabolite occurs in patients with renal impairment and for this reason morphine is normally avoided in patients with renal failure.

Fentanyl is a synthetic opioid that is commonly used in anaesthetic practice. In single doses, fentanyl has a short duration of action. However, redistribution rather than the clearance determines duration of action. Thus, after a prolonged infusion, recovery from fentanyl can take a considerable time. Alfentanil is shorter acting than fentanyl. The action of alfentanil is terminated by clearance rather than distribution, thus following a prolonged infusion accumulation is less likely. However, in critically ill patients even the clearance of alfentanil can be variable. Remifentanil is ultra-short acting, but as yet there are limited data on its use in critical care.

Assessment of sedation

It may be possible to simply ask the patient whether or not their sedation is adequate. In most cases, however, the patient's illness, the presence of a tracheal tube, and the effects of sedation itself may make this impossible. There are a variety of sedation scoring systems but the most widely used is that described by Ramsay:

Awake levels

1. Patient anxious and agitated or restless, or both.
2. Patient co-operative, orientated and tranquil.
3. Patient responds to commands only.

Asleep levels dependent on response to glabellar tap or loud auditory stimulus

4. Brisk response.
5. Sluggish response.
6. No response.

Levels 2–4 are appropriate for most patients. The level of sedation must be assessed regularly, particularly when the sedatives are given by infusion. Physical methods of measuring sedation have been described. Most are used primarily for assessing depth of anaesthesia and many are based on electroencephalography. None of these systems are in routine clinical use.

Neuromuscular blocking drugs

In most critical care units neuromuscular blocking drugs are used only occasionally, typically for those patients who are otherwise difficult to ventilate or to prevent rise of intracranial pressure with coughing in head-injured patients. Atracurium and cisatracurium are non-cumulative and are the neuromuscular blockers of choice in the critically ill. Serious myopathies and neuropathies have been described with prolonged infusions of aminosteroid drugs (e.g., vecuronium).

Drugs used for sedation, analgesia and paralysis

Drug	Bolus	Infusion	Comments
Midazolam	$25–50 \ \mu g \ kg^{-1}$	$50–100 \ \mu g \ kg^{-1} \ h^{-1}$	Prolonged effects in the critically ill
Propofol	$0.5–2 \ mg \ kg^{-1}$	$1–3 \ mg \ kg^{-1} \ h^{-1}$	Causes hypotension
Morphine	$0.1–0.2 \ mg \ kg^{-1}$	$40–80 \ \mu g \ kg^{-1} \ h^{-1}$	Active metabolites accumulate in renal failure
Fentanyl	$1–5 \ \mu g \ kg^{-1}$	$2–7 \ \mu g \ kg^{-1} \ h^{-1}$	Cumulative with prolonged infusion
Alfentanil	$15–30 \ \mu g \ kg^{-1}$	$20–120 \ \mu g \ kg^{-1} \ h^{-1}$	Relatively expensive
Atracurium	$0.5 \ mg \ kg^{-1}$	$0.1–0.5 \ mg \ kg^{-1} \ h^{-1}$	Metabolized independently of renal/hepatic function

Further reading

Park GR, Gempler F. *Sedation and Analgesia*. London: WB Saunders, 1993.

Related topics of interest

Analgesia – basic, p. 14; Psychological aspects of critical care, p. 183

SICKLE CELL DISEASE

Sickle cell disease is a haemoglobinopathy with autosomal dominant inheritance found in people of African origin, people from around the Mediterranean, and in parts of India. The β chain of haemoglobin A (HbA) has valine substituted for glutamine in position 6 to produce HbS. In the heterozygous form (sickle cell trait) this provides some protection against falciparum malaria. Ten per cent of people of African origin in the UK have sickle cell trait. This is associated with a normal life expectancy, a Hb greater than 11 g dl^{-1}, no clinical signs or symptoms, and sickling only if the SaO$_2$ is less than 40%. There is, however, an increased risk of pulmonary infarcts. Co-dominant expression of the haemoglobin gene allows normal and abnormal haemoglobin to coexist. Haemoglobin S may be produced with mutant haemoglobins such as haemoglobin C (giving SC disease), and with β thalassaemia. In the homozygote, deoxygenated HbS becomes insoluble and causes red blood cells to become rigid and sickle shaped. This is more likely if hypoxia, acidosis, low temperature or cellular dehydration occurs. Sickling is initially reversible, but when potassium and water are lost from the cell it becomes irreversible. Sickled cells result in decreased microvascular blood flow causing further local hypoxia, acidosis and thus more sickling. Local infarction causes the symptoms and signs of a sickle cell crisis. Chest symptoms (pleuritic pain, cough and fever), musculoskeletal complaints (bone pain, muscle tenderness, erythema), abdominal pain, splenic sequestration (acute anaemia and aplastic crisis), haematuria, priapism and cerebral vascular events [transient ischaemic attacks (TIAs) and strokes] may occur during a crisis. Chronic haemolytic anaemia, increased infection risk and specific organ damage such as 'auto-splenectomy', gall stones, renal and pulmonary damage occur as the result of long term sickling. Osteomyelitis and meningitis are more common and prophylactic antibiotics are often given. Homozygotes usually present in early childhood when HbF levels fall and HbS predominates. Survival beyond the fourth or fifth decade is rare.

Problems

1. **Anaemia** may present as an acute illness in the very young. Children as young as 10 weeks may suffer acute splenic sequestration. The spleen enlarges rapidly and traps large numbers of red blood cells. This may result in a sudden and progressive anaemia and circulatory failure. Death may ensue in as little as 5 hours. Episodes are frequently recurrent with the third or fourth ending in death. The child must be resuscitated with blood and fluid to maintain tissue oxygenation. This may then be followed by release of the sequested red cells from the spleen and subsequent polycythaemia as the spleen returns to its normal size. Acute sequestration is increasingly uncommon after 5 years of age by which age children who survive have usually undergone autosplenectomy and rendered the spleen functionally useless.

2. **Infection risk.** Below the age of 2 years there is an increased risk of pneumococcal septicaemia and meningitis. The increased risk of pneumococcal meningitis may be between 20 and 600 times normal. Splenomegally suggests an at-risk child. Prophylactic penicillin and pneumococcal vaccine should be given.

Prevention of sickle crisis

Normothermia, good hydration and oxygenation prevent the development of a sickle crisis. A high FiO_2 is used. Hyperventilation (respiratory alkalosis) shifts the oxygen dissociation curve to the left and oxygen is more readily bound to haemoglobin thus preventing sickling. Cardiac output is maintained to prevent microvascular sludging and vasoconstrictors are avoided. Monitoring includes pulse oximetry, temperature, urine output and the state of hydration. Regional anaesthesia may be used for patients in post-operative pain or those in an acute crisis. Tourniquets are avoided and patients nursed carefully to prevent venous stasis. Sedation with the risk of hypoventilation and hypoxia, should be avoided.

At-risk patients should have a Sickledex test which detects HbS by causing sickling when the cells are exposed to sodium metabisulphite. It does not differentiate between the homozygote and the heterozygote and, if positive, formal electrophoresis must be performed. This will quantify the types and amounts of each haemoglobin. In the homozygote HbA concentrations $> 40\%$ with a total Hb > 10 g dl^{-1} but < 12 g dl^{-1} should be achieved by exchange transfusion. This optimizes oxygen delivery and blood viscosity. Patients are assessed for pre-existing organ damage and other pathologies consequent upon tissue infarction.

Further reading

Harrison JF, Davies SC. Acute problems in sickle cell disease. *Hospital Update* 1992; **18**: 709–716 and 751.
Vijay V, Cavenagh JD, Yate P. The anaesthetists role in acute sickle cell crisis. *British Journal of Anaesthesia* 1998; **80**: 820–828.

Related topics of interest

Blood transfusion, p. 43; Hypothermia, p. 136

SIRS, SEPSIS AND MULTIPLE ORGAN FAILURE

The systemic inflammatory response syndrome (SIRS), sepsis, shock and other related terms have been defined precisely by consensus:

(a) Infection is the inflammatory response to micro-organisms or the invasion of normally sterile host tissue by those organisms.
(b) Bacteraemia is the presence of viable bacteria in the blood.
(c) SIRS occurs in response to a variety of clinical insults. The response is manifested by two or more of the following conditions:

- Temperature $> 38°C$ or $< 36°C$.
- Heart rate > 90 beats min^{-1}.
- Respiratory rate > 20 breaths min^{-1} or $PaCO_2 < 4.3kPa$.
- White blood count $> 12\,000$ cells mm^{-3}, < 4000 cells mm^{-3}, or $> 10\%$ immature (band) forms.

(d) Sepsis is the systemic response to infection as defined by the presence of two or more of the SIRS criteria (above).
(e) Severe sepsis is sepsis associated with organ dysfunction, hypoperfusion, or hypotension.
(f) Septic shock is sepsis-induced hypotension (systolic blood pressure < 90 mmHg or a reduction of > 40 mmHg from the baseline, or the need for vasopressors) despite adequate fluid resuscitation, along with the presence of perfusion abnormalities.
(g) Multiple organ dysfunction syndrome (MODS) is the presence of altered organ function in an acutely ill patient such that homeostasis cannot be maintained without intervention.

There are no universally agreed definitions of organ system failure largely because severity will be influenced strongly by treatment.

Pathophysiology of the inflammatory cascade

An initial insult (e.g., infection or trauma) triggers the production of pro-inflammatory cytokines [e.g., tumour necrosis factor (TNF), interleukin-1 (IL-1), interleukin-8 (IL-8)]. These cytokines activate leukocytes and endothelium, and promote neutrophil-endothelial-cell adhesion and migration into tissues. The trapped leukocytes discharge a series of secondary inflammatory mediators, including other cytokines, prostaglandins, and proteases. Ischaemia-reperfusion injury is also implicated in the inflammatory process. It generates toxic oxygen free radicals that cause cell membrane lipid peroxidation and increased membrane permeability. Depending on the severity of the initial insult and ischaemia-reperfusion injury, the inflammatory response will generate a SIRS and MODS. The arachidonic acid metabolites thromboxane A_2, prostacyclin, and prostaglandin E_2 contribute to the generation of fever, tachycardia, tachypnoea, and lactic acidosis. Anti-inflammatory mediators, such as IL-6 and IL-10, are also released and serve as negative feedback on the inflammatory process. They inhibit the generation of TNF, enhance the action of immunoglobulins, and inhibit T-lymphocyte and macrophage function.

Tissue hypoxia

Some organs are particularly susceptible to ischaemia and hypoxia and may then form the trigger for MOF. Blood flow to the gut is not autoregulated for pressure; gut blood flow falls in response to reductions in cardiac output. Furthermore, plasma skimming of the blood in the gut mucosa results in a haematocrit of only 10%, which reduces oxygen content substantially. Hepatic blood flow also has a limited capacity for autoregulation, thus the splanchnic organs are at particular risk from a systemic reduction in oxygen supply. Ischaemia-reperfusion injury increases gut permeability probably because of increased synthesis of nitric oxide by gut epithelium or vascular endothelium. The subsequent translocation of bacteria and endotoxin was thought to be a primary mechanism for the initiation of sepsis and MOF. However, there is little evidence that translocation causes systemic symptoms in humans. Instead, translocation is probably part of the normal physiological process of immune sampling by gut-associated lymphoid tissue (GALT).

Oxygen supply and demand

Severe sepsis and SIRS are associated with a marked increase in oxygen demand. Although systemic vascular resistance is low, hypovolaemia secondary to leaky capillaries and relative myocardial depression may result in a global reduction in oxygen delivery. The activation of leukocytes and other cellular elements causes capillary obstruction, endothelial cell injury and microvascular shunting. Thus, even after fluid resuscitation and the institution of inotropic therapy, oxygen utilization may be significantly depressed. The persistent tissue dysoxia will be manifest by a lactic acidosis.

Gastric tonometry

The development of lactic acidosis is a global indicator of tissue hypoxia. Early warning of tissue ischaemia and hypoxia at a regional level may provide the opportunity for earlier intervention with the possibility of improving patient outcome. The precarious nature of gut mucosal blood flow makes this an appropriate organ to monitor for early evidence of global inadequate oxygen supply or utilization. Gastric tonometry is a method of monitoring the gastric mucosa for evidence of ischaemia. At equilibrium, the partial pressure of diffusible carbon dioxide in the lumen of the stomach is the same as that in the gastric endothelium. The gastric tonometer comprises a sampling tube with a distal semi-permeable silicone balloon. The balloon is filled with saline and after allowing 90 minutes for equilibration, the regional PCO_2 ($PrCO_2$) is measured in a blood gas analyser. The $PrCO_2$ is converted into an intramucosal pH (pHi) using a modified Henderson–Hasselbach equation. This calculation is based on the controversial assumption that tissue bicarbonate concentration is the same as that in arterial blood. A recent development of gastric tonometry, continuous air tonometry, is more convenient to use. Air is cycled through the balloon and the PCO_2 of the gas is measured. Calculation of the gastrointestinal-end-tidal PCO_2 gap provides a convenient method of trending the status of the gastric mucosa.

Treatment of SIRS and sepsis

1. ***General principles.*** The management of these inflammatory processes involves treating the cause and supporting vital organ function. Treatment of sepsis requires aggressive antimicrobial therapy and, where appropriate, surgical eradication of the focus of infection. Oxygen delivery is optimized through fluid resuscitation, supplemental oxygen and, if necessary, inotropes and mechanical ventilation. Enteral nutrition will increase gut blood flow and help to preserve gastric mucosal integrity. The maintenance of adequate mean arterial pressure and cardiac output will maximize renal blood flow. Dopamine or frusemide will help to maintain urine output but will not influence renal function per se. The onset of oliguric renal failure will require the institution of renal replacement therapy.

2. ***Goal directed therapy.*** In the past, the management of SIRS and sepsis has involved aggressively increasing oxygen delivery (DO_2) (using fluid and inotropes) and oxygen consumption (VO_2) until certain empirically derived goals were achieved. Earlier evidence had suggested that this strategy would reduce mortality. More recent evidence indicates that this approach either makes no difference or increases mortality. It is possible that global indices are not the best goals to aim for and, in theory, splanchnic focused resuscitation may be better. Whilst pHi appears to be a good predictor of outcome, efforts to use it as a target for goal directed therapy have so far been unsuccessful. Thus, gastric tonometry remains largely a research tool. The commonest approach to resuscitation is to ensure normo-volaemia and, using moderate inotropic support, increase cardiac output with the goal of minimizing the base deficit and/or serum lactate.

3. ***Specific therapies for septic shock.*** Considerable resource has been invested into developing a specific therapy for septic shock. Various therapies have been used in an effort to neutralize circulating endotoxin, TNF or IL-1. None of these studies have demonstrated significant beneficial effect. These disappointing results are a reflection of the complexity of the inflammatory cascade; individual cytokines are likely to have both protective and harmful effects. Clinical trials of nitric oxide synthase blockers have also produced disappointing results.

Further reading

Davies MG, Hagen PO. Systemic inflammatory response syndrome. *British Journal of Surgery* 1997; **84:** 920–935.
Wheeler AP, Bernard GR. Treating patients with severe sepsis. *New England Journal of Medicine* 1999; **340:** 207–214.

Related topics of interest

Cardiac failure, p. 73; Nutrition, p. 159; Renal failure – rescue therapy, p 192.

SODIUM

Sodium is the principle extracellular cation. Normal plasma values are in the range 133–145 mmol l^{-1} with a requirement of 1–2 mmol kg^{-1} day^{-1}.

Hyponatraemia

Hyponatraemia is the most common electrolyte abnormality seen in hospitalized patients. It is most commonly associated with an increased total body water and sodium and is compounded by the administration of hypotonic intravenous fluids.

Pathophysiology

Hyponatraemia may occur in the presence of low, normal or high total body sodium and may be associated with a low, normal or high serum osmolality. Basic mechanisms involve:

- Shift of water out of cells secondary to osmotic shifts (hyperglycaemia, mannitol, alcohol).
- Shift of sodium into cells to maintain electrical neutrality (hypokalaemia).
- Excessive water retention [renal failure, oedematous states (congestive heart failure, nephrotic syndrome, cirrhosis, hypoalbuminaemia), SIADH].
- Excessive water administration (glucose infusions, absorption of irrigation solutions).
- Excessive sodium loss (renal, bowel loss).
- Translocational hyponatraemia.
- Hyperglycaemia accounts for up to 15% of cases of hyponatraemia, every 5.6 mmol l^{-1} increase in serum glucose causes the serum sodium to fall by 1.6 mmol l^{-1}.

Causes of hyponatraemia associated with volume depletion are:

- Renal loss: diuretics, osmotic diuresis (glucose, mannitol), renal tubular acidosis, salt losing nephropathy, mineralocorticoid deficiency / antagonist.
- Non-renal loss: vomiting, diarrhoea, pancreatitis, peritonitis, burns.

Causes of hyponatraemia associated with normal or increased circulating volume include:

- Water intoxication: post-operative 5% glucose administration, TURP syndrome, inappropriate ADH syndrome, renal failure.
- Oedematous states (congestive heart failure, cirrhosis, nephrotic syndrome).
- Glucocorticoid deficiency, hypothyroidism.

Clinical features of hyponatraemia

The rate of change of serum sodium is more important than the absolute concentration. Symptoms are rare with serum sodium > 125 mmol l^{-1}.

- Mild: confusion, nausea, cramps, weakness.
- Severe (sodium usually < 120 mmol l^{-1}): headache, ataxia, muscle twitching, convulsions, cerebral oedema, coma, respiratory depression.

Diagnosis

The patient's urine volume and level of hydration (circulating volume) should be assessed. The nature of any intravenous fluid replacement should be noted as should the recent administration of diuretics. Hyperglycaemia should be excluded and simultaneous urine and plasma osmolalities measured. The urine osmolality is inappropriately high with the syndrome of inappropriate ADH secretion (SIADH) and advanced renal failure.

In order to diagnose SIADH there must be a serum osmolality < 270 mosmol kg^{-1} and a urine osmolality inappropriately high (> 100 mosmol kg^{-1}). There should also be an absence of renal disease and no recent diuretic administration. The urine sodium will be increased despite a normal salt and water intake. The signs of SIADH improve with fluid restriction.

Management

This follows the ABC priorities. The underlying disorder should be treated. The rate of correction of the hyponatraemia depends on the underlying condition and the clinical features. In chronic causes with mild or no symptoms, hyponatraemia should be corrected slowly over a period of days because of the risk of osmotic demyelination with rapid correction. Increased risk of demyelination is seen in association with malnutrition, alcoholism, hypokalaemia, severe burns and elderly females taking thiazides.

Rapid partial correction of hyponatraemia may be accomplished by:

- Stopping all hypotonic fluids.
- Fluid restriction.
- Giving demeclocycline or lithium (ADH antagonists).
- Administration of frusemide.

The rate of correction of acute and symptomatic hyponatraemia is more difficult to dictate. The morbidity from acute cerebral oedema is worse in children, females (particularly during menstruation and elderly females on thiazides), and psychiatric patients. Acute hyponatraemia developing over less than 48 hours carries a high risk of permanent neurological damage and rapid partial correction of the hyponatraemia is indicated. Depending on the underlying cause, rapid partial correction of hyponatraemia may be accomplished by :

- Stopping all hypotonic fluids.
- Hypertonic saline (3% sodium chloride solution at 1 ml kg^{-1} h^{-1}).
- Use of diuretics (frusemide is best given by low dose infusion).
- Frequent measurement of electrolytes with adjustment of therapy.

For acute symptomatic hyponatraemia the aim is to increase the serum sodium by 2 mmol l^{-1} h^{-1} until symptoms resolve (correction may need to be more rapid if severe neurological signs are present). For chronic symptomatic hyponatraemia aim for a correction rate of < 1 mmol l^{-1} h^{-1}.

The main causes of morbidity associated with hyponatraemia are cerebral oedema, respiratory failure and hypoxia. The relation and risk of central pontine myelinolysis associated with rapid correction is unclear. The risks of rapid correction must be weighted against the risk of continued symptomatic hyponatraemia.

Hypernatraemia

Hypernatraemia results from inadequate urine concentration, losses of hypotonic fluids by various routes, or from excessive administration of sodium. Patients who are unable to drink have lost their major defence against hypernatraemia. High-risk groups include infants and the elderly, patients on hypertonic infusions and osmotic diuretics.

Pathophysiology

Hypernatraemia may be seen in the context of low, normal or high total body sodium.

Low total body sodium and hypernatraemia results from loss of both sodium and water but the water loss is proportionately greater. It is caused by hypotonic fluid loss via kidney or gut and is accompanied by signs of hypovolaemia.

Increased total body sodium and hypernatraemia usually follows administration of hypertonic sodium containing solutions.

Normal total body sodium and hypernatraemia results from the predominant loss of water without sodium loss. This usually results from renal losses due to central or nephrogenic diabetes insipidus (DI). Initially euvolaemia is maintained but uncorrected water loss will eventually lead to severe dehydration and hypovolaemia.

Diabetes insipidus

DI results from the impaired reabsorption of water by the kidney. Water reabsorbtion is regulated by anti-diuretic hormone (ADH) which is secreted by the posterior pituitary. Cranial DI results from a lack of ADH production or release while nephrogenic DI results from renal insensitivity to the effects of circulation ADH.

Causes of cranial DI

- Head injury.
- Neurosurgery.
- Pituitary tumour (primary: pituitary, craniopharyngioma, pinealoma; secondary: breast).
- Pituitary infiltration (sarcoid, histiocytosis, tuberculosis).
- Meningitis/encephalitis.
- Guillain-Barré syndrome.
- Raised intracranial pressure.
- Drugs (ethanol, phenytoin).
- Idiopathic.

Causes of nephrogenic DI

- Drugs (lithium, demeclocycline).
- Congenital nephrogenic DI.
- Chronic renal failure.

- Sickle cell disease.
- Hypokalaemia.
- Hypercalaemia.

Diagnosis

Polyuria (may be > 400 ml h^{-1}) in the presence of a raised serum osmolality (> 300 mosmol kg^{-1}). Simultaneous osmolalities will demonstrate an inappropriately low urine osmolality (often < 150 mosmol kg^{-1}) in the presence of an abnormally high serum osmolality. The effects of osmotic and loop diuretics must be excluded.

Psychogenic polydipsia (compulsive water drinking) is differentiated by the presence of a low serum osmolality (< 280 mosmol kg^{-1}).

Clinical features

Signs and symptoms of hypernatraemia are often non-specific and include: lethargy, irritability, confusion, nausea and vomiting, muscle twitching, hyper-reflexia and spasticity, seizures and coma.

Management

Treatment of DI follows the ABC priorities. Treat the underlying pathology and replace water (usually as 5% glucose i.v.). Vasopressin may be given (caution in coronary artery disease and peripheral vascular disease). DDAVP has a longer half-life and less vasoconstrictor effect.

In nephrogenic DI administration of the causative drug should be stopped. Thiazides (e.g., chlorthalidone) have a paradoxical anti-diuretic effect. Other agents (e.g., chlorpropamide and carbamazepine) may also be of use.

Morbidity and mortality tend to be higher in acute severe hypernatraemia when compared to chronic hypernatraemia. Mortality associated with chronic severe hypernatraemia (serum sodium > 160 mmol l^{-1}) can be as high as 60% while acute severe hypernatraemia is associated with mortality rates of up to 75%. Neurological damage is common in those surviving severe hypernatraemia. Correction should be slow (< 2 mmol l^{-1} h^{-1}) to avoid the risk of cerebral oedema.

Further reading

Arieff AI, Ayus JC. Pathogenein and management of hypernatraemia. *Current Opinion in Critical Care* 1996; 2: 418–423.
Kumar S, Berl T. Sodium. *Lancet* 1998; 352: 220–228.

Related topics of interest

Calcium, magnesium and phosphate, p. 56; Convulsions, p. 100; Fluid therapy, p. 122; Potassium, p. 180

SPINAL INJURY

Claire Fouque

Management of patients who have sustained multiple trauma or localized spinal trauma requires careful assessment for spinal injury. Failure to immobilize, investigate and manage these patients may result in the worsening of existing spinal cord injury or the production of a cord injury.

The incidence of spinal cord injuries is around 15–20 per million population per year. Most often men aged 15–35 years are affected. The usual mechanisms of trauma are road traffic accidents (RTAs) (45%), falls (20%), sports injuries (15%), and physical violence (stabbing, gunshot wounds) (15%).

Injury to the cord can be expected in 1–3% of major trauma victims with the risk increasing to approximately 8% if the victim is ejected from a vehicle. The majority of spinal injuries (55%) involve the cervical region. The commonest sites in adults are C_5/C_6 and T_{12}/L_1.

Pathophysiology

Primary neural damage results directly from the initial insult.

Secondary neural injury may result from mechanical disruption after failure to immobilize, hypoxia (may be due to ventilatory impairment from cord damage or chest trauma), hypotension (hypovolaemia, sympathetic blockade, myocardial dysfunction), oedema, haemorrhage into the cord, and hyper/hypoglycaemia.

Types of injury

1. **Complete cord lesion.** All motor function, sensation and reflexes are lost below the level of the lesion. Only 1% of patients who continue to have no cord function after 24 hours will achieve functional recovery.

2. **Incomplete cord lesion.** There are four main clinical syndromes:

- Anterior cord syndrome. Occurs as a result of ischaemic damage to the cord following aortic trauma or cross-clamping where blood supply from the anterior spinal artery is disrupted. There is damage to the cortico-spinal and spino-thalamic tracts with paralysis and abnormal touch, pain and temperature sensation. The posterior columns are unaffected with preservation of joint position and vibration sense.
- Central cord syndrome. The central grey matter is damaged. Paralysis with variable sensory loss is greater in the upper limbs than the lower limbs because these fibres are arranged towards the centre of the cord. Bladder dysfunction presents as urinary retention.
- Brown–Sequard syndrome. Refers to hemisection of the cord, usually due to penetrating trauma. There is ipsilateral paralysis and loss of vibration and joint position sense with contralateral loss of pain and temperature sensation.
- Cauda equina syndrome. Presents with loss of bowel and bladder function with lower motor neurone signs in the legs following a lumbar fracture. Sensory changes are unpredictable.

Pattern of events

The initial injury causes an immediate massive sympathetic outflow with sudden rise in systemic vascular resistance and blood pressure. Patients may suffer acute myocardial infarction, cerebrovascular accidents and fatal arrhythmias.

Spinal shock. All voluntary and reflex activity ceases below the level of the lesion. Recovery to chronic state over a period of months with abnormal reflex activity.

Problems

1.   Airway. There is increased risk of aspiration due to impaired upper airway reflexes and gastric stasis. There may be no pre-monitory sign of vomiting.

2.   Breathing. Cord injury above C_4 leads to loss of diaphragmatic function, apnoea and death if artificial ventilation is not commenced. T_2–T_{12} innervate the intercostal muscles and patients with fractures above this level are reliant on diaphragmatic breathing with limited expansion, decreased tidal volumes and impaired cough. Residual volume is increased and the FRC falls. Muscle power is reduced and there is poor sputum clearance. Bronchopneumonia is common. Other respiratory problems include neurogenic pulmonary oedema, ARDS, Ondine's curse and pulmonary emboli.

As spinal shock resolves, lung function improves with increasing muscle tone. Vital capacity may increase by 65–80% and the patient may be weaned from mechanical ventilation.

3.   Circulation. Loss of sympathetic vasoconstrictor tone results in neurogenic shock. Cord damage above T_1 disrupts the sympathetic innervation of the heart resulting in loss of reflex tachycardia, impaired LV function and the risk of severe bradycardia or asystole following unopposed vagal stimulation.

4.   Neurology. Spinal shock refers to the muscle flaccidity and areflexia seen after spinal injury. It may last for 48 hours to 9 weeks. Following the acute phase of spinal shock, 50–80% of patients with lesions above T_7 will demonstrate episodes of autonomic dysreflexia. Stimulation below the level of the lesion causes a mass spinal sympathetic reflex that would normally be inhibited from above. Patients develop a sudden marked rise in blood pressure and compensatory severe brady-cardia, with flushing and sweating above the level of the lesion. This may be so extreme as to cause fitting, cerebrovascular accidents or cardiac arrest. Triggering factors include distended bladder or bowel, cutaneous irritation from pressure sores, and medical procedures.

5.   Temperature. Hypothermia may be precipitated by heat loss due to peripheral vasodilation.

6.   G.I.T. Paralytic ileus may last for several days.

7.   G.U. Bladder atony necessitates catheterization.

8.   Biochemical and endocrine. Increased ADH secretion leads to water retention with a dilutional hyponatraemia. Glucose intolerance may occur. This must be avoided as it causes worsening of the neurological injury by providing energy substrate that is then metabolized anaerobically in the absence of sufficient oxygen delivery. Nasogastric losses may lead to a metabolic alkalosis. Hypoventilation results in a respiratory acidosis. There is chronic loss of bone mass and osteoporosis. There may be associated hypercalcaemia.

9. *Skin.* Prone to pressure sores.

10. *Thromboembolism.* High incidence of DVT and PE.

11. *Musculoskeletal.* May develop contractures and muscle spasms after resolution of spinal shock

12. *Psychological.* Reactive depression is common.

Management

Primary survey and resuscitation

Fifty per cent of patients with damage to the spinal cord have other injuries. Secondary damage to the cord is reduced by immobilization, minimizing spinal hypoxia and hypoperfusion and by ensuring the patient is fully resuscitated prior to transfer to a specialist centre.

1. *Airway with cervical spine control.* Manual in-line stabilization of the neck is maintained until a correctly sized hard collar and lateral support and tape are fitted.

Early intubation should be undertaken if consciousness is depressed. Manual in-line stabilization must be maintained throughout a rapid sequence induction of anaesthesia. An awake fibreoptic intubation or blind nasal techniques are possible alternatives but require experience.

2. *Breathing.* The patient is given sufficient oxygen to maintain $SaO_2 > 95\%$ and mechanical ventilation instituted as required.

3. *Circulation.* An adequate blood pressure must be maintained to perfuse the damaged cord and decrease secondary injury. Most patients will stabilize with fluid loading alone but some may require vasopressors and inotropic support.

Secondary survey and diagnosis

Spinal injury must be suspected in all severely injured patients.

1. *History – mechanism of injury.* The risk of cervical spine injury is 10–15% if the patient is unconscious and injury is due to a fall or RTA.

2. *Examination.* A careful neurological examination with meticulous documentation is essential. Spinal cord injury may be demonstrated without radiographic abnormality. It is also important to determine the presence of any motor or sensory function below the level of a lesion since this has important prognostic implications. Log-roll to assess for local tenderness and palpable 'step-off' deformity.

Patients may demonstrate:

- Flaccid anal sphincter.
- Areflexia.
- Diaphragmatic breathing.

- Hypotension without tachycardia (if lesion above level of cardioaccelerator sympathetic outflow ~T_2).
- Priapism.

3. Investigations
- Cervical spine X-rays; lateral, AP, and open mouth views.
- Thoracic and lumbar X-rays; AP and lateral.
- CT scanning is targeted at those areas of the spine in which there is suspicion of injury or that are not seen clearly on plain X-rays.
- MRI. This is the definitive investigation but it is difficult to use in the acute phase. MRI will demonstrate soft-tissue and ligamentous injury and give an indication of the severity of the cord injury.

Definitive care

Most specialist centres advocate early fixation therefore early referral to a spinal injuries unit is essential. Surgeons should be contacted for application of halo frame to stabilize the neck as an interim measure.

1. Airway. Tracheostomy is performed for long term ventilation. This should be performed after any surgery to the cervical spine is completed.

2. Breathing. Close monitoring of ventilation is essential as deterioration may be insidious over a number of days. Early intubation must be considered since respiratory complications account for the majority of deaths post-spinal injury. Suxamethonium must be avoided after the first 24 hours for a year following injury since it may precipitate severe hyperkalaemia.

3. Circulation. Invasive blood pressure and central venous pressure monitoring is essential.

4. Minimizing secondary injury
- Prevent hypotension and hypoxia.
- Steroids given within 8 hours of injury have been shown to improve long-term neurological outcome. An immediate loading dose of methylprednisolone 30 mg kg^{-1} i.v. over 15 min is followed 45 min later by a continuous infusion of 5.4 mg kg^{-1} h^{-1} for 23 hours.
- Treat hyper/hypothermia.

5. Autonomic dysreflexia. Management is preventive. Avoid precipitating stimuli and ensure good bowel and bladder care. Regional or general anaesthesia may be required to avoid crises precipitated by surgery.

6. G.I.T. Early enteral feeding is important in maintaining the integrity of the gut mucosa. Percutaneous gastrostomy (PEG) may be used for long term feeding if swallowing is inadequate. Bowel management with lactulose, rectal glycerine and manual evacuation may be needed.

7. G.U. Patients with indwelling catheters are predisposed to urinary infections.

8. Skin. Meticulous nursing and 2 hourly turning are needed to prevent pressure sores.

9. *Thromboembolism.* Prophylaxis with TED stockings, calf compression devices and s/c LMWH for minimum of 8 weeks.

10. *Psychological.* Multidisciplinary team support and guidance is essential. Clear advice and honesty are paramount. Support groups will help the relatives.

Spinal injuries in children

This low incidence of bony spinal injury (0.2% of all paediatric fractures and dislocations) is due to the mobility of the spine in children that can dissipate forces over a larger area. Treatment is similar to adults. Infants and children less than 8 years may require padding placed under the back to achieve the neutral position in which to immobilize the cervical spine.

SCIWORA (Spinal Cord Injury WithOut Radiological Abnormality)
There is no obvious injury to the spine in up to 55% of children with complete cord injuries. The upper cervical cord where there is greatest mobility is usually affected. It occurs almost exclusively in children under 8 years old.

Further reading

Chiu WT, Liu A, Chen SY. Recent developments in the management of spinal cord injuries. *Current Opinion in Critical Care* 1995; **1**: 494–502.
Tator CH. Biology of neurological recovery and functional restoration after spinal cord injury. *Neurosurgery* 1998; **42**: 696–707.

Related topics of interest

Head injury, p. 128; Trauma – primary survey and resuscitation, p. 257; Trauma – secondary survey, p. 260; Trauma – anaesthesia and critical care, p. 263

STRESS ULCERATION

Stress ulceration or stress-related mucosal damage is distinct from peptic ulcer disease. Ulcers arising from critical illness are superficial, well demarcated, often multiple, and not associated with surrounding oedema. They are usually located in the fundus of the stomach or the first part of the duodenum. Stress ulceration occurs in critically ill patients as a result of major physiological disturbances. The incidence of stress ulceration is poorly understood but has been quoted as ranging from 52% to 100% of all patients admitted to ICU, depending on the diagnostic criteria used. The finding of occult blood on testing of either gastric aspirate or faecal material produces an unacceptably high incidence of false positive results when looking for stress ulceration. Adopting the stricter diagnostic criteria of overt bleeding or a decrease in haemoglobin of more than 2 g dl^{-1} and complicated by either haemodynamic instability or the need for transfusion of red cells produces an incidence < 5%.

Upper gastrointestinal endoscopy remains the gold standard for the diagnosis of stress ulceration.

Pathogenesis

This was originally thought to be due to an excess of gastric acid production. It may be the explanation for those ulcers occurring in head injured patients (Cushing's ulcer) or patients who have suffered burns (Curling's ulcer). Critically ill patients usually, however, suffer gastric exocrine failure and do not produce an excess of gastric acid. Reduced gastric mucosal defences may thus be more important. Gastric mucosal ischaemia occurs following shock or sepsis and may result in a failure of protective mucosal secretion. Damaging free radicals may also be formed. These mechanisms may be exacerbated by reperfusion injury following resuscitation. The mucosal barrier may also be disrupted by reflux of bile or pancreatic juice.

Complications

These are similar to those of peptic ulceration and include bleeding, perforation, and obstruction, the latter two being rare from stress ulceration.

Risk factors for bleeding from stress ulceration

- Sepsis.
- Respiratory failure.
- Multi-organ failure.
- Head injury.
- Severe burns.
- Coagulopathy.
- Anticoagulation therapy.

Management

Treatment of the underlying critical illness.

Enteral nutrition

This may decrease the incidence of stress ulceration by buffering gastric acid and improving the nutritional status of the catabolic patient.

Antacids

Antacids have been shown to decrease the incidence of both microscopic and macroscopic bleeding from the upper GI tract. The aim is to maintain the pH of the gastric content above 4. This is tedious to do, requiring regular measurement of pH by either aspiration of gastric content from a gastric tube or using a pH probe. Antacids must be given frequently (every 2–4 hours). They may produce hyper-magnesaemia, hyperaluminaemia, alkalosis, hypernatraemia, constipation or diarrhoea. Frequent administration of antacids may represent a large volume load to a non-functioning gut.

H$_2$-receptor antagonists

These include cimetidine, ranitidine, famotidine, and nizatidine. They are as effective as antacids in reducing clinically significant bleeding by comparison to placebo. There are a wide range of potential side effects with each of these agents. The most important clinical side effect is the risk of nosocomial pneumonia due to the loss of the bacteriocidal effect of gastric acid. This results in colonization of the stomach and subsequently the nasopharynx followed by aspiration in to the trachea.

There is no logic in giving H$_2$-receptor antagonists to patients with gastric exocrine failure and an already elevated gastric pH.

Sucralfate

This is the basic aluminium salt of sucrose octasulphate. It is administered via a nasogastric tube. It does not raise intragastric pH but appears to polymerize and adhere to damaged ulcerated mucosa. It also binds bile salts and increases mucosal production of mucus and bicarbonate. Sucralfate is as effective as H$_2$-receptor antagonists in preventing stress ulceration in endoscopic studies and costs less. Theoretically it should be associated with a lower incidence of nosocomial pneumonia. This remains to be proved.

Omeprazole

This is a hydrogen-potassium ATPase receptor antagonist. It binds irreversibly to the gastric parietal cell proton pump, markedly reducing the secretion of hydrogen ions. It may be less effective in fasting patients but has proven able to maintain the gastric pH above 4.0 in critically ill patients.

Misoprostol

An analogue of prostaglandin E$_1$ which inhibits basal and stimulated gastric acid secretions and increases gastric mucus and bicarbonate production. Its role in the prevention of stress ulceration has yet to be established.

Further reading

Cook DJ, *et al.* Stress ulcer prophylaxis in critically ill patients: resolving discordant metanalysis. *JAMA* 1996; **275**: 308–314.

Levy MJ, DiPalma JA. Stress ulcer prophylaxis may not be for everyone. *Current Opinion in Critical Care* 1996; **2**: 129–133.

Related topics of interest

Blood coagulation, p. 34; Pulmonary aspiration, p. 185

STROKE

A stroke is defined as a focal neurological deficit of abrupt onset, of non-traumatic origin which lasts more than 24 hours. A TIA is qualitatively the same but signs and symptoms resolve within 24 hours. Stroke is the leading cause of brain injury in adults. It has an incidence of 200 per 100 000 population per annum. The incidence shows marked age variation, being 2000 per 100 000 in those aged over 85 years. Acute stroke lacks a specific treatment but management of patients in a critical care environment improves outcome.

Pathogenesis

1. Ischaemic stroke. This comprises thrombotic and embolic disease and accounts for > 80% of cases. Mechanisms of injury include:

- Atherothrombosis of large and medium sized cerebral vessels (50%).
- Intracranial small vessel disease (25%).
- Cardiac embolism (20%).

2. Haemorrhagic stroke. 20% of all strokes.

Investigation

The physical signs of the stroke should be documented. Serial blood pressure measurements should be made and a cardiac rhythm other than sinus rhythm sought. Stroke following an ischaemic event and that following haemorrhage cannot be differentiated clinically. A CT scan of the brain will help differentiate them and exclude stroke from other causes such as tumour or abscess.

Management

The aims of acute management of stroke are:

1. Maintain cerebral perfusion. The blood pressure should not be allowed to fall or be actively lowered except in the presence of severe hypertension. A low cardiac output state (e.g. heart failure, atrial fibrillation) should be treated. Additional oxygen should be given by facemask. The patient should be nursed with 30° of head up tilt (aids cerebral venous drainage). ICP monitoring may be considered for those with evidence of raised ICP on CT scan.

2. Restore blood flow to cerebral tissue at risk of infarction. The role of thrombolytic therapy in acute stroke has been investigated. Two large placebo-controlled studies of acute carotid artery territory stroke showed that thrombolysis with rt-PA produced a better neurological outcome in those who survived. There was, however, a higher overall mortality in those given thrombolysis (secondary to intracranial haemorrhage).

3. Anticoagulation. Aspirin 300 mg given as soon as a CT scan has excluded intracranial haemorrhage results in a small but significant improvement in neurological outcome. This dose should be given daily for 2–4 weeks before being reduced to a maintenance dose of 75 mg. The use of heparin in acute stroke has not been shown to produce benefit.

4. *Commence acute stroke rehabilitation.*

Outcome

Outcome from acute stroke is improved if the patient is admitted to and managed in an acute unit rather than a general ward. The role of thrombolytic therapy requires further refinement.

Further reading

Bath P. Alteplase not yet proven for acute ischaemic stroke. *The Lancet* 1998; **352**: 1238–1239.

Hacke W, Kaste M, Fieschi C, *et al.* Randomised double-blind placebo-controlled trial of thrombolytic therapy with intravenous alteplase in acute ischaemic stroke (ECAS II). *The Lancet* 1998; **352**: 1245–1251.

Related topics of interest

Head injury, p. 128; Subarachnoid haemorrhage, p. 245

SUBARACHNOID HAEMORRHAGE

Kim Gupta

Blood is commonly found in the subarachnoid space following intracranial haemorrhage of any cause (e.g., after trauma). The term subarachnoid haemorrhage (SAH) is usually reserved for spontaneous haemorrhage from either intracranial aneurysms (85%) or arteriovenous malformations (15%).

Aneurysmal SAH haemorrhage

The incidence of SAH from intracranial aneurysms is 10 per 100 000 population per year. Mortality is high; 20–30% die before surgery, 30% within 1 month of surgery and 30% of survivors are left with major neurological deficit. Up to 5% of adults are found to have intracranial aneurysms as an incidental finding at autopsy. Intracranial vessels lack an external elastic lamina and so form aneurysms more readily than extracranial vessels. Around 80% of aneurysms occur on the anterior cerebral circulation and 20% on the posterior circulation. Approximately 25% of patients with a SAH are found to have multiple aneurysms.

For surgically treated patients vasospasm accounts for 28% of mortality and 39% of morbidity (delayed ischaemic deficits).

Risk factors

Intracranial aneurysms are associated with polycystic renal disease, neurofibromatosis type I, Marfan's syndrome, and Ehlers–Danlos syndrome type IV. Cigarette smoking produces a ten fold increase in the risk of aneurysm formation. Hypertension is also a risk factor as is a family history of SAH. First degree relatives of a SAH patient have a four times greater risk of aneurysm development than the general population.

Clinical features

Aneurysms are clinically silent until they rupture. About one third of patients admit to symptoms attributable to a warning leak in the weeks before their major SAH. Haemorrhage may occur at any time but is more common during stress or physical exercise. It presents as an abrupt onset, severe headache with nausea, vomiting or even loss of consciousness. Neck stiffness takes hours to develop. Intraocular (subhyaloid) haemorrhage occurs in 25% of cases. Focal signs such as third nerve palsy, brain stem dysfunction or lateralizing signs may develop from either a mass effect from a haematoma or ischaemia from arterial spasm, embolus, or vessel dissection. The prognosis following SAH correlates closely with the clinical state at presentation, the combination of a motor deficit and a low GCS score (see p. 219) predicting the worst outcome. Grading of SAH commonly follows the World Federation of Neurological Surgeons scale (WFNS) or the Hunt and Hess scale.

Investigations

1. Detection of subarachnoid blood. A non-contrast computerized tomographic (CT) scan of the brain is the investigation of choice. It will detect blood in 95% of patients with a SAH within 24 hours of the bleed. Lumbar puncture is indicated if

WFNS scale

	Motor deficit	GCS score
Grade 1	Absent	15
Grade 2	Absent	13–14
Grade 3	Present	13–14
Grade 4	Present or absent	7–12
Grade 5	Present or absent	3–6

The Hunt and Hess scale

Grade 1	Asymptomatic or minimal headache or neck stiffness
Grade 2	Moderate to severe headache, neck stiffness, no neurological deficit of cranial nerve palsy
Grade 3	Drowsy, confusion, mild focal deficit
Grade 4	Stupor, moderate to severe hemiparaesis
Grade 5	Deep coma, decerebrate rigidity, moribund

SAH is clinically likely but the CT scan is normal. Uniform blood staining with a yellow supernatant (xanthochromia) is diagnostic but may not appear until 12 hours after the haemorrhage.

2. Aneurysm location. Four vessel (bilateral carotid and vertebral) digital subtraction angiography is the investigation of choice. It can detect aneurysms < 3 mm in diameter and is superior to non-invasive techniques using MRI or spiral CT for surgical planning. It has an associated mortality of 0.1%.

Management

Patients who are older than 75 years old, or who have a GCS < 5 without significant hydrocephalus or intracerebral haematoma are unlikely to benefit from aggressive management.

1. Medical
- Airway and breathing. Ensure adequate oxygenation, SpO_2 > 95%, intubation if airway compromise.
- Fluid resuscitation. Sodium and water excretion by the kidney is enhanced following SAH (which may include cerebral salt wasting). Treatment is with salt and water replacement, with CVP and electrolyte monitoring. A systolic blood pressure of 120–150 mmHg (in the absence of vasospasm) is aimed for.
- Analgesia.
- Treat convulsions.
- Prevent vasospasm. Nimodipine is the calcium channel blocker of choice for the prevention of vasospasm. Nimodipine can reduce the incidence of delayed ischaemic deficit and angiographic vasospasm. Intravenous nimodipine is probably more effective than oral. An intravenous infusion dose of at least 20 mg kg^{-1} h^{-1} should be given. Intravenous or oral treatment is continued for

21 days. Early surgery may also be of benefit in preventing vasospasm. Angiographically proven vasospasm is seen in 67% of patients with aneurysmal SAH. Vasospasm causes ischaemic deficit in 32%. Established vasospasm is managed by continuing nimodipine. Some centres advocate the induction of hypertension, hypervolaemia and haemodilution [referred to as HHH (triple H) therapy]. To maintain a positive fluid balance 0.9% sodium chloride at 1.7 ml kg^{-1} h^{-1} is used as maintenance fluid. The volume loss that follows intravenous contrast induced diuresis will also need replacement. Chemical angioplasty with papaverine or balloon angioplasty may be of benefit.

Cardiac arrhythmias may occur following SAH (in particular supraventricular tachycardias). Patients should be monitored appropriately and treated in the event of haemodynamically significant arrhythmias. Reversible cardiac depression is a recognized complication of subarachnoid haemorrhage.

2. *Surgery.* The aim of surgery is to exclude the aneurysm sac from the circulation whilst preserving the parent artery.

- Aneurysm clipping. A clip is placed across the neck of the aneurysm. Early surgery (within 48–72 hours) is technically more difficult due to oedema and clot around the aneurysm. It does, however, abolish the high risk of rebleeding and allows aggressive management of vasospasm.
- Endovascular surgery. Some aneurysms may be managed with insertion of soft metallic coils which thrombose and obliterate the aneurysmal sac.

Hydrocephalus

Hydrocephalus is present in 19% of patients with SAH at presentation and develops in an additional 3% within the first week. It usually presents as an acute neurological deterioration and requires urgent CSF drainage. Of those who survive a SAH, 20% require permanent CSF shunting.

Non-aneurysmal SAH

This may result from a venous or capillary bleed around the midbrain, particularly the interpeduncular fossa (peri-mesencephalic haemorrhage). Arteriovenous malformations are a common cause of haemorrhage in normotensive young patients. The mortality from the latter is around 10% (i.e., much lower than aneurysmal SAH).

Further reading

Gupta KJ, Finfer SR, Morgan MK. Intensive care for subarachnoid haemorrhage; the state of the art. *Current Anaesthesia and Critical Care* 1998; **9**: 202–208.
Schierink WI. Intracranial aneurysms. *New England Journal of Medicine* 1997; **336**: 28–40.

Related topics of interest

THYROID EMERGENCIES

The thyroid gland concentrates iodide and produces tetraiodothyronine (T4) and triiodothyronine (T3). Triiodothyronine has more metabolic activity than T4. Thyroid gland function is regulated by thyroid stimulating hormone (TSH) which is secreted by the anterior pituitary gland. The secretion of TSH is partly controlled by higher centres such as the hypothalamus via thyrotropin releasing hormone (TRH).

Thyroid crisis

1. Pathogenesis. Thyroid crises occur more commonly in women than men. They may be precipitated in patients with poorly controlled hyperthyroidism by an intercurrent illness, especially an infection, trauma, thyroid surgery, poorly controlled diabetes mellitus, or labour. A thyroid crisis may also occur in eclamptic patients with otherwise well controlled thyroid function.

2. Clinical features. These are those of extreme hyperthyroidism and may be confused in the critically ill with sepsis or malignant hyperthermia. The signs include:

- Pyrexia.
- Confusion, restlessness and delirium.
- Tachycardia, atrial fibrillation and high output cardiac failure.
- Flushing, sweating and abdominal pain.
- Dehydration and ketosis.

Even with appropriate treatment, the risk of death remains high.

3. Management. This should be both supportive and specific. Supportive measures include the administration of supplementary oxygen (the metabolic rate is high) and treatment of the precipitating cause of the crisis. Attention to hydration is essential and the patient may require cooling and sedating. Dantrolene has been used to good effect in those cases characterized by extreme muscle activity. Assisted ventilation may be required.

Specific therapy aims at reducing the synthesis, release, and peripheral effects of thyroid hormones.

- Beta-blockade. Propranolol given i.v. remains the drug of choice providing there are no contraindications to a poorly selective beta-blocker (e.g., reactive airways, heart failure). Beta-blockade will reduce the heart rate, fever, tremor and agitation. Propranolol also reduces the peripheral conversion of T4 to T3.
- Thiourea derivatives. Propylthiouracil must be given enterally. It blocks the iodination of tyrosine and partially inhibits the peripheral conversion of T4 to T3. Carbimazole is metabolized to methimazole and is slower in onset though longer acting. It is often associated with a temporary reduction in the white cell count.
- Iodine and lithium both inhibit the synthesis and release of thyroid hormones.
- Digoxin may be required to treat atrial fibrillation once any hypokalaemia has been corrected. Amiodarone is an alternative though may itself alter thyroid function.

Myxoedema coma

1. **Pathogenesis.** This occurs more frequently in the winter and typically in elderly female patients. It is the endstage of untreated hypothyroidism and is associated with a high mortality. It may occur secondary to autoimmune thyroiditis, radioiodine therapy, following the administration of antithyroid drugs, iodine, lithium, or amiodarone, or after thyroidectomy. The following laboratory results are indicative of the associated conditions:

- Primary hypothyroidism – ↑ TSH and ↓ T3/T4.
- Secondary hypothyroidism – ↓ TSH and ↓ T3/T4.
- Tertiary (hypothalamic) – ↓ TRH.

2. **Clinical features.** The clinical presentation is that of coma associated with depressed thyroid function. Coma may be precipitated by a low body temperature, CNS depressant agents, infection, trauma, or heart failure. The coma is often associated with seizures as well as the following features:

- Hypothermia.
- Hypoventilation (causing hypercarbia and hypoxia).
- Hypotension.
- ECG changes – low heart rate, low voltage recording, prolonged QT interval, flat or inverted T waves.
- Hypoglycaemia.
- Hyponatraemia, with increased total body water (TBW) but low circulating volume.
- Hypophosphataemia.
- Reduced gut and bladder function.

3. **Management.** The management is both supportive and specific. Supportive measures will include control of the airway and assisted ventilation with warmed, humidified gases. Hypoglycaemia should be corrected. The circulating compartment should be expanded with fluid administration guided by measurement of the CVP. Fluid management should include water restriction in those patients with hyponatraemia. External warming may also be required.

Specific management will aim at treating the underlying cause of the hypothyroidism. Thyroid hormones may be administered in small incremental doses over a period of time. Some advocate the use of steroids as there may be a reduced adrenal glucocorticoid response.

Related topics of interest

Hyperthermia, p. 133; Hypothermia, p. 136

TRACHEOSTOMY

Tracheostomy has always been fundamental to the airway management of patients requiring long-term mechanical ventilation on ICU. However, the widespread introduction of percutaneous dilatational tracheostomy (PDT) techniques over the last decade has increased the use of tracheostomy in the 'medium-term' critical care patient.

Indications

The main indications for tracheostomy are prolonged ventilation, weaning from ventilatory support, bronchial toilet and upper airway obstruction. Translaryngeal tracheal intubation may cause laryngeal damage in two ways: (a) abrasion of the laryngeal mucosa from tube movement during coughing etc; (b) pressure necrosis from the round tracheal tube as it passes through the pentagonal shaped larynx. However, whether early conversion of tracheal tube to tracheostomy alters the incidence of laryngotracheal damage is controversial. Recent guidelines have recommended that a tracheostomy be performed when it is estimated that the patient will be ventilator-dependent for at least 2–3 weeks. The advent of percutaneous techniques has encouraged many intensivists to considerably reduce this threshold for performing tracheostomies. The advantages of tracheostomy over prolonged translaryngeal tracheal intubation include:

- Less dead space and work of breathing.
- Less sedation required.
- Airway fixed more securely allowing greater patient mobility.
- Better oral hygiene.
- Improved efficiency of airway suctioning.
- Allows patient to eat and speak.
- Faster weaning from mechanical ventilation.
- Reduced ICU length of stay.

Modern mechanical ventilators have very sensitive flow triggers. In combination with tracheostomy, the need for sedation is virtually eliminated and weaning is much more efficient. The removal of sedation improves the success of enteral feeding.

Percutaneous dilatational tracheostomy

PDT has been popularised by Ciaglia who described his technique of serial dilatation over a wire in 1985. The other commonly used technique comprises a single forceps dilatation (Griggs technique) over a wire placed percutaneously. The more complex technique of translaryngeal tracheostomy (Fantoni) has been introduced very recently. In comparison with surgical tracheostomy PDT has many advantages and relatively few disadvantages:

1. Advantages of PDT
- No need for the patient to go to the operating theatre.
- Short operating time.

- Less cost.
- Low incidence of wound infection.
- Small, cosmetically more acceptable scar.
- Low incidence of tracheal stenosis.
- Less bleeding

2. Disadvantages to PDT

- More difficult to replace in an emergency.
- Loss of airway during procedure.
- Deskills surgeons.

The list of absolute contraindications to PDT has become shorter with increasing experience of the technique. The addition of fibreoptic guidance improves safety and is essential in patients with more difficult anatomy. Routine bronchoscopy during PDT should probably be standard.

3. Contraindications to PDT

(a) Absolute

- The need for immediate airway access (where intubation is impossible in an emergency, cricothyroidotomy remains the technique of choice).
- Children – this may change as more data become available.

(b) Relative

- Ill defined anatomy (inability to feel cricoid, obesity, thyroid enlargement).
- Coagulopathy.
- Haemodynamic instability.
- Neck extension contraindicated.
- High oxygen, PEEP and ventilatory requirement.

4. Complications of PDT.

Comparative studies have shown that the incidence of early complications with PDT is lower than those associated with surgical tracheostomy. The minimal tissue damage makes infection (0–4% vs. 10–30%) and secondary haemorrhage less likely. The limited data available on long term complications also suggest that PDT is less likely to cause tracheal stenosis than conventional, surgical tracheostomy.

(a) Immediate complications

- Hypoxia due to failure of ventilation during procedure (accidental extubation or puncture of the tracheal tube cuff).
- Misplacement: too high, paratracheal, through posterior wall of trachea, into oesophagus.
- Bleeding: minor – common, major – rare.

(b) Intermediate complications

- Early displacement of the tracheostomy tube – very small tracheal stoma makes replacement very difficult without dilators.
- Obstruction from blood or secretions.
- Infection.
- Secondary haemorrhage.

(c) Late complications
- Tracheal stenosis (26% when defined by a tracheal stenosis of > 10%).
- Subglottic stenosis – rare.

5. *The technique of PDT.* Different techniques require specific approaches. All patients for PDT should be given 100% O_2. The tracheal tube is withdrawn until the top of the cuff is across the cords. Alternatively, the tracheal tube can be replaced with a laryngeal mask airway (LMA) or intubating laryngeal mask airway (ILMA). A cannula is inserted between the 1st and 2nd or 2nd and 3rd tracheal rings and a guidewire passed through it. The use of a bronchoscope to observe and confirm entry of the needle and guidewire into the trachea is highly recommended. After the guidewire has been inserted the stoma is enlarged with a series of dilators (Ciaglia) or with forceps (Griggs). A size 8.0 mm tracheostomy tube will be adequate in most patients.

Further reading

Bishop G, Hillman K, Bristow P. Tracheostomy. In: Vincent JL (ed.), *Yearbook of Intensive Care and Emergency Medicine.* Berlin: Springer-Verlag, 1997, pp. 457–469.
Soni N. Percutaneous tracheostomy: how to do it. *British Journal of Hospital Medicine* 1997; **57**: 339–345.

Related topics of interest

Respiratory support – non-invasive, p. 200; Respiratory support – invasive, p. 205; Respiratory support – weaning from ventilation, p. 210

TRANSFER OF THE CRITICALLY ILL

David Lockey

As hospital specialist services become more centralized, the transfer of critically ill patients between hospitals becomes more frequent. Transfers may be primary (to hospital from the site of the incident/accident) or secondary (between hospitals). Patients are also frequently transferred within a hospital. Since relatively few doctors practice pre-hospital care, most medically supervised transfers are secondary. Transfer can be hazardous for the patient and, rarely, for accompanying personnel. Attention is increasingly being given to designated transfer teams and the development of transfer guidelines. Key points to consider when transferring the critically ill include:

- Communication between hospitals.
- Detailed patient assessment.
- Pre-transfer physiological stabilization.
- Anticipation of likely problems during transfer.
- Pre-transfer interventions.
- Equipment checks.
- Comprehensive handover.

General principles

Prior to transferring any critically ill patient the risks should be weighed against the potential benefits of treatment at the receiving unit. Transfer should be arranged if the appropriate level of care is not available at the original location. Early communication between senior clinical staff at the referring and the receiving hospital is essential. Ideally, the receiving hospital should take responsibility for the transfer and provide a team to perform it. Patients should be resuscitated and physiologically stable (unless the patient has a condition which can only be stabilized at the receiving hospital).

Potential hazards of transfer

- Removal of patient from secure hospital environment.
- Reduced number of carers who may lack experience.
- Reduced or less effective monitoring.
- Reduced access to patient.
- No access to additional equipment.
- Difficulty in performing resuscitation or other practical procedures.
- Hostile environment: limited space, noise, motion sickness, fatigue.

The clinician supervising the transfer is responsible for assessment of the patient at the referring hospital. This must include a primary survey and a review of the history. When it is decided to sedate a patient with a head injury the neurological status before sedation should be carefully recorded. The neurological status of patients with suspected spinal injuries should be recorded before and after the transfer.

Unconscious patients should always be intubated before transfer. Virtually all head-injured patients with an altered level of consciousness will require intubation.

The inspired oxygen concentration is noted and a current arterial blood gas analysis obtained. If a transfer ventilator is to be used, check an arterial blood gas 10 min after the patient is connected to it. Haemodynamic normality and stability should be achieved pre-transfer. Adequate intravenous lines should be inserted and fixed securely. Intravenous fluids should be warmed if necessary. Blood and blood products should be available if required. If infusions of inotropes are required spare infusions should be drawn up and labelled properly.

Potential problems

Fractures should be splinted to prevent neurovascular damage. A comprehensive written referral should accompany the patient. On departure, the receiving hospital should be contacted with an estimated time of arrival.

Personnel

Personnel accompanying a critically ill patient should be able to cope with all common problems. Ideally a transfer team should retrieve the patient from the referring hospital. Such teams are well established in paediatric practice but are not always available for adult patients. An appropriately trained doctor skilled in resuscitation and support of organ systems should always accompany the patient, along with at least one appropriately trained assistant. The doctor supervising the transfer will often be an anaesthetist or intensive care doctor. Adequate death and injury insurance should be provided for the transfer team.

Equipment

All equipment should be checked before collecting the patient. Ideally it should be reliable, simple, and durable.

The following basic equipment should accompany all critically ill patients:

- Mechanical ventilator (with facility for airway pressure monitoring, minute volume measurement and disconnect alarm).
- Oxygen – enough for the transfer plus enough for unforeseen delays, preferably with an independent alternative supply.
- Airway equipment – intubation and surgical airway equipment.
- Self inflating bag-valve-mask device.
- Effective suction apparatus.
- Intravenous access and infusion equipment and a stock of intravenous fluids.
- Syringe pumps (with fully charged batteries).
- Volumatic intravenous fluid pumps (infusion by gravity is unreliable during transfer).
- Defibrillator.
- Spare batteries.

Drugs

The following should always be carried:

- Resuscitation drugs (adrenaline and atropine).
- Cardiovascular drugs e.g., nitrates, anti-arrhythmics, inotropes.

- Anticonvulsants e.g., diazepam, thiopentone.
- Analgesics.
- Hypnotic agents e.g., midazolam, propofol.
- Muscle relaxants.
- Respiratory drugs e.g., salbutamol.
- Other drugs such as naloxone, mannitol, glucose.

Monitoring

The ideal monitoring for critically ill patients during transfer is the same as would be used on the critical care unit. This may not always be possible but modern multifunction monitors allow several pressure waves to be displayed in addition to standard functions.

Non-invasive blood pressure monitoring is susceptible to vibration artefact as well as inaccuracy due to arrhythmias (e.g., atrial fibrillation). Where haemodynamic instability is a possibility intra-arterial pressure monitoring is the only reliable method of measurement. Pulse oximetry is mandatory, as is capnography in ventilated patients. Temperature should be measured, particularly in children. All critically ill patients should be catheterized and hourly urine output should be recorded. Central venous pressure should be monitored if necessary.

Modes of transport

The majority of interhospital transfers are carried out by ground ambulance. The problems of ground ambulance transfers are excessive movement, noise, lack of space, motion sickness and occasionally extended transfer times (either due to long distances or traffic congestion). If the patient deteriorates en route the ambulance should be stopped to allow effective resuscitation, intervention or examination of the patient.

Air ambulance transfers may be appropriate in certain circumstances. The usual indications are that the patient needs to be transferred a long distance or in a short period of time. Transfer may be by fixed wing aircraft or by helicopter. Fixed wing aircraft are used for long distances. Helicopters can travel moderate distances quickly and often land at, or very close to, the receiving hospital.

Air transfers are expensive. Problems en route include poor patient access, limited space, motion sickness, high noise levels and vibration. Cabins are pressurized only to the equivalent of approximately 2000 m above sea level so supplementary oxygen should always be administered. The expansion of gases at altitude can be a problem where a patient has a pneumothorax or excessive gas in the bowel (e.g., in bowel obstruction) and where a tracheal tube is filled with air (saline should be substituted).

Transfers within hospitals

The general principles of transfers between hospitals are equally applicable to transfers within hospitals. The patient should not be moved until the receiving department is ready to commence the investigation or procedure. At least two people should accompany the patient on the transfer, a doctor and a nurse.

Further reading

Oakley PA. Interhospital transfer of the trauma patient. *Trauma* 1999; 1: 61–70.
Runci CJ, Reeve WG, Reidy J, Dougall JR. A comparison of measurements of blood pressure, heart rate and oxygenation during interhospital transfer of the critically ill. *Intensive Care Medicine* 1990; 16: 317–322.

Related topics of interest

TRAUMA – PRIMARY SURVEY AND RESUSCITATION

Trauma is the leading cause of death in the first four decades of life. Hypoxia and hypovolaemia are common causes of preventable trauma deaths. The Advanced Trauma Life Support (ATLS) Course teaches a structured approach to the management of trauma. Severely injured patients admitted to an Accident and Emergency department will require the immediate attention of the critical care team.

Prehospital management

Time spent at the scene must be minimized. Treatment at the scene should be limited to stabilizing the airway and spine and ensuring adequate ventilation. Unless the patient is trapped, attempts at i.v. cannulation should be deferred until en route to hospital.

Communication

Wherever possible, ambulance personnel should provide the hospital with advance warning of the impending arrival of a seriously injured patient. Accident department staff can prepare the resuscitation room and call the trauma team. The appropriate drugs, fluids, and airway equipment should be prepared before the patient's arrival.

The trauma team

Trauma patient resuscitation is most efficiently undertaken by a team of medical and nursing staff. The team leader co-ordinates the activities of the whole team.

Resuscitative procedures can be undertaken simultaneously. The initial management of the trauma patient is divided into four phases:

- Primary survey.
- Resuscitation.
- Secondary survey.
- Definitive care.

The primary survey

1. **Airway and cervical spine control.** High concentration oxygen is given by facemask with a reservoir bag. The cervical spine is stabilized with manual in-line cervical stabilization (MILS) or a rigid cervical collar with lateral blocks. Tracheal intubation will be required if the airway is at risk (comatose, haemorrhage, or oedema). Unless the patient is in extremis, intubation will necessitate rapid sequence induction of anesthesia, MILS and cricoid pressure. Induction of general anesthesia will cause profound hypotension in the presence of hypovolaemia.

2. **Breathing.** Immediately life threatening chest injuries require urgent treatment at this stage:

    - **Tension pneumothorax.** Reduced chest movement reduced breath sounds, and a resonant percussion note on the affected side, along with respiratory distress, hypotension and tachycardia, indicate a tension pneumothorax. Deviation of the trachea to the opposite side is a late sign, and neck veins may not be distended in the presence of hypovolaemia. Treatment is immediate decompression with a large cannula placed in the 2nd inter-costal space, in the mid-clavicular line on the affected side. Once intra-venous access has been obtained, a large chest drain (36 F) should be placed in the 5th intercostal space in the anterior axillary line, and connected to an under-water seal drain.

- **Open pneumothorax.** Any open pneumothorax should be covered with an occlusive dressing and sealed on three sides.
- **Flail chest.** The underlying pulmonary contusion may cause immediately life threatening hypoxia with the need for intubation and mechanical ventilation.
- **Massive haemothorax.** This is defined by > 1500 ml blood in a hemithorax and will result in reduced chest movement and dull percussion note, in the presence of hypoxaemia and hypovolaemia. A chest drain is inserted once volume resuscitation has been started.
- **Cardiac tamponade.** Distended neck veins in the presence of hypotension are suggestive of cardiac tamponade, although after rapid volume resus-citation myocardial contusion will also present in this way. If cardiac tamponade is suspected, and the patient is deteriorating despite all resus-citative efforts, pericardiocentesis should be performed. In the presence of a suitably experienced surgeon, open pericardiotomy is the more effective procedure.

3. **Circulation.** Control any major external haemorrhage with direct pressure. Rapidly assess the patient's haemodynamic state and attach ECG leads. Until proven otherwise, hypotension is caused by hypovolaemia. Less likely causes include myocardial contusion, cardiac tamponade, tension pneumothorax, neurogenic shock and sepsis. Hypovolaemic shock can be conveniently divided into four classes according to the percentage of the total blood volume lost, and the associated symptoms and signs.

- Class 1, 15%   Minimal signs
- Class 2, 30%   Narrowed pulse pressure and tachycardia.
- Class 3, 30–40%   Fall in systolic pressure and oliguria
- Class 4, > 40%   Pre-terminal

Intravenous access is best obtained with two large-bore peripheral cannulae. Alternatives include the subclavian, internal jugular or femoral veins. The proximal or distal saphenous vein can be cannulated by cutdown. The response to an initial fluid challenge (2 l of crystalloid or 1 l colloid) will indicate the degree of hypovolaemia. All fluid must be warmed. Hypothermia will increase bleeding, and independently increases mortality. In the seriously injured a transfusion trigger of 10 g dl^{-1} is appropriate.

4. **Disability.** The size of the pupils and their reaction to light is checked and the Glasgow Coma Scale (GCS) is assessed rapidly (see p. 219).
5. **Exposure/environment.** The patient should be undressed completely and then protected from hypothermia with warm blankets.

X-rays

The chest X-ray and pelvic X-ray are obtained immediately after the primary survey. Cervical spine X-rays can be deferred until the secondary survey. A cervical spine injury is assumed in all trauma patients until a reliable clinical examination and appropriate X-rays (lateral, AP, through mouth) have been obtained.

Tubes

Having excluded urethral injury, a urinary catheter should be inserted. Urine output is a guide to renal blood flow. A nasogastric tube will decompress the stomach. If there is any suspicion of a basal skull fracture the oro-gastric route should be used.

Further reading

Nolan JP, Parr MJA. Aspects of resuscitation in trauma. *British Journal of Anaesthesia* 1997; 79: 226–240.

Related topics of interest

Acute respiratory distress syndrome, p. 5; Burns, p. 51; Head injury, p. 128; Hypothermia, p. 136; Transfer of the critically ill, p. 253; Trauma – secondary survey, p. 260; Trauma – anaesthesia and critical care, p. 263;

TRAUMA – SECONDARY SURVEY

The detailed head-to-toe examination is not undertaken until resuscitation is underway and the patient's vital signs are relatively stable. Continual re-evaluation is essential. Those patients with exsanguinating haemorrhage may need a laparotomy as part of the resuscitation phase.

Head and neck

1. **The head** is inspected for lacerations, haematomas or depressed fractures. Check for signs of a basal skull fracture:

- Racoon eyes.
- Battle's sign (bruising over the mastoid process).
- Subhyaloid haemorrhage.
- Scleral haemorrhage without a posterior margin.
- Haemotympanium.
- Cerebrospinal fluid rhinorrhoea and otorrhoea.

Brain injury is discussed elsewhere (see Head injury p. 128).

2. **Face and neck.** The orbital margins and zygoma are inspected. Check for mobile segments in the mid-face or mandible and inspect the neck for swelling, lacerations, tenderness or deformities.

Thorax

There are six potentially life threatening injuries that may be identified by careful examination of the chest during the secondary survey:

1. **Pulmonary contusion.** Even in the absence of rib fractures, pulmonary contusion is the commonest potentially lethal chest injury. The earliest indication of pulmonary contusion is hypoxaemia (reduced PaO_2/FiO_2 ratio). Patchy infiltrates may not develop until later. Increasing the FiO_2 alone may be insufficient. Mask CPAP or tracheal intubation and positive pressure ventilation may be required to maintain adequate oxygenation.

2. **Cardiac contusion.** Cardiac contusion must be considered in any patient with severe blunt chest trauma, particularly those with sternal fractures. Cardiac arrhythmias, ST changes, and elevated CPK-MB isoenzymes may indicate contusion but these signs are very non-specific. Echocardiography is the most useful investigation. The right ventricle is most frequently injured, as it is pre-dominantly an anterior structure. The severely contused myocardium is likely to require inotropic support.

3. **Aortic rupture.** The thoracic aorta is at risk in any patient sustaining a significant decelerating injury. Only 10–15% of these patients will reach hospital alive and of these survivors, without surgery two thirds will die of delayed rupture within 2 weeks. The commonest site for aortic injury is just distal to the origin of the left subclavian artery at the level of the ligamentum arteriosum. In survivors the

haematoma is contained by an intact aortic adventitia or mediastinal pleura. Patients sustaining traumatic aortic rupture usually have multiple injuries and may be hypotensive at presentation. However, upper extremity hypertension is present in 40% of cases. The supine CXR will show a widened mediastinum in the vast majority of cases. However, 90% of widened mediastinums are due to venous bleeding. An erect CXR will provide a clearer view of the thoracic aorta. Other signs suggesting possible rupture of the aorta are:

- Wide mediastinum.
- Pleural capping.
- Left haemothorax.
- Deviation of the trachea to the right.
- Depression of the left mainstem bronchus.
- Loss of the aortic knob.
- Deviation of the nasogastric tube to the right.
- Fracture of the thoracic spine.

CT scan or transoesophageal echocardiography is often used to screen the aorta but the definitive investigation is angiography. On diagnosis, the patient's blood pressure should be maintained at 80–100 mmHg systolic (using a drug such as esmolol). The patient must be transferred immediately to the nearest cardiothoracic unit. Thirty per cent of patients with blunt aortic injury reaching hospital alive will die.

4. *Diaphragmatic rupture.* Rupture of the diaphragm occurs in about 5% of patients sustaining severe blunt trauma to the trunk. The diagnosis is often made late. Approximately 75% of ruptures occur on the left side. The stomach or colon commonly herniates into the chest and strangulation of these organs is a significant complication. Plain X-ray may reveal an elevated hemidiaphragm, gas bubbles above the diaphragm, shift of the mediastinum to the opposite side, or the nasogastric tube in the chest.

5. *Oesophageal rupture.* A severe blow to the upper abdomen may result in a torn lower oesophagus as gastric contents are forcefully ejected. The conscious patient will complain of severe chest and abdominal pain and mediastinal air may be visible on the CXR. Gastric contents may appear in the chest drain. The diagnosis is confirmed by contrast study of the oesophagus or endoscopy. Urgent surgery is essential since accompanying mediastinitis carries a high mortality.

6. *Rupture of the tracheobronchial tree.* Laryngeal fractures are rare. Signs of laryngeal injury include hoarseness, subcutaneous emphysema, and palpable fracture crepitus. Tracheostomy, rather than cricothyroidotomy, may be indicated. Transections of the trachea or bronchi proximal to the pleural reflection cause massive mediastinal and cervical emphysema. Injuries distal to the pleural sheath lead to pneumothoraces. The bronchopleural fistula causes an air leak. Most bronchial injuries occur within 2.5 cm of the carina and the diagnosis is confirmed by bronchoscopy. Tracheobronchial injuries will require urgent repair through a thoracotomy.

Abdomen

The priority is to determine the need for laparotomy and not to spend considerable time trying to define precisely which viscus is injured. The abdomen is inspected for bruising, lacerations, and distension. Careful palpation may reveal tenderness. A rectal examination is performed to assess sphincter tone and to exclude the presence of pelvic fracture or a high prostate. Diagnostic peritoneal lavage (DPL), ultrasound or CT is indicated whenever abdominal examination is unreliable:

- Patients with a depressed level of consciousness (head injury, drugs, or alcohol).
- In the presence of lower rib or pelvic fractures.
- When the examination is equivocal, particularly if prolonged general anaesthesia for other injuries will make reassessment impossible.
- The surgeon who will be responsible for any subsequent laparotomy should perform the DPL.

Major pelvic trauma resulting in exsanguinating haemorrhage should be dealt with during the resuscitative phase.

Extremities

All limbs must be inspected for bruising, wounds, and deformities, and examined for vascular and neurological defects. Neurovascular impairment may be corrected by appropriate realignment of any deformity and splintage of the limb.

Spinal column

A detailed neurological examination at this stage should detect any motor or sensory deficits. The patient will need to be log-rolled to enable a thorough inspection and palpation of the whole length of the spine. A safe log-roll requires a total of five people: three to control and turn the patient's body, one to maintain the cervical spine in neutral alignment with the rest of the body, and one to examine the spine.

Analgesia

Effective analgesia should be given to the severely injured patient as soon as practically possible. If the patient needs surgery imminently, then immediate induction of general anaesthesia is a logical and very effective solution to the patient's pain. If not, an intravenous opioid (e.g., fentanyl or morphine) should be titrated to the desired effect. A thoracic epidural will provide excellent analgesia for multiple rib fractures and will help the patient to tolerate physiotherapy and reduce the requirement for intubation and mechanical ventilation.

Further reading

Nolan JP, Parr MJA. Aspects of resuscitation in trauma. *British Journal of Anaesthesia* 1997; **79**: 226–240.

Related topics of interest

Acute respiratory distress syndrome, p. 5; Burns, p. 51; Head injury, p. 128; Hypothermia, p. 136; Trauma – primary survey and resuscitation, p. 257; Trauma – anaesthesia and critical care, p. 263

TRAUMA – ANAESTHESIA AND CRITICAL CARE

A smooth induction of anaesthesia and neuromuscular blockade provides optimal conditions for intubation in high-risk trauma patients. All anaesthetic induction agents are vaso-depressors and respiratory depressants and have the potential to produce or worsen hypo-tension. There is no evidence that the choice of induction agent alters survival in major trauma patients. Their appropriate use during resuscitation involves a careful assessment of the clinical situation and a thorough knowledge of their clinical pharmacology. Severely injured patients requiring intubation generally fall into three groups:

(a) Patients who are stable and adequately resuscitated; they should receive a standard or slightly reduced dose of induction agent.
(b) Patients who are unstable or inadequately resuscitated but require immediate intubation; they should receive a reduced, titrated dose of induction agent.
(c) Patients who are in extremis, and are severely obtunded and hypotensive; here induction agents would be inappropriate but muscle relaxants may be used to facilitate intubation. As soon as adequate cerebral perfusion is achieved anaesthetic and analgesic drugs should be administered.

Suxamethonium remains the neuromuscular blocker with the fastest onset of action, and is the first choice relaxant for intubation of the acute trauma patient.

Intraoperative management

The following considerations are of relevance to the anaesthetist during surgery for the severely injured patient:

- Prolonged surgery – the patient will be at risk from heat loss and the develop-ment of pressure sores. Anaesthetists (and surgeons) should rotate to avoid exhaustion. Avoid nitrous oxide in those cases expected to last more than 6 hours.
- Fluid loss – be prepared for heavy blood and 'third space' losses. The combina-tion of hypothermia and massive transfusion will result in profound coagu-lopathy. Expect to see a significant metabolic acidosis in patients with major injuries. This needs frequent monitoring (arterial blood gases) and correction with fluids and inotropes, as appropriate.
- Multiple surgical teams – it is more efficient if surgical teams from different specialties are able to work simultaneously. However, this may severely restrict the amount of space available to the anaesthetist.
- Acute lung injury – trauma patients are at significant risk of hypoxia resulting from acute lung injury. This may be secondary to direct pulmonary contusion or due to fat embolism from orthopaedic injuries. Advanced ventilatory modes may be required to maintain appropriate oxygenation.

Management of the trauma patient on the ICU

The initial management of the trauma patient on ICU comprises continuation of resuscitation and correction of metabolic acidosis. Once haemodynamic stability has been achieved the focus shifts to the prevention of complications and exclusion of injuries missed in the accident department. Major trauma patients will develop SIRS. Secondary infection will compound the risk of developing multiple organ failure. Ventilation strategies aim to minimize barotrauma (see ARDS). Early fracture fixation permits the patient to be mobilized and reduces respiratory complications. Enteral nutrition (possibly with immune-enhanced feed) reduces the risk of septic complications.

Further reading

Nolan JP. Care for trauma patients in the intensive care unit. *Current Anaesthesia and Critical Care* 1996; 7: 139–145.

Related topics of interest

Acute respiratory distress syndrome, p. 5; Burns, p. 51; Head injury, p. 128; Hypothermia, p. 136; Transfer of the critically ill, p. 253; Trauma – primary survey and resuscitation, p. 257

Index

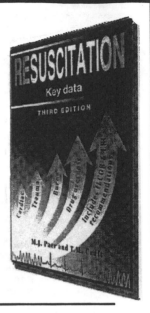

Clinical Intensive Care

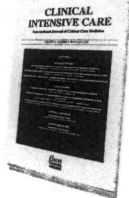

an International Journal of Critical Care Medicine

BIOS Scientific Publishers Ltd is pleased to announce the acquisition of the journal *Clinical Intensive Care* from Castle House Publications. The journal will enhance further the profile of BIOS in the medical field, building on the success of our medical book programme. The first issue to appear under the BIOS imprint is Volume 10, number 1, February 1999.

Immediate changes are being made to revitalise the journal. To reflect the widening scope of intensive care medicine and increase the breadth of coverage of the journal, the *Editor*, Professor David Bennett, will now be assisted by an expanded Editorial Board, as follows:

Deputy Editor - Andrew Rhodes, St Georges Hospital
US Editor - Thomas Higgins, Baystate Medical Center
Reviews Editor - Steve Brett, Hammersmith Hospital
Paediatric Editor UK - Ian Murdoch, Guy's Hospital
Paediatric Editor USA - Brahm Goldstein, Oregon Health Sciences University
Nursing Editor - Sue Osborne, St George's Hospital

These new appointments are responsible for commissioning high profile articles and encouraging a broader range of submissions to ensure that the journal caters for the requirements of its increasing readership. The new Editorial Board will work with an Advisory Panel comprising approximately 20 international intensive care specialists.

Authors, subscribers and other readers of *Clinical Intensive Care* will all benefit from these and other changes currently being implemented:

· articles will be refereed and published more rapidly (under 10 weeks from acceptance)
· even broader coverage of the issues that matter in clinical practice
· electronic access for subscribers planned for 2000
· it is anticipated that the changes will ensure that the journal will be included in all appropriate indexing services in the near future
· an extra 100 pages in 1999 compared to 1998 for no increase in subscription charges
· exposure at international meetings will be significantly increased, as will advertising and promotion, as befits one of Europe's leading critical care journals
· a complete redesign is planned for the first issue in 2000, to give the journal a clear modern look and new features internally to make it more reader-friendly

For all subscription enquiries please contact us immediately using the details below.

BIOS Scientific Publishers Ltd
9 Newtec Place, Magdalen Road, Oxford OX4 1RE, UK
T: (+44) 1865 726286; F: (+44) 1865 200386; E: sales@bios.co.uk
BIOS on the web: www.bios.co.uk